Pediatric Fractures—Volume II

Pediatric Fractures—Volume II

Christiaan J. A. van Bergen
Joost W. Colaris

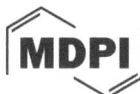

Basel • Beijing • Wuhan • Barcelona • Belgrade • Novi Sad • Cluj • Manchester

Editors
Christiaan J. A. van Bergen
Dept. Orthopedic Surgery
Amphia
Breda
Netherlands

Joost W. Colaris
Orthopedics & Sports Medicine
Erasmus MC
Rotterdam
Netherlands

Editorial Office
MDPI AG
Grosspeteranlage 5
4052 Basel, Switzerland

This is a reprint of articles from the Special Issue published online in the open access journal *Children* (ISSN 2227-9067) (available at: www.mdpi.com/journal/children/special_issues/K73507NT3S).

For citation purposes, cite each article independently as indicated on the article page online and as indicated below:

Lastname, A.A.; Lastname, B.B. Article Title. *Journal Name* **Year**, *Volume Number*, Page Range.

ISBN 978-3-7258-2324-6 (Hbk)
ISBN 978-3-7258-2323-9 (PDF)
doi.org/10.3390/books978-3-7258-2323-9

© 2024 by the authors. Articles in this book are Open Access and distributed under the Creative Commons Attribution (CC BY) license. The book as a whole is distributed by MDPI under the terms and conditions of the Creative Commons Attribution-NonCommercial-NoDerivs (CC BY-NC-ND) license.

Contents

Preface vii

Christiaan J. A. van Bergen and Joost W. Colaris
Shedding Light on Pediatric Fractures: Bridging the Knowledge Gap
Reprinted from: *Children* **2024**, *11*, 565, doi:10.3390/children11050565 1

Tim F. F. Saris, Denise Eygendaal, Bertram The, Joost W. Colaris and Christiaan J. A. van Bergen
Lateral Humeral Condyle Fractures in Pediatric Patients
Reprinted from: *Children* **2023**, *10*, 1033, doi:10.3390/children10061033 4

Laura Lewallen, Marilyn E. Elliott, Amy McIntosh and Christine A. Ho
Pediatric Elbow Dislocations and Associated Fractures
Reprinted from: *Children* **2023**, *10*, 993, doi:10.3390/children10060993 16

Özgür Kaya, Batuhan Gencer, Ahmet Çulcu and Özgür Doğan
Extra Lateral Pin or Less Radiation? A Comparison of Two Different Pin Configurations in the Treatment of Supracondylar Humerus Fracture
Reprinted from: *Children* **2023**, *10*, 550, doi:10.3390/children10030550 25

Christy Graff, George Dennis Dounas, Maya Rani Louise Chandra Todd, Jonghoo Sung and Medhir Kumawat
Management of Traumatic Nerve Palsies in Paediatric Supracondylar Humerus Fractures: A Systematic Review
Reprinted from: *Children* **2023**, *10*, 1862, doi:10.3390/children10121862 34

Mark F. Siemensma, Christiaan J.A. van Bergen, Eline M. van Es, Joost W. Colaris and Denise Eygendaal
Indications and Timing of Guided Growth Techniques for Pediatric Upper Extremity Deformities: A Literature Review
Reprinted from: *Children* **2023**, *10*, 195, doi:10.3390/children10020195 45

Kasper Roth, Eline van Es, Gerald Kraan, Denise Eygendaal, Joost Colaris and Filip Stockmans
Accuracy of 3D Corrective Osteotomy for Pediatric Malunited Both-Bone Forearm Fractures
Reprinted from: *Children* **2022**, *10*, 21, doi:10.3390/children10010021 63

Roman Michalik, Frank Hildebrand and Heide Delbrück
Stabilisation of Pathologic Proximal Femoral Fracture near the [-25]Growth Plate with Use of a Locking Plate and Transphyseal Screws
Reprinted from: *Children* **2022**, *9*, 1932, doi:10.3390/children9121932 73

Mehak Chandanani, Raian Jaibaji, Monketh Jaibaji and Andrea Volpin
Tibial Spine Avulsion Fractures in Paediatric Patients: A Systematic Review and Meta-Analysis of Surgical Management
Reprinted from: *Children* **2024**, *11*, 345, doi:10.3390/children11030345 83

Te-Feng Arthur Chou, Ting-Yu Liu, Matthew N. Wang and Chen-Yuan Yang
Treatment of Refractory Congenital Pseudoarthrosis of Tibia with Contralateral Vascularized Fibular Bone Graft and Anatomic Distal Tibial Locking Plate: A Case Series and Literature Review
Reprinted from: *Children* **2023**, *10*, 503, doi:10.3390/children10030503 111

Albert T. Anastasio, Emily M. Peairs, Caitlin Grant, Billy I. Kim, Anthony Duruewuru and Samuel B. Adams
Fracture through Pre-Existing Tarsal Coalition: A Narrative Review
Reprinted from: *Children* **2022**, *10*, 72, doi:10.3390/children10010072 . . . . **123**

Lucca B. Palavani, Raphael Bertani, Leonardo de Barros Oliveira, Sávio Batista, Gabriel Verly and Filipi Fim Andreão et al.
A Systematic Review and Meta-Analysis on the Management and Outcome of Isolated Skull Fractures in Pediatric Patients
Reprinted from: *Children* **2023**, *10*, 1913, doi:10.3390/children10121913 . . . . **134**

Raluca Iulia Juncar, Abel Emanuel Moca, Mihai Juncar, Rahela Tabita Moca and Paul Andrei Țenț
Clinical Patterns and Treatment of Pediatric Facial Fractures: A 10-Year Retrospective Romanian Study
Reprinted from: *Children* **2023**, *10*, 800, doi:10.3390/children10050800 . . . . **147**

Preface

Fractures are extremely common in children. The fracture risk is 40% in boys and 28% in girls. Although many pediatric fractures are frequently regarded as "innocent" or "forgiving", typical complications do occur in this precious population, including premature physeal closure and post-traumatic deformity, which may cause life-long disability.

Despite the high incidence of pediatric injuries, there is still much debate regarding optimal treatment regimes. Although non-operative and surgical treatment techniques have been extensively developed during the past several decades, current management is still more eminence-based rather than evidence-based because of limited scientific evidence. For example, the recently developed comprehensive Dutch clinical practice guidelines on the diagnosis and treatment of the most common pediatric fractures included almost solely "low"- or "very low"-level recommendations based on the Grading of Recommendations Assessment, Development, and Evaluation (GRADE) criteria. The only exceptions were some forearm fracture recommendations, which received "moderate" GRADEs. There is a clear lack of data and a need for higher-level science in pediatric trauma.

Considering the success and popularity of the previous Special Issue, entitled "Pediatric Fractures" published in the journal *Children*, we have published a second Special Issue where we aimed to gather original research papers and review articles related to pediatric fractures, including the diagnosis, treatment, or follow-up of common fractures. This is a reprint of the second Special Issue on "Pediatric Fractures" and contains all 13 articles.

Christiaan J. A. van Bergen and Joost W. Colaris
Editors

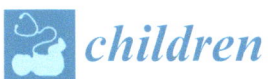

Editorial

Shedding Light on Pediatric Fractures: Bridging the Knowledge Gap

Christiaan J. A. van Bergen [1,2,*] and Joost W. Colaris [2]

1. Department of Orthopedic Surgery, Amphia Hospital, 4818 CK Breda, The Netherlands
2. Department of Orthopaedics and Sports Medicine, Erasmus University Medical Center—Sophia Children's Hospital, 3015 GD Rotterdam, The Netherlands; j.colaris@erasmusmc.nl
* Correspondence: cvanbergen@amphia.nl

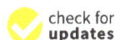

Citation: van Bergen, C.J.A.; Colaris, J.W. Shedding Light on Pediatric Fractures: Bridging the Knowledge Gap. *Children* **2024**, *11*, 565. https://doi.org/10.3390/children11050565

Received: 3 April 2024
Accepted: 26 April 2024
Published: 8 May 2024

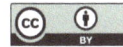

Copyright: © 2024 by the authors. Licensee MDPI, Basel, Switzerland. This article is an open access article distributed under the terms and conditions of the Creative Commons Attribution (CC BY) license (https://creativecommons.org/licenses/by/4.0/).

After the great success of the printed edition of the Special Issue "Pediatric Fractures—Volume I", which was published in 2023 containing 24 high-quality papers [1], we are proud to present our new printed edition of the Special Issue "Pediatric Fractures—Volume II".

Pediatric fractures, though commonplace, often find themselves in the shadows of adult orthopedic research. Despite their high prevalence [2–4], there remains a stark deficiency in comprehensive studies dedicated to understanding and effectively treating pediatric fractures. This is not merely a matter of academic interest, but carries significant implications for the health and well-being of children.

It is important to mention that children should not be treated as "miniature adults". Unlike adults, children's bones are still in the process of growth and development [5], making their fracture management markedly distinct. Children possess a remarkable ability to correct improperly healed fractures through growth—a phenomenon where nature itself acts as a friend in the healing process. However, there are instances where nature's hand is less forgiving, particularly when fractures involve the growth plates. The physes are particularly vulnerable in children and must be carefully considered during treatment and follow-up [6]. Neglecting these factors can have far-reaching implications, potentially leading to growth disturbances and functional deficits in the affected limb [7–9].

Because of the unique potential of growth in pediatric bones, long-term follow-up is important to detect and address any potential complications that may arise over time, especially nowadays, to study the effects of the more aggressive treatment of pediatric fractures without substantiated evidence [10].

To address the gaps in knowledge concerning pediatric fractures, the Special Issue "Pediatric Fractures—Volume II" features eleven high-quality, peer-reviewed articles focusing on the comprehensive care of a variety of pediatric fractures.

This Special Issue places particular emphasis on fractures around the elbow and the associated complications that may arise. Saris et al. (1) focused on lateral humeral condyle fractures, which occur often in children but have potential pitfalls in treatment. The article describes classifications, treatment strategies, and handles on how to prevent complications. In line with this, Lewallen et al. (2) discuss acute elbow dislocation and their associated fractures in children and deliberate on conservative versus surgical treatment.

Even more frequent are pediatric supracondylar humerus fractures, which are often treated with closed reduction methods and percutaneous K-wire fixation. However, the configuration of the pins used to stabilize the fracture remains a point of debate. Therefore, Kaya et al. (3) conducted a randomized trial to determine the most effective pin configuration while also considering the potential risks associated with radiation exposure. Moreover, supracondylar humerus fractures are frequently associated with traumatic nerve injury. To unravel the best diagnostics and treatment of traumatic nerve palsies in these fractures, Graff et al. (4) wrote a review article of the current literature.

If nature does not behave like a friend in pediatric fractures and growth disturbances arise, clinicians are challenged to assess the indications and value of different treatment options. Siemensma et al. (5) dove into the unique treatment options of growth disturbances of the upper limb in children, which consist of a wait-and-see policy or surgical techniques, including physeal bar resection, (hemi-)epiphysiodesis, and osteotomies to correct the deformity. The pearls and pitfalls of these treatment strategies are discussed to guide clinicians.

In contrast with malunited wrist fractures, which remodel relatively quickly due to their proximity to the physis, diaphyseal forearm fractures are notorious for their malalignment and subsequent impairment of forearm rotation. In such a pathology, a corrective osteotomy is often performed. Roth et al. (6) assessed the accuracy of three-dimensional corrections and studied the relation between the precision of anatomic correction and functional outcome.

Moving from the upper to the lower extremity, interesting contributions were received that studied a spectrum of injuries from hip to foot. Michalik et al. (7) unraveled the treatment of aneurysmal bone cysts in the femoral neck and its relation to a pathological fracture in children.

Chandanani et al. (8) performed a comprehensive meta-analysis on the treatment of children with tibial spine avulsion fractures. Based on the results of 38 studies, they found that arthroscopic-assisted reduction and internal fixation with a suture seems to be the preferred treatment.

Patients with congenital tibial pseudoarthrosis are treated in different ways. Chou et al. (9) described three previously treated patients with congenital pseudoarthrosis of the tibia using a contralateral vascularized fibular bone graft and stabilization with a distal tibial locking plate.

Abnormal fibrous or bony connections between the tarsal bones of the foot occur in children and are known as tarsal coalitions. Although these coalitions do not always become symptomatic, some may cause pain and changes in morphology and biomechanics. Anastasio et al. (10) reviewed the foot biomechanics seen in tarsal coalitions and concomitant fractures. Furthermore, diagnostic and treatment options are discussed.

Finally, two studies on head trauma in children were published. Although these are common injuries, there is relatively little literature available on the subject. Palavani et al. (11) conducted a systematic review to unveil the state of the evidence concerning acute neurosurgical intervention, hospitalizations after injury, and neuroimaging in isolated skull fractures in children. In line with this research, Juncar et al. (12) studied the main clinical characteristics of pediatric facial fractures (such as fracture location, fracture pattern, treatment, complications, and evolution).

In conclusion, this Special Issue comprises a wide array of studies, all of which are aimed at enhancing the care of pediatric fractures. The editors are optimistic that this compilation will contribute significantly to closing knowledge gaps surrounding pediatric fractures. Furthermore, this Issue provides inspiration for further study and improved care for this challenging population.

Acknowledgments: The authors would like to thank all the editors for their invaluable assistance in composing this Special Issue.

Conflicts of Interest: The authors declare no conflicts of interest.

List of Contributions:

1. Saris, T.F.F.; Eygendaal, D.; The, B.; Colaris, J.W.; van Bergen, C.J.A. Lateral Humeral Condyle Fractures in Pediatric Patients. *Children* **2023**, *10*, 1033. https://doi.org/10.3390/children10061033.
2. Lewallen, L.; Elliott, M.E.; McIntosh, A.; Ho, C.A. Pediatric Elbow Dislocations and Associated Fractures. *Children* **2023**, *10*, 993. https://doi.org/10.3390/children10060993.
3. Kaya, Ö.; Gencer, B.; Çulcu, A.; Doğan, Ö. Extra Lateral Pin or Less Radiation? A Comparison of Two Different Pin Configurations in the Treatment of Supracondylar Humerus Fracture. *Children* **2023**, *10*, 550. https://doi.org/10.3390/children10030550.

4. Graff, C.; Dounas, G.D.; Todd, M.R.L.C.; Sung, J.; Kumawat, M. Management of Traumatic Nerve Palsies in Paediatric Supracondylar Humerus Fractures: A Systematic Review. *Children* **2023**, *10*, 1862. https://doi.org/10.3390/children10121862.
5. Siemensma, M.F.; van Bergen, C.J.; van Es, E.M.; Colaris, J.W.; Eygendaal, D. Indications and Timing of Guided Growth Techniques for Pediatric Upper Extremity Deformities: A Literature Review. *Children* **2023**, *10*, 195. https://doi.org/10.3390/children10020195.
6. Roth, K.; van Es, E.; Kraan, G.; Eygendaal, D.; Colaris, J.; Stockmans, F. Accuracy of 3D Corrective Osteotomy for Pediatric Malunited Both-Bone Forearm Fractures. *Children* **2023**, *10*, 21. https://doi.org/10.3390/children10010021.
7. Michalik, R.; Hildebrand, F.; Delbrück, H. Stabilisation of Pathologic Proximal Femoral Fracture near the Growth Plate with Use of a Locking Plate and Transphyseal Screws. *Children* **2022**, *9*, 1932. https://doi.org/10.3390/children9121932.
8. Chandanani, M.; Jaibaji, R.; Jaibaji, M.; Volpin, A. Tibial Spine Avulsion Fractures in Paediatric Patients: A Systematic Review and Meta-Analysis of Surgical Management. *Children* **2024**, *11*, 345. https://doi.org/10.3390/children11030345.
9. Chou, T.-F.A.; Liu, T.-Y.; Wang, M.N.; Yang, C.-Y. Treatment of Refractory Congenital Pseudoarthrosis of Tibia with Contralateral Vascularized Fibular Bone Graft and Anatomic Distal Tibial Locking Plate: A Case Series and Literature Review. *Children* **2023**, *10*, 503. https://doi.org/10.3390/children10030503.
10. Anastasio, A.T.; Peairs, E.M.; Grant, C.; Kim, B.I.; Duruewuru, A.; Adams, S.B. Fracture through Pre-Existing Tarsal Coalition: A Narrative Review. *Children* **2023**, *10*, 72. https://doi.org/10.3390/children10010072.
11. Palavani, L.B.; Bertani, R.; de Barros Oliveira, L.; Batista, S.; Verly, G.; Andreão, F.F.; Ferreira, M.Y.; Paiva, W.S. A Systematic Review and Meta-Analysis on the Management and Outcome of Isolated Skull Fractures in Pediatric Patients. *Children* **2023**, *10*, 1913. https://doi.org/10.3390/children10121913.
12. Juncar, R.I.; Moca, A.E.; Juncar, M.; Moca, R.T.; Țenț, P.A. Clinical Patterns and Treatment of Pediatric Facial Fractures: A 10-Year Retrospective Romanian Study. *Children* **2023**, *10*, 800. https://doi.org/10.3390/children10050800.

References

1. van Bergen, C.J.A. Advances in Pediatric Fracture Diagnosis and Treatment Are Numerous but Great Challenges Remain. *Children* **2022**, *9*, 1489. [CrossRef] [PubMed]
2. Farrell, C.; Hannon, M.; Monuteaux, M.C.; Mannix, R.; Lee, L.K. Pediatric Fracture Epidemiology and US Emergency Department Resource Utilization. *Pediatr. Emerg. Care* **2022**, *38*, e1342–e1347. [CrossRef] [PubMed]
3. Lempesis, V.; Rosengren, B.E.; Nilsson, J.Å.; Landin, L.; Tiderius, C.J.; Karlsson, M.K. Time trends in pediatric fracture incidence in Sweden during the period 1950-2006. *Acta Orthop.* **2017**, *88*, 440–445. [CrossRef] [PubMed]
4. Brazell, C.J.; Carry, P.M.; Holmes, K.S.; Salton, R.L.; Hadley-Miller, N.; Georgopoulos, G. Pediatric and Adult Fracture Incidence: A Decreasing Trend with Increasing Hospital Admissions. *Orthopedics* **2023**, *46*, e369–e375. [CrossRef] [PubMed]
5. Lindaman, L.M. Bone healing in children. *Clin. Podiatr. Med. Surg.* **2001**, *18*, 97–108. [CrossRef]
6. Sepúlveda, M.; Téllez, C.; Villablanca, V.; Birrer, E. Distal femoral fractures in children. *EFORT Open Rev.* **2022**, *7*, 264–273. [CrossRef] [PubMed]
7. Golshteyn, G.; Katsman, A. Pediatric Trauma. *Clin. Podiatr. Med. Surg.* **2022**, *39*, 57–71. [CrossRef]
8. Basener, C.J.; Mehlman, C.T.; DiPasquale, T.G. Growth disturbance after distal femoral growth plate fractures in children: A meta-analysis. *J. Orthop. Trauma* **2009**, *23*, 663–667. [CrossRef] [PubMed]
9. Kallini, J.R.; Fu, E.C.; Shah, A.S.; Waters, P.M.; Bae, D.S. Growth Disturbance Following Intra-articular Distal Radius Fractures in the Skeletally Immature Patient. *J. Pediatr. Orthop.* **2020**, *40*, e910–e915. [CrossRef] [PubMed]
10. Eismann, E.A.; Little, K.J.; Kunkel, S.T.; Cornwall, R. Clinical research fails to support more aggressive management of pediatric upper extremity fractures. *J. Bone Joint Surg. Am.* **2013**, *95*, 1345–1350. [CrossRef] [PubMed]

Disclaimer/Publisher's Note: The statements, opinions and data contained in all publications are solely those of the individual author(s) and contributor(s) and not of MDPI and/or the editor(s). MDPI and/or the editor(s) disclaim responsibility for any injury to people or property resulting from any ideas, methods, instructions or products referred to in the content.

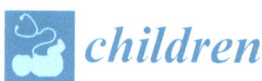

Review

Lateral Humeral Condyle Fractures in Pediatric Patients

Tim F. F. Saris [1,2], Denise Eygendaal [2], Bertram The [1], Joost W. Colaris [2] and Christiaan J. A. van Bergen [1,2,*]

1. Department of Orthopedic Surgery, Amphia Hospital, 4818 CK Breda, The Netherlands
2. Department of Orthopaedics and Sports Medicine, Erasmus University Medical Center—Sophia Children's Hospital, 3015 GD Rotterdam, The Netherlands
* Correspondence: cvanbergen@amphia.nl

Abstract: Lateral humeral condyle fractures are frequently seen in pediatric patients and have a high risk of unfavorable outcomes. A fall on the outstretched arm with supination of the forearm is the most common trauma mechanism. A physical examination combined with additional imaging will confirm the diagnosis. Several classifications have been described to categorize these fractures based on location and comminution. Treatment options depend on the severity of the fracture and consist of immobilization in a cast, closed reduction with percutaneous fixation, and open reduction with fixation. These fractures can lead to notable complications such as lateral condyle overgrowth, surgical site infection, pin tract infections, stiffness resulting in decreased range of motion, cubitus valgus deformities, 'fishtail' deformities, malunion, non-union, avascular necrosis, and premature epiphyseal fusion. Adequate follow-up is therefore warranted.

Keywords: lateral humeral condyle; fracture; children; diagnosis; treatment; surgery

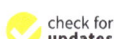

Citation: Saris, T.F.F.; Eygendaal, D.; The, B.; Colaris, J.W.; van Bergen, C.J.A. Lateral Humeral Condyle Fractures in Pediatric Patients. *Children* **2023**, *10*, 1033. https://doi.org/10.3390/children10061033

Academic Editor: Johannes Mayr

Received: 4 May 2023
Revised: 25 May 2023
Accepted: 7 June 2023
Published: 8 June 2023

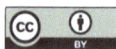

Copyright: © 2023 by the authors. Licensee MDPI, Basel, Switzerland. This article is an open access article distributed under the terms and conditions of the Creative Commons Attribution (CC BY) license (https://creativecommons.org/licenses/by/4.0/).

1. Introduction

The occurrence rate of any fracture during childhood (0–17 years) is between 12–34% for boys and 6–34% for girls [1,2]. Elbow fractures account for 28.4% of this number [3]. Lateral humeral condyle fractures in children are the second most frequent type of elbow fracture [4–7]. In most cases, standard radiographs will visualize the fracture. However, in 5.2–16.6% of all cases, nondisplaced fractures are overlooked on conventional radiographs, which could result in an unfavorable outcome or long-term complication [8–10]. Therefore, early recognition and adequate treatment are necessary to optimize outcomes [8]. The objective of this narrative review is to provide an overview of the epidemiology, anatomy, diagnosis, treatment options, and complications of pediatric lateral humeral condyle fractures based on the most recent literature.

2. Epidemiology

Lateral humeral condyle fractures account for 9.6–22.3% of all elbow fractures [1,2,4–7,11–14]. The majority (63–67.4%) of pediatric patients are male [8,9,13–15]. Most lateral humeral condyle fractures are seen between the ages of four and ten, but cases as early as 1.9 years have been reported [5–9,11,13,16,17]. Lateral humeral condyle fractures are typically a result of playground activities (53.7%) and/or sports (49.6%) [6,8,9], and as a consequence, they do occur more than twice as much during the summer period [5]. The handedness of the patient has an effect on fracture occurrence in the elbow: the non-dominant side fractures more often than the dominant side [18]. A slight majority (51.5%) of lateral humeral condyle fractures are nondisplaced fractures or show minor displacement (<2 mm) in plain radiography [8,9].

2.1. Anatomy

The capitulum of the humerus and the lateral condyle demarcate the anatomical region of the lateral side of the elbow [19]. The ossification center of the capitulum develops first at the age of one, and the ossification center of the lateral condyle develops last at the age range between eight and thirteen [20]. The ossification process toward the total osseous fusion of the lateral side of the elbow is completed between the ages of twelve and fourteen. The blood supply for the tissue on the lateral side originates posterior from the branched variation of the radial collateral artery over the lateral condyle and the brachial artery between the capitulum and the humeral trochlea. The cephalic vein and accompanying lymph vessels traverse the capitulum toward the radial head as seen in Figure 1. The radial fossa is a slight anatomical depression of the humerus just above the capitulum, where the brachial artery (Figure 1) and radial nerve track are located.

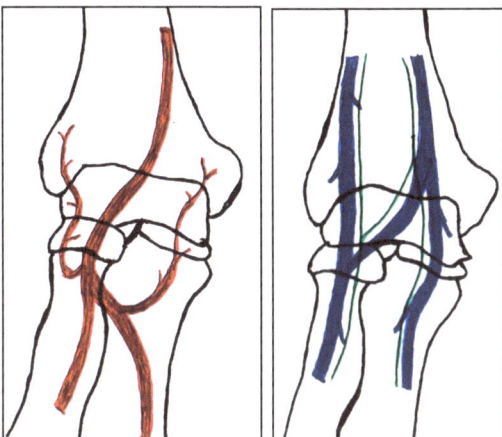

Figure 1. Simple schematic visualization of the anatomy of the arteries (**left**) and the veins with their respective lymphatic vessels (**right**) of the elbow as seen from an anterior view.

2.2. Trauma Mechanism and Associated Injuries

The most common trauma mechanism resulting in a lateral humeral condyle fracture is a fall on an outstretched arm with the wrist in full supination [16]. Another common trauma mechanism is a direct hit to the lateral side of the elbow [6,9]. These mechanisms result in either a varus injury with an avulsion fracture of the lateral condyle and possible concomitant fracture of the capitulum or direct impact of the radial head into the lateral condyle resulting in an impaction fracture.

2.3. Classification of Fractures

Several classifications have been described to categorize the different fracture patterns. Most of these classifications use anatomical landmarks of the elbow and the amount of displacement to determine the severity of the fracture. The most commonly used classifications, presented in Table 1, in historical chronology are Milch (1956), Jakobs (1975), Finnbogason (1995), Weiss (2009), and Song (2010).

The Milch Classification [16], designed in 1956, is a classification that uses the anatomical regions within the elbow to define the different types of lateral humeral condyle fractures. Milch type 1, with an occurrence of 11.4–50.7% [8,9,21], is a fracture through the capitulum humeri with or without the involvement of the lateral side of the trochlear groove. This fracture type occurs after an axially loaded trauma to the elbow. Milch type 2, with an occurrence of 49.3–88.6% [8,9,21], is a fracture of the lateral condyle and part of the medial trochlear groove in the capitulum humeri. This fracture results from ulnar outward rotation with lateral displacement of the distal fragment.

The Jakobs Classification [21], designed in 1975, is a classification that differentiates lateral humeral condyle fractures based on the anatomical region and the extent of displacement of the fractures seen on conventional radiographs. Jakobs type 1, with an occurrence of 8–51.5% [8,9], is a fracture with minimal displacement (<2 mm) and without discontinuation of the articular surface of the capitulum/trochlea (incomplete fracture). Jakobs type 2, with an occurrence of 29.9–65% [8,9], is a fracture with minimal displacement (between 2 and 4 mm) and a discontinuation of the articular surface. Jakobs type 3, with an occurrence of 18.7–27% [8,9], is a displaced fracture with discontinuation of the articular surface and displacement measuring > 4 mm.

The Finnbogason classification [22], designed in 1995, is a modified version of the Jakobs classification based on anatomy and displacement of the articular surface as seen using conventional radiographs. Type A is a lateral humeral condyle fracture with a small gap without displacement or discontinuation of the articular surface. Type B is a fracture with a small gap without displacement but with discontinuation of the articular surface. Type C is a fracture with a considerable gap, displacement, and discontinuation of the articular surface.

The Weiss classification [23], designed in 2009, is a modified version of the Milch classification. Weiss et al. found that the Milch classification inadequately divided fractures based on their potential treatment options. More focus was placed on articular congruity and the potential to guide within the treatment options. Weiss type 1 is a lateral humeral condyle fracture with an intact articular surface and displacement of <2 mm. Weiss type 2 is a fracture with an intact articular surface and displacement of >2 mm. Weiss type 3 is a fracture with the incongruity of the articular surface and displacement of >2 mm.

The Song classification [4] is the most recent updated classification, focusing on conventional radiographs, especially the internal oblique view. Song type 1 is a stable lateral humeral condyle fracture confined to the metaphyseal bone on all radiographical views with a displacement of <2 mm. Song type 2 is a potentially unstable fracture with <2 mm displacement through the cartilaginous layer but showing no intra-articular fracture. Song type 3 is an unstable intra-articular fracture with a displacement of <2 mm. Song type 4 is an unstable intra-articular fracture with a lateral displacement of >2 mm. Finally, Song type 5 is an unstable intra-articular fracture with a rotational displacement of >2 mm.

Table 1. Visual summarization of the most commonly used classifications for lateral humeral condyle fractures in pediatric patients in historical chronology. The Finnbogason classification type is described with alphabetical numeration within brackets.

Classification	Type 1 (A)	Type 2 (B)	Type 3 (C)	Type 4	Type 5
Milch. [16]					
Jacobs et al. [21]					

Table 1. *Cont.*

Classification	Type 1 (A)	Type 2 (B)	Type 3 (C)	Type 4	Type 5
Finnbogason et al. [22]					
Weiss et al. [23]					
Song et al. [4]					

Rarely is the Milch classification used to identify lateral humeral condyle fractures, mainly because it focuses on the anatomical position of the fracture and does not direct the user toward treatment options [24,25]. The Song classification compiles the positives taken from Weiss and Jakobs's classifications. The Song classification divides fractures based on the indication criteria for surgical interventions or non-surgical treatment. Ramo et al. have extensively tested and validated the interobserver reliability of the Song classification and its ability to determine the correct treatment option accurately [26]. The Song classification might therefore be preferred.

2.4. Diagnosis

Children with an elbow injury suspected of an elbow fracture usually present with an adequate trauma mechanism, localized pain, possible deformity, swelling, limitation in elbow range of motion, and inability to use the injured arm. Although standard radiographs in the anterior–posterior and lateral direction can confirm the diagnosis, additional diagnostic imaging, such as an internal oblique view, X-rays of the contralateral elbow, computed tomography (CT), and magnetic resonance imaging, are helpful in selected cases. A physician should also assess the possibility of child abuse as a trauma mechanism for the elbow fracture and look for potential additional injuries.

2.4.1. Medical History and Physical Examination

A patient's medical history should include detailed information on identifiable risk factors for an elbow fracture. These risk factors include but are not limited to age, gender, physical activities leading to trauma, trauma mechanism, external visual deformity, and sensorimotor function. During a physical examination, visible deformity of the elbow joint and localized ecchymosis due to tearing blood vessels or hematoma from articular capsular bleeding are solid indicators of a potential fracture. Other strong indicators are a reduced range of motion or inability to move, sharp pain, and crepitations felt during palpation [27]. A full assessment of the forearm's sensory and motor function and a vascular examination of the radial and ulnar arteries will complete the physical examination.

2.4.2. Diagnostic Imaging

If the suspicion of a lateral humeral condyle fracture or other elbow fracture is raised, diagnostic imaging will be the next step. First, conventional radiographs will be taken from two angles: an anterior–posterior view with the arm in supination and as much extension as possible, and a lateral view with the elbow in a 90-degree flexion and neutral rotation. Recent studies have shown that fractures and/or displacement of the lateral humeral condyle are often missed with the conventional approach [10,28,29]. Therefore, it is suggested to perform additional imaging by taking a conventional radiograph of the uninjured elbow or by taking an internal oblique view (anterior–posterior position with hand in full pronation) [10]. Furthermore, a fat-pad sign is a radiographic finding that suggests hydrops or hematoma of the joint and, thus, a possible fracture. A radiograph with a fat-pad sign and no evident fracture is usually considered as no fracture [30,31]. However, recent studies showed that 44.6% (confidence interval: 30.4% to 59.7%) of children with a positive fat-pad sign and no evident fracture visible on conventional radiographs have an occult fracture [31]. In total, 14% of these occult fractures consisted of lateral humeral condyle fractures [31]. Therefore, when in doubt, it is advised to perform additional CT-imaging to appreciate the extent of injury to the elbow joint fully, define the proper classification, and execute the suitable treatment method [32]. Historically, elbow surgeons have used 2 mm and 4 mm as the cut-off values to determine conservative or surgical treatment. The literature does not accurately describe the origin of these margins and whether or not these margins are optimal. Nevertheless, the 2 mm and 4 mm values are now common practice. The distance is measured between the most lateral gap between the fracture site and the fractured bone piece. It is the biggest measurable distance between bone and fractured bone. This measurement is susceptible to measurement errors due to the thick cartilaginous layer surrounding the articular surface of the bone in children and the inability to visualize the cartilage on fluoroscopy and/or radiography. If a fracture shows displacement and rotation, the protrusion of a thick cartilage layer between the fracture site and the bone piece could overestimate the distance of the gap and have significant implications for the correct treatment option.

3. Treatment Options

Non-operative treatment is the preferred option for fractures with a minor (<2 mm) displacement and no other additional injuries [33]. Closely regulated follow-up is mandatory to rule out secondary displacement in the cast. Follow-up should be performed within one week after trauma in the outpatient clinic and should include conventional X-rays in AP and lateral and oblique views. If the fracture is >2 mm displaced, with a disruption of the articular surface, reduction and fixation of the fracture are recommended [33,34]. The authors of each classification system for lateral humeral condyle fractures have made recommendations concerning treatment options based on the severity of the fractures; these recommendations can be found in Table 2. In cases with a successful fracture union and without complications, the success rate for non-operative and operative lateral humeral condyle fracture, as described in meta-analyses, is between 89.8–91.5% [8,33,35,36]. A delayed diagnosis of these fractures (>3 weeks after injury) should initially be given based on the time between the injury and presentation and the amount of displacement, in accordance with the above-described options [37,38]. Unfortunately, a malunion or nonunion of these fractures with a delayed diagnosis is quite common after 3 months [37]. Treatment of these complications requires a different approach depending on displacement, elbow alignment, and a stable condylar fragment (see Sections 3.2.1 and 3.2.2).

Table 2. Classification of lateral humeral condyle fractures and their respective preferred treatment options for the pediatric patient.

	1 (A)	2 (B)	3 (C)	4	5
Milch [16]	Cast/CRPP	CRPP/ORIF	-	-	-
Jakobs [21]	Cast/CRPP	CRPP	ORIF	-	-
Finnbogason [22]	Cast/CRPP	CRPP	CRPP/ORIF	-	-
Weiss [23]	Cast/CRPP	CRPP	ORIF	-	-
Song [29]	Cast	Cast/CRPP	CRPP	CRPP	ORIF

Cast = above elbow cast, CRPP = closed reduction and percutaneous pinning with Kirschner wires, ORIF = open reduction internal fixation with Kirschner wires and/or cannulated screw.

3.1. Non-Surgical/Operative Treatment Options: Plastered Cast Therapy

The non-operative treatment option for lateral humeral condyle fractures in children is an above-elbow cast. This applies to a fracture with no displacement, an intact articular surface, and no additional injury [11,16,17,21,33,34]. The elbow should be positioned in a 90-degree flexion, and the wrist and hands should be in a neutral position (Figure 2). Patients will return after 4 weeks for cast removal if non-operative treatment shows no secondary fracture displacement on the X-ray in a long arm cast within the first week after injury [8,10,11,33,34,39,40]. If the physician, after removal, doubts whether cast therapy for 4 weeks has been enough, an additional X-ray should be made. If the X-ray shows no callus around the fracture, treatment with plastered cast therapy should be continued for another 2 weeks [8,10,11,33,34,39,40]. Secondary fracture displacement, which warrants an operative treatment [34,41] (unstable fracture, see classifications Table 1), occurs most frequently between three and seven days after injury [33,41]. Secondary displacement of lateral humeral condyle fractures treated with a cast occurs in 4.8–29.4% of all pediatric cases [4,10,33–35,39,41,42].

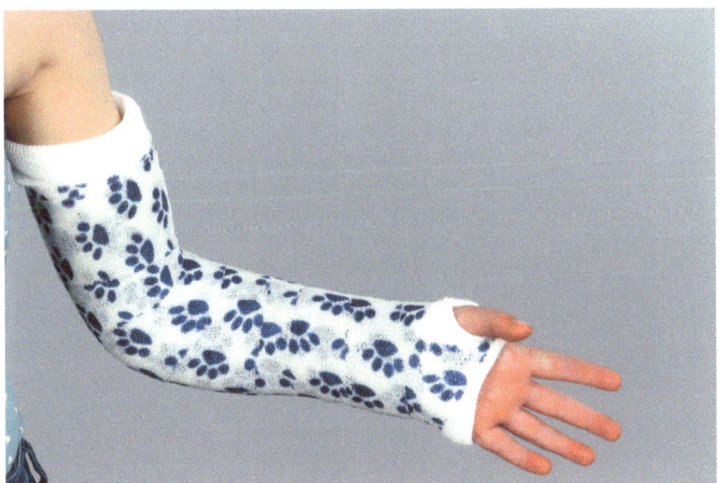

Figure 2. Digital picture of a left arm in an above-elbow cast in the recommended position (90-degree flexion and neutral rotation).

Plastered cast therapy for a patient with a malunion or nonunion after >3 months and after an initial delayed diagnosis is only viable if the displacement is less than 5 mm, shows a stable condylar fragment, and shows evidence of bony bridging on a CT scan [37].

3.2. Surgical/Operative Treatment Options

3.2.1. Closed Reduction and Internal Fixation

The minimally invasive surgical technique to reduce and stabilize the lateral humeral condyle fracture is called closed reduction and internal fixation (CRIF), or closed reduction and percutaneous pinning (CRPP). This technique is generally used for unstable/displaced fractures with 2 mm–4 mm displacement [43]. Most fractures that do not show signs of rotation of the fragment and/or additional fractures of the elbow are treated with CRPP. Fracture reduction through CRPP is achieved by flexing the elbow and supinating the wrist while applying pressure to the lateral side of the elbow. Simultaneous imaging should be performed to deduce the effects of the closed reduction. Successful reduction shows an anatomical articular surface during imaging. Fluoroscopy and ultrasound-guided reduction are suitable options to provide basic imaging during surgery.

Ultrasound-assisted reduction creates the opportunity to provide basic imaging of good quality while negating the negative effects of fluoroscopy radiation [44]. The image quality and ability to perform the surgery is linked to the imaging capabilities of the surgeon when using ultrasound. Ultrasound-assisted closed reduction is a relatively new technique with a learning curve for the surgeon. Nevertheless, recent results show comparable complication rates to closed reduction with fluoroscopy and/or ORIF [44].

Through simultaneous fluoroscopy, one can deduce the effects of the reduction. However, the diagnostic accuracy of joint reduction appreciated on two-dimensional fluoroscopy used in the operating theater shows inferior results compared to a CT scan [45]. The subjective image quality of fluoroscopy is the main contributing factor toward inferior diagnostic accuracy. The imaging quality is affected by the degree of image focus achieved during surgery. The most notable factor which directly impacts the quality of the image is the presence of osteosynthesis material, which results in scattering and artifacts. A secondary factor influencing the image quality is the relative thickness of the cartilage, which is more prominent in children than adults, compared to bone thickness. The cartilage and articular surface of the elbow in children are not as visible using fluoroscopy as they would be through arthrotomy since fluoroscopy does not show cartilaginous tissue as clearly as bone. Considering these factors, and combined with the over-estimation in the measurement of displacement seen in radiography prior to surgery, it is best to visualize a joint reduction through arthrography, arthroscopy, or arthrotomy.

Next, the surgeon performs a percutaneous fixation of the reduced fracture by placing two smooth Kirschner wires perpendicular to the fracture line. Crossed Kirschner wires may reduce fracture stability [46]. A third Kirschner wire can be placed through the condyles, parallel to the joint, to increase fracture stability and minimize rotation. Kirschner wires can be buried underneath the skin or exposed for easy removal. Both methods show similarly low complication rates, low infection rates, and high successful union rates. Kirschner wires are left in place for 4 weeks after surgery. In addition, the patient receives a long arm cast with elbow back slab support for 4 weeks.

CRPP for a patient with a malunion or nonunion after >3 months and after an initial delayed diagnosis is only viable if the displacement is less than 5 mm, shows an unstable condylar fragment, and shows no evidence of bony bridging on a CT scan [37].

3.2.2. Open Reduction and Internal Fixation

Open reduction and internal fixation (Figure 3) is the preferred surgical treatment option for a fracture showing more than 4-mm displacement and/or rotation of the fragment. It is also the next step-up surgical option when CRPP fails to reduce the fracture to an anatomic situation. A small incision is made on the anterolateral side of the elbow. Subsequent careful dissection of the subcutaneous tissue, fascia, and articular capsule is performed. The malrotation of the fracture's fragment and size warrants careful dissection not to disrupt the distal humerus's blood supply and/or harm the radial nerve bundle. Like with CRPP, the surgeon will fix the fracture by placing two smooth Kirschner wires perpendicular to the fracture line. The postoperative treatment is similar to that of the

CRPP. Surgeons can opt for screw fixation with a small AO bone screw combined with K-wires for rotational stability of the fragment. However, studies show screw fixation results in comparable quality of life and range of motion postoperatively while having disadvantages such as second surgery to remove the screw, impairment of the range of motion, delayed union, and wound infections [36,43].

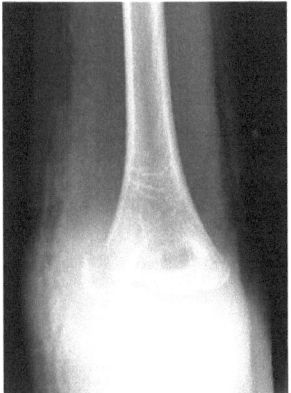 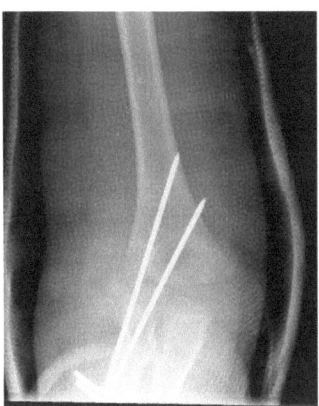 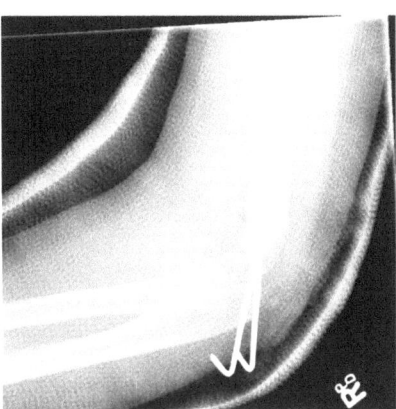

Figure 3. (**Left**) Anterior–posterior view of a lateral humeral condyle fracture. (**Middle**) Anterior–posterior and (**right**) lateral radiographic view of the elbow after open reduction and internal k-wire fixation.

ORIF for a patient with a malunion or nonunion after >3 months and after an initial delayed diagnosis is viable if the displacement is greater than 5 mm or is less than 5 mm with a normal elbow alignment [37,38]. If the patient has an elbow malalignment, a corrective osteotomy with simultaneous anterior transposition of the ulnar nerves can be performed [37,38].

4. Complications

Complications can occur during and after treatment. One in ten patients with lateral humeral condyle fractures has severe complications of the fracture and/or treatment [8,33,36]. Unsuccessful treatment of this complicated and menacing fracture may lead to a long-term loss in quality of life for pediatric patients. To minimize the risk of complications during treatment, the attending physician benefits from consulting an experienced pediatric elbow surgeon when discussing treatment options. The most notable complications are lateral condyle overgrowth, surgical site infection, pin tract infections, stiffness resulting in decreased range of motion, cubitus valgus deformities, 'fishtail' deformities, malunion, non-union, avascular necrosis, and premature epiphyseal fusion.

4.1. Lateral Overgrowth

Lateral overgrowth or lateral 'spurring' is a hypertrophic bony overgrowth on the lateral side of the elbow due to overstimulation of osteoblasts during the normal bone healing process [47,48]. Lateral overgrowth can be appreciated on conventional radiographs and felt during a physical examination of the elbow [10,29]. The occurrence rate of this complication is comparable between both treatment groups (non-surgical, 4.5–74%; and surgical, 4.5–73.7%) and between surgical techniques (CRPP, 4.5–73.7%; ORIF K-wires, 22.1–73.7%; and ORIF cannulated screw, 10.1–74%) [4,29,34,36,42,49–51].

4.2. Infections

Infections are an infrequent complication of surgical interventions and can be divided into two groups: superficial surgical site infections and deep infections of the osteosynthesis material. Treatment options for these infections can differ, ranging from local topical (antibiotic) treatment to extensive revision surgery. The occurrence rate of infections as a complication of lateral humeral condyle elbow surgery is 0.01–19.3% [10,36,39,42,43,50,51].

4.3. Malunion and Non-Union

A malunion of the bone describes the situation in which a patient's bone does not heal properly and creates an abnormally shaped joint with possible impaired function of the extremity as a result. A delayed or even non-union of the bone is a failure of a fracture to heal properly after three to nine months [52]. Malunion can cause structural deformities with a cubitus varus or, more commonly, cubitus valgus or impairment in the range of motion. Non-union or malunion of lateral humeral condyle fractures often require revision surgery to attempt to repair shortcomings and improve clinical outcomes for the patient [38,53–57]. Non-union or malunion, as a complication after revision surgery, occurred between 0–13% [54–56]. The physical performance score of the elbow, measured using the mayo performance score, increased in more than 80% of patients [54–56]. Non-union and malunion of the fracture occur more frequently in the cast therapy group [10,33,42]. The occurrence rate of non-union and malunion of the fracture is between 0–11.8% and 1.3–11.8%, respectively [4,8,10,36,39,40,42,43,49–51,53,58]. This rate of occurrence is exceptionally high, demonstrating the unforgiving nature of fracture healing for lateral humeral condyle fractures.

4.4. Avascular Necrosis

Avascular necrosis, or osteonecrosis, is a complication that causes ischemic damage to bone cells and, eventually, necrosis of bone due to the loss of blood supply. This can occur to bones after trauma because of the increased swelling, decreased range of motion of the elbow, and rotation of the broken fragment with subsequent tearing of the arteries [40]. The capitulum and lateral condyle are supplied solely with blood from a couple of small end arteries on the lateral side of the elbow. Hence, the capitulum and lateral condyle are considered to be relatively avascular. Therefore, one can appreciate how a slight traumatic injury or surgical operation through a posterior dissection approach can cause permanent damage to the small arteries supplying the lateral side, causing avascular necrosis [59]. The occurrence rate of avascular necrosis after lateral condyle fractures is 0.9–3.1% [8,39,40,49,51,58]. No study has reported the difference in occurrence rates of avascular necrosis between a non-operative and surgical treatment option. The elbow's functionality, stability, and range of motion are highly impeded after avascular necrosis. As a result, the patient will have a long-term disability when it comes to daily function.

5. Conclusions

Lateral humeral condyle fractures are frequently seen in pediatric patients. The Song's classification is the best validated and most recommended method out of all classification systems developed in the past. Treatment options vary from non-operative treatment with a cast to an open reduction and internal fixation. The success rate for these treatments, i.e., patients with successful fracture healing and without complications, is between 89.8–91.5%. The most notable complications are malunion or non-union, avascular necrosis, postoperative infections, and decreased mobility. Most important, the complications of lateral humeral condyle fractures are quite severe and, if untreated, could lead to a disproportionate loss in the quality of life.

Author Contributions: Conceptualization, T.F.F.S. and C.J.A.v.B.; writing—original draft preparation, T.F.F.S.; writing—review and editing, J.W.C., B.T., D.E. and C.J.A.v.B.; visualization, T.F.F.S. and C.J.A.v.B.; artwork, T.F.F.S.; supervision, D.E. and C.J.A.v.B.; project administration, J.W.C., C.J.A.v.B. All authors have read and agreed to the published version of the manuscript.

Funding: This research received no external funding.

Institutional Review Board Statement: Not applicable.

Informed Consent Statement: Not applicable.

Data Availability Statement: No new data were created or analyzed in this study. Data sharing is not applicable to this article.

Conflicts of Interest: The authors declare no conflict of interest.

References

1. Hedström, E.M.; Svensson, O.; Bergström, U.; Michno, P. Epidemiology of fractures in children and adolescents: Increased incidence over the past decade: A population-based study from northern Sweden. *Acta Orthop.* **2010**, *81*, 148–153. [CrossRef] [PubMed]
2. Naranje, S.M.; Erali, R.A.; Warner, W.C.; Sawyer, J.R.; Kelly, D.M. Epidemiology of Pediatric Fractures Presenting to Emergency Departments in the United States. *J. Pediatr. Orthop.* **2016**, *36*, e45–e48. [CrossRef] [PubMed]
3. Hussain, S.; Dar, T.; Beigh, A.Q.; Dhar, S.; Ahad, H.; Hussain, I.; Ahmad, S. Pattern and epidemiology of pediatric musculoskeletal injuries in Kashmir valley, a retrospective single-center study of 1467 patients. *J. Pediatr. Orthop. Part B* **2015**, *24*, 230–237. [CrossRef] [PubMed]
4. Hwan Koh, K.; Wook Seo, S.; Mu Kim, K.; Sup Shim, J. Clinical and Radiographic Results of Lateral Condylar Fracture of Distal Humerus in Children. *J. Pediatr. Orthop.* **2010**, *30*, 425–429.
5. Landin, L.A.; Danielsson, L.G. Elbow fractures in children. *Acta Orthop. Sand.* **1986**, *57*, 309–312. [CrossRef]
6. Houshian, S.; Mehdi, B.; Larsen, M.S. The epidemiology of elbow fracture in children: Analysis of 355 fractures, with special reference to supracondylar humerus fractures. *J. Orthop. Sci.* **2001**, *6*, 312–315. [CrossRef]
7. Emery, K.H.; Zingula, S.N.; Anton, C.G.; Salisbury, S.R.; Tamai, J. Pediatric elbow fractures: A new angle on an old topic. *Pediatr. Radiol.* **2016**, *46*, 61–66. [CrossRef]
8. Tan, S.H.S.; Dartnell, J.; Lim, A.K.S.; Hui, J.H. Paediatric lateral condyle fractures: A systematic review. *Arch. Orthop. Trauma Surg.* **2018**, *138*, 809–817. [CrossRef]
9. James, V.; Chin, A.; Chng, C.; Lim, F.; Ting, M.; Chan, Y.H.; Ganapathy, S. Lateral Condyle Fracture of the Humerus Among Children Attending a Pediatric Emergency Department; A 10-Year Single-Center Experience. *Pediatr. Emerg. Care* **2021**, *37*, e1339–e1344. [CrossRef]
10. Kwang, S.; Song, H.; Kang, B.; Woo, M.; Chul Bae, K.; Cho, C.H. Internal Oblique Radiographs for Diagnosis of Nondisplaced or Minimally Displaced Lateral Condylar Fractures of the Humérus in Children. *J. Bone Jt. Surg.* **2007**, *89*, 58–63.
11. Hill, C.E.; Cooke, S. Common Paediatric Elbow Injuries. *Open Orthop. J.* **2017**, *11*, 1380–1393. [CrossRef] [PubMed]
12. Shaerf, D.A.; Vanhegan, I.S.; Dattani, R. Diagnosis, management and complications of distal humerus lateral condyle fractures in children. *Shoulder Elb.* **2018**, *10*, 114–120. [CrossRef] [PubMed]
13. Okubo, H.; Nakasone, M.; Kinjo, M.; Onaka, K.; Futenma, C.; Kanaya, F. Epidemiology of paediatric elbow fractures: A retrospective multi-centre study of 488 fractures. *J. Child Orthop.* **2019**, *13*, 516–521. [CrossRef] [PubMed]
14. Rennic, L.; Court-Brown, C.M.; Mok, J.Y.Q.; Beattie, T.F. The epidemiology of fractures in children. *Injury* **2007**, *38*, 913–922. [CrossRef]
15. Sananta, P.; Sintong, L.; Prasetio, B.; Putera, M.A.; Andarini, S.; Kalsum, U.; Dradjat, R.S. Elbow fracture in children at saiful anwar general hospital, nine years experiences. *Open Access Maced. J. Med. Sci.* **2019**, *7*, 4069–4071. [CrossRef]
16. Milch, H. Fractures and fracture dislocations of the humeral condyles. *J. Trauma* **1964**, *4*, 592–607. [CrossRef] [PubMed]
17. Abzug, J.M.; Dua, K.; Kozin, S.H.; Herman, M.J. Current Concepts in the Treatment of Lateral Condyle Fractures in Children. *J. Am. Acad. Orthop. Surg.* **2020**, *28*, E9–E19. [CrossRef]
18. Herdea, A.; Ulici, A.; Toma, A.; Voicu, B.; Charkaoui, A. The relationship between the dominant hand and the occurrence of the supracondylar humerus fracture in pediatric orthopedics. *Children* **2021**, *8*, 51. [CrossRef]
19. Bryce, C.D.; Armstrong, A.D. Anatomy and Biomechanics of the Elbow. *Orthop. Clin. N. Am.* **2008**, *39*, 141–154. [CrossRef]
20. Paulsen, F.; Waschke, J. (Eds.) *Sobotta Atlas of Human Anatomy*, 15th ed.; Elsevier: Amsterdam, The Netherlands, 2011.
21. Jakob, R.; Fowles, J.V.; Rang, M.; Kassab, M.T. Observations concerning fractures of the lateral humeral condyle in children. *J. Bone Jt. Surg. Br.* **1975**, *57*, 430–436. [CrossRef]
22. Finnbogason, T.; Karlsson, G.; Lindberg, L.; Mortensson, W. Nondisplaced and minimally displaced fractures of the lateral humeral condyle in children: A prospective radiographic investigation of fracture stability. *J. Pediatr. Orthop.* **1995**, *15*, 422–425. [CrossRef] [PubMed]

23. Weiss, J.M.; Graves, S.; Yang, S.; Mendelsohn, E.; Kay, R.M.; Skaggs, D.L. A new classification system predictive of complications in surgically treated pediatric humeral lateral condyle fractures. *J. Pediatr. Orthop.* **2009**, *29*, 602–605. [CrossRef] [PubMed]
24. Mirsky, E.C.; Karas, E.H.; Weiner, L.S. Lateral condyle fractures in children: Evaluation of classification and treatment. *J. Orthop. Trauma* **1997**, *11*, 117–120. [CrossRef]
25. Pennington, R.G.C.; Corner, J.A.; Brownlow, H.C. Milch's classification of paediatric lateral condylar mass fractures: Analysis of inter- and intraobserver reliability and comparison with operative findings. *Injury* **2009**, *40*, 249–252. [CrossRef]
26. Ramo, B.A.; Funk, S.S.; Elliott, M.E.; Jo, C.H. The Song Classification Is Reliable and Guides Prognosis and Treatment for Pediatric Lateral Condyle Fractures: An Independent Validation Study with Treatment Algorithm. *J. Pediatric Orthop.* **2020**, *40*, E203–E209. [CrossRef] [PubMed]
27. Appelboam, A.; Reuben, A.D.; Benger, J.R.; Beech, F.; Dutson, J.; Haig, S.; Higginson, I.; Klein, J.A.; Le Roux, S.; Saranga, S.S.; et al. Elbow extension test to rule out elbow fracture: Multicentre, prospective validation and observational study of diagnostic accuracy in adults and children. *BMJ* **2009**, *338*, 31–33. [CrossRef] [PubMed]
28. Knutsen, A.; Avoian, T.; Borkowski, S.L.; Ebramzadeh, E.; Zionts, L.E.; Sangiorgio, S.N. Accuracy of radiographs in assessment of displacement in lateral humeral condyle fractures. *J. Child Orthop.* **2014**, *8*, 83–89. [CrossRef]
29. Soon Song, K.; Woon Shin, Y.; Wug, C.O.; Choer Bae, K.; Hyun Cho, C. Closed Reduction and Internal Fixation of Completely Displaced and Rotated Lateral Condyle Fractures of the Humerus in Children. *J. Orthop. Trauma* **2010**, *24*, 434–438. [CrossRef]
30. Poppelaars, M.A.; Eygendaal, D.; The, B.; van Oost, I.; van Bergen, C.J.A. Diagnosis and Treatment of Children with a Radiological Fat Pad Sign without Visible Elbow Fracture Vary Widely: An International Online Survey and Development of an Objective Definition. *Children* **2022**, *9*, 950. [CrossRef]
31. Kappelhof, B.; Roorda, B.L.; Poppelaars, M.A.; The, B.; Eygendaal, D.; Mulder, P.G.H.; Van Bergen, C.J. Occult Fractures in Children with a Radiographic Fat Pad Sign of the Elbow: A Meta-Analysis of 10 Published Studies. *JBJS Rev.* **2022**, *10*, e22. [CrossRef]
32. Chapman, V.M.; Grottkau, B.E.; Albright, M.; Salamipour, H.; Jaramillo, D. Multidetector computed tomography of pediatric lateral condylar fractures. *J. Comput. Assist. Tomogr.* **2005**, *29*, 842–846. [CrossRef] [PubMed]
33. Knapik, D.M.; Gilmore, A.; Liu, R.W. Conservative Management of Minimally Displaced ($\leq$2 mm) Fractures of the Lateral Humeral Condyle in Pediatric Patients: A Systematic Review. *J. Pediatr. Orthop.* **2017**, *37*, e83–e87. [CrossRef] [PubMed]
34. Marcheix, P.S.; Vacquerie, V.; Longis, B.; Peyrou, P.; Fourcade, L.; Moulies, D. Distal humerus lateral condyle fracture in children: When is the conservative treatment a valid option? *Orthop. Traumatol. Surg. Res.* **2011**, *97*, 304–307. [CrossRef]
35. Zhang, S.; Tan, S.H.S.; Lim, A.K.S.; Hui, J.H.P. Surgical outcomes in paediatric lateral condyle non-union: A systematic review and meta-analysis. *Orthop. Traumatol. Surg. Res.* **2022**, *108*, 102933. [CrossRef]
36. Eckhoff, M.D.; Tadlock, J.C.; Nicholson, T.C.; Wells, M.E.; Garcia, E.s.J.; Hennessey, T.A. Open reduction of pediatric lateral condyle fractures: A systematic review. *Shoulder Elb.* **2022**, *14*, 317–325. [CrossRef] [PubMed]
37. Trisolino, G.; Antonioli, D.; Gallone, G.; Stallone, S.; Zarantonello, P.; Tanzi, P.; Olivotto, E.; Stilli, L.; Di Gennaro, G.L.; Stilli, S. Neglected fractures of the lateral humeral condyle in children; which treatment for which condition? *Children* **2021**, *8*, 56. [CrossRef]
38. Prakash, J.; Mehtani, A. Open reduction versus in-situ fixation of neglected lateral condyle fractures: A comparative study. *J. Pediatr. Orthop. Part B* **2018**, *27*, 134–141. [CrossRef]
39. Pace, J.L.; Arkader, A.; Sousa, T.; Broom, A.M.; Shabtai, L. Incidence, Risk Factors, and Definition for Nonunion in Pediatric Lateral Condyle Fractures. *J. Pediatr. Orthop.* **2018**, *38*, e257–e261. [CrossRef]
40. Shabtai, L.; Lightdale-Miric, N.; Rounds, A.; Arkader, A.; Pace, J.L. Incidence, risk factors and outcomes of avascular necrosis occurring after humeral lateral condyle fractures. *J. Pediatr. Orthop. Part B* **2020**, *29*, 145–148. [CrossRef]
41. Pirker, M.E.; Weinberg, A.M.; Höllwarth, M.E.; Haberlik, A. Subsequent displacement of initially nondisplaced and minimally displaced fractures of the lateral humeral condyle in children. *J. Trauma Inj. Infect. Crit. Care* **2005**, *58*, 1202–1207. [CrossRef]
42. Gaston, M.S.; Irwin, G.J.; Huntley, J.S. Lateral condyle fracture of a child's humerus: The radiographic features may be subtle. *Scott Med. J.* **2012**, *57*, 1–4. [CrossRef] [PubMed]
43. Wendling-Keim, D.S.; Teschemacher, S.; Dietz, H.G.; Lehner, M. Lateral Condyle Fracture of the Humerus in Children: Kirschner Wire or Screw Fixation? *Eur. J. Pediatr. Surg.* **2021**, *31*, 374–379. [CrossRef] [PubMed]
44. Li, X.; Shen, X.; Wu, X.; Wang, S. Ultrasound-assisted closed reduction and percutaneous pinning for displaced and rotated lateral condylar humeral fractures in children. *J. Shoulder Elbow Surg.* **2021**, *30*, 2113–2119. [CrossRef] [PubMed]
45. Beerekamp, M.S.H.; Sulkers, G.S.I.; Ubbink, D.T.; Maas, M.; Schep, N.W.L.; Goslings, J.C. Accuracy and consequences of 3D-fluoroscopy in upper and lower extremity fracture treatment: A systematic review. *Eur. J. Radiol.* **2012**, *81*, 4019–4028. [CrossRef]
46. Colton, C.; Monsell, F.; Slongo, T. AO General K-Wires Principles. 2023. Available online: https://surgeryreference.aofoundation.org/orthopedic-trauma/pediatric-trauma/basic-technique/general-k-wire-principles (accessed on 23 May 2023).
47. Hasler, C.C.; von Laer, L. Prevention of growth disturbances after fractures of the lateral humeral condyle in children. *J. Pediatr. Orthop. B* **2001**, *10*, 123–130.
48. Pribaz, J.R.; Bernthal, N.M.; Wong, T.C.; Silva, M. Lateral spurring (overgrowth) after pediatric lateral condyle fractures. *J. Pediatr. Orthop.* **2012**, *32*, 456–460. [CrossRef]

49. Ganeshalingam, R.; Donnan, A.; Evans, O.; Hoq, M.; Camp, M.; Donnan, L. Lateral condylar fractures of the humerus in children: Does the type of fixation matter? *Bone Jt. J.* **2018**, *100-B*, 387–395. [CrossRef]
50. Leonidou, A.; Chettiar, K.; Graham, S.; Akhbari, P.; Antonis, K.; Tsiridis, E.; Leonidou, O. Open reduction internal fixation of lateral humeral condyle fractures in children. A series of 105 fractures from a single institution. *Strateg. Trauma Limb Reconstr.* **2014**, *9*, 73–78. [CrossRef]
51. Pennock, A.T.; Salgueiro, L.; Upasani, V.V.; Bastrom, T.P.; Newton, P.O.; Yaszay, B. Closed Reduction and Percutaneous Pinning Versus Open Reduction and Internal Fixation for Type II Lateral Condyle Humerus Fractures in Children Displaced >2 mm. *J. Pediatr. Orthop.* **2016**, *36*, 780–786. [CrossRef]
52. Thomas, J.D.; Kehoe, J.L. *Bone Nonunion*; StatPearls: Tampa, FL, USA, 2023.
53. Launay, F.; Leet, A.I.; Jacopin, S.; Jouve, J.-L.; Bollini, G.; Sponseller, P.D. Lateral humeral condyle fractures in children: A comparison of two approaches to treatment. *J. Pediatr. Orthop.* **2004**, *24*, 385–391. [CrossRef]
54. Toh, S.; Tsubo, K.; Nishikawa, S.; Inoue, S.; Nakamura, R.; Narita, S. Osteosynthesis for Nonunion of the Lateral Humeral Condyle. *Clin. Orthop. Relat. Res.* **2002**, *405*, 230–241. [CrossRef]
55. Eamsobhana, P.; Kaewpornsawan, K. Should we repair nonunion of the lateral humeral condyle in children? *Int. Orthop.* **2015**, *39*, 1579–1585. [CrossRef]
56. Park, H.; Hwang, J.H.; Kwon, Y.U.; Kim, H.W. Osteosynthesis In Situ for Lateral Condyle Nonunion in Children. *J. Pediatr. Orthop.* **2015**, *35*, 334–340. [CrossRef]
57. Salgueiro, L.; Roocroft, J.H.; Bastrom, T.P.; Edmonds, E.W.; Pennock, A.T.; Upasani, V.V.; Yaszay, B. Rate and Risk Factors for Delayed Healing Following Surgical Treatment of Lateral Condyle Humerus Fractures in Children. *J. Pediatr. Orthop.* **2017**, *37*, 1–6. [CrossRef]
58. Silva, M.; Cooper, S.D. Closed Reduction and Percutaneous Pinning of Displaced Pediatric Lateral Condyle Fractures of the Humerus. *J. Pediatr. Orthop.* **2015**, *35*, 661–665. [CrossRef]
59. Eygendaal, D.; Bain, G.; Pederzini, L.; Poehling, G. Osteochondritis dissecans of the elbow: State of the art. *J. ISAKOS* **2017**, *2*, 47–57. [CrossRef]

Disclaimer/Publisher's Note: The statements, opinions and data contained in all publications are solely those of the individual author(s) and contributor(s) and not of MDPI and/or the editor(s). MDPI and/or the editor(s) disclaim responsibility for any injury to people or property resulting from any ideas, methods, instructions or products referred to in the content.

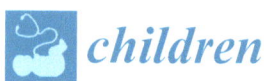 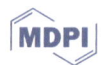

Article

Pediatric Elbow Dislocations and Associated Fractures

Laura Lewallen [1], Marilyn E. Elliott [2], Amy McIntosh [3,4] and Christine A. Ho [3,4,*]

1. Department of Orthopaedic Surgery, University of Chicago Medicine, Chicago, IL 60637, USA
2. Scottish Rite for Children, Dallas, TX 75219, USA
3. Department of Orthopaedic Surgery, Children's Medical Center of Dallas, Dallas, TX 75235, USA
4. Department of Orthopaedic Surgery, University of Texas Southwestern, Dallas, TX 75390, USA
* Correspondence: christine.ho@childrens.com; Tel.: +1-(214)-456-6050

Abstract: The objective was to evaluate pediatric patients with acute elbow dislocation and/or associated fracture to determine which were indicated for surgical intervention, using a single institution, Institutional Review Board (IRB) approved retrospective review of patients who presented to the Emergency Department (ED) with an acute elbow dislocation. Inclusion criteria were age ≤ 18 years, acute elbow dislocation injury, and appropriate imaging. A total of 117 patients were included 37 had a simple elbow dislocation, 80 had an associated fracture (medial epicondyle 59, lateral condyle 9, radial head/neck 7, other 5). A total of 62% (73/117) were male. The average age was 10.3 years (range 4–17). Mechanisms of injury included: falls from height/playground equipment (46), trampoline (14), and sports (57). All 37 patients with a simple elbow dislocation were successfully treated with closed reduction. Of the 80 patients with an associated fracture, 30 (38%) went on to open reduction internal fixation (ORIF). A total of 59 patients had an associated medial epicondyle fracture; 24 (41%) of whom went on to ORIF. Nine patients had an associated lateral condyle fracture, five (56%) of whom went on to ORIF. Patients with a simple elbow dislocation can be successfully treated with a closed reduction in the ED. However, 30/80 patients with an associated fracture (medial epicondyle, lateral condyle, or radial neck) required operative management.

Keywords: elbow dislocation; medial epicondyle fracture; pediatric elbow injury

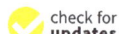

Citation: Lewallen, L.; Elliott, M.E.; McIntosh, A.; Ho, C.A. Pediatric Elbow Dislocations and Associated Fractures. *Children* **2023**, *10*, 993. https://doi.org/10.3390/children10060993

Academic Editors: Johannes Mayr, Cinzia Maspero, Christiaan J. A. van Bergen and Joost W. Colaris

Received: 7 March 2023
Revised: 7 April 2023
Accepted: 30 May 2023
Published: 1 June 2023

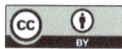

Copyright: © 2023 by the authors. Licensee MDPI, Basel, Switzerland. This article is an open access article distributed under the terms and conditions of the Creative Commons Attribution (CC BY) license (https://creativecommons.org/licenses/by/4.0/).

1. Introduction

Upper extremity injuries are common in the pediatric population. Elbow dislocations account for approximately 3–6% of elbow injuries in the pediatric population [1,2]. These injuries most often occur in children between 10–15 years of age [2]. Boys have a higher incidence compared to girls, by a ratio of 3:1 [3].

The mechanism of injury typically involves a fall on an outstretched arm, most often with the elbow extended. These types of injuries often occur as a result of a fall from playground equipment, bicycles, trampolines, or sporting activities. Posterolateral displacement is the most frequent pattern of dislocation. A valgus force may result in the avulsion of the ulnar collateral ligament (UCL) and/or an associated medial epicondyle fracture. Direct force may also cause a medial epicondyle fracture [4].

Various types of fractures about the elbow may occur in association with a dislocation event. The majority of associated injuries in the pediatric population involve simple fracture patterns, though more complex fracture patterns do occur [5]. Medial epicondyle fractures are the most common; associated with an elbow dislocation in 30–60% of pediatric cases [2,6]. These fractures account for approximately 12–20% of elbow injuries in the pediatric population [4,7]. Other fractures associated with pediatric elbow dislocations include lateral condyle, radial head/neck, coronoid process, or olecranon.

The standard of treatment for an acute elbow dislocation is urgent closed reduction, followed by brief immobilization and early active range of motion [1,6]. Reduction maneuvers including hyperextension, longitudinal traction, forearm supination, and elbow flexion are usually successful. Patients with an open injury, associated neurovascular injury, or persistent instability typically require open reduction and exploration. Open reduction internal fixation (ORIF) is indicated for those with an incarcerated fracture fragment (i.e., medial epicondyle) [8]. However, controversy exists regarding the amount of fracture displacement which is acceptable for non-operative management [9,10].

Our hypothesis was that a subset of patients with these injuries (elbow dislocation and associated fracture) may be safely managed with reduction/surgery in a delayed fashion, rather than acute reduction in the Emergency Department. The objective of this study was to evaluate pediatric patients with an acute elbow dislocation, and/or associated elbow fracture, to further characterize which patients were indicated for surgical intervention.

2. Materials and Methods

2.1. Study Design

This was an Institutional Review Board (IRB) approved retrospective review of patients who presented to our Emergency Department (ED) with an acute elbow dislocation between 1 January 2008 and 31 December 2016. The study's IRB number is STU-092016-039 and was approved on 12 October 2016. The study was performed at a single institution, a pediatric level-1 trauma center.

2.2. Population

Patients with an acute elbow injury who were treated with closed reduction were first identified from paper fluoroscopy logs kept by the radiology department. In total, 303 elbow injuries were identified in this manner. The type of elbow injury was confirmed through a chart review of the orthopedic consult notes and radiology reports, as well as a radiographic review of the images.

2.3. Inclusion/Exclusion Criteria

Patients were included in the final analysis if they met the following criteria: (1) acute elbow dislocation with or without an associated elbow fracture, (2) age 18 years or younger at the time of injury, and (3) appropriate imaging to characterize the injury. Patients were excluded from the final analysis if they (1) had any acute elbow injury that did not include an elbow dislocation (i.e., radial head dislocation, supracondylar or other distal humerus fracture, Monteggia injury), (2) were over the age of 18 years at the time of injury, or (3) did not have appropriate imaging.

2.4. Data Collection/Analysis

The following data were collected: age, gender, laterality, mechanism of injury, treatment at an outside hospital (if any), nature of associated fracture (if any), amount of displacement at the fracture site, whether the closed reduction was attempted, whether surgery was necessary, time from initial treatment (closed reduction) to surgery, indication for surgery, a surgical procedure performed, and length of follow up. Outside treatment was collected from either Emergency Medical Services (EMS) reports or initial ED documentation. The mechanism of injury was grouped into the following categories: fall from height or playground activity, sporting activity, or trampoline. Initial closed reduction data were obtained from the orthopedic consult notes and procedure notes. Surgical indications and procedures performed were determined from the operative notes. The maximum amount of displacement at the fracture site was measured on post-reduction radiographs, for those patients with an associated fracture (medial epicondyle, lateral condyle, radial head/neck). Length of follow-up was collected from the clinic progress notes.

3. Results

3.1. Demographic Data

In total, 303 patients with acute elbow injuries were identified. A total of 117 met our inclusion criteria. A total of 31.6% (37/117) of patients had a simple elbow dislocation. A total of 68.4% (80/117) had an associated fracture, with the medial epicondyle being the most common (73.8%, 59/80). Nine patients had an associated lateral condyle fracture, seven patients had a radial head/neck fracture, and five patients had other fractures (coronoid, olecranon) (Figure 1). There were more males than females (62.4% versus 37.6%). The average age at the time of injury was 10.3 years (range 4–17 years).

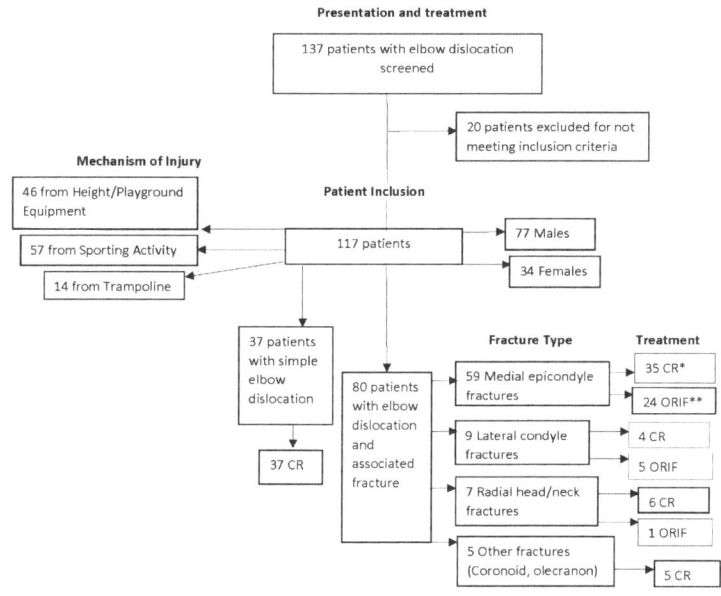

Figure 1. Flow chart of patient presentation and treatment.

3.2. Mechanism of Injury

As shown in Table 1, the most common mechanisms of injury were a fall from height/playground equipment (39.3%, 46/117) or sporting activity (48.7%, 57/117). Trampoline injuries were less common (12%, 14/117).

Table 1. Demographic Data.

		n = 117
Sex	Male	73
	Female	44
Mechanism of Injury	Fall from height/playground equipment	46
	Sporting Activity	57
	Trampoline	14

3.3. Treatment

All 117 patients underwent closed reduction under sedation in the ED. Reductions were performed by resident physicians or advanced practice providers (APPs), including orthopedic nurse practitioners and orthopedic physician assistants. Standard closed reduction maneuvers were performed, including a combination of longitudinal traction, supination, and elbow flexion, anteriorly directed force on the olecranon.

The 37 patients with a simple elbow dislocation (i.e., no associated fractures) were all successfully treated with closed reduction.

The number of associated fractures, as well as the treatment summary, are shown in Table 2. Of the 80 patients with an associated fracture, 73.8% (59/80) had a medial epicondyle fracture. A total of 40.7% (24/59) of the medial epicondyle fractures were treated with open reduction internal fixation after reduction of the elbow dislocation (Figure 2).

Table 2. Injury Pattern and Treatment Summary.

	n	CR * Attempted?	CR * Successful?	ORIF **	Indication for ORIF **
TOTAL INCLUDED	117	117	85	30	
Simple dislocation	37	37	37	0	
Associated fracture	80	80	50	30	
Medial epicondyle fracture	59	59	35	24 (40.7%)	fracture displacement—19 (79.2%)
					incarcerated fracture fragment—5 (20.8%)
Lateral condyle fracture	9	9	4	5 (55.6%)	fracture displacement—5 (100%)
Radial head/neck fracture	7	7	6	1 (14.3%)	fracture displacement—1
Other (coronoid, olecranon)	5	5	5	0	

CR *—Closed Reduction. ORIF **—Open Reduction Internal Fixation.

The indication for surgery was the amount of fracture displacement per the attending surgeon's operative notes in 79.2% (19/24), and an incarcerated fracture fragment in 20.8% (5/24).

Nine patients had a lateral condyle fracture. A total of 55.6% (5/9) of these patients underwent open reduction internal fixation after reduction of the elbow dislocation (Figure 3).

The indication for surgery in all five patients was the amount of fracture displacement. One patient was treated with closed reduction in the operating room (OR), due to ongoing instability after initial reduction in the ED.

Seven patients had a radial head/neck fracture. One of these patients was treated with open reduction internal fixation, due to displacement of the fracture fragment.

Five patients had various other associated fractures (coronoid, olecranon). None of these patients were treated surgically.

For those patients with an associated fracture (medial epicondyle, lateral condyle, or radial head/neck), the maximum amount of displacement was measured on post-reduction radiographs. Several patients did not have appropriate imaging to measure the maximum displacement. Comparisons were made between patients treated non-operatively and those treated with ORIF. The results are shown in Table 3.

Table 3. Comparisons of Post-Reduction Maximum Displacement between Open Reduction/Internal Fixation (ORIF) and No-ORIF groups.

Variables	Overall		No-ORIF Group		ORIF Group		p-Value
	n	Mean ± Std *, Med (Range)	n	Mean ± Std *, Med (Range)	n	Mean ± Std *, Med (Range)	
Fracture displacement (mm)	51	6.52 ± 5.28, 5.00 (0, 21.10)	33	4.30 ± 3.50, 4.00 (0, 11.00)	18	10.58 ± 5.66, 11.05 (1.50, 21.10)	0.0004
Fracture displacement (mm)—with medial epicondyle fracture	47	6.85 ± 5.37, 6.80 (0, 21.10)	33	4.30 ± 3.50, 4.00 (0, 11.00)	14	12.85 ± 4.07, 12.75 (6.80, 21.10)	<0.0001
Fracture displacement (mm)—with lateral condyle fracture	4	2.63 ± 1.11, 2.50 (1.50, 4.00)	0		4	2.63 ± 1.11, 2.50 (1.50, 4.00)	

Std *—standard deviation.

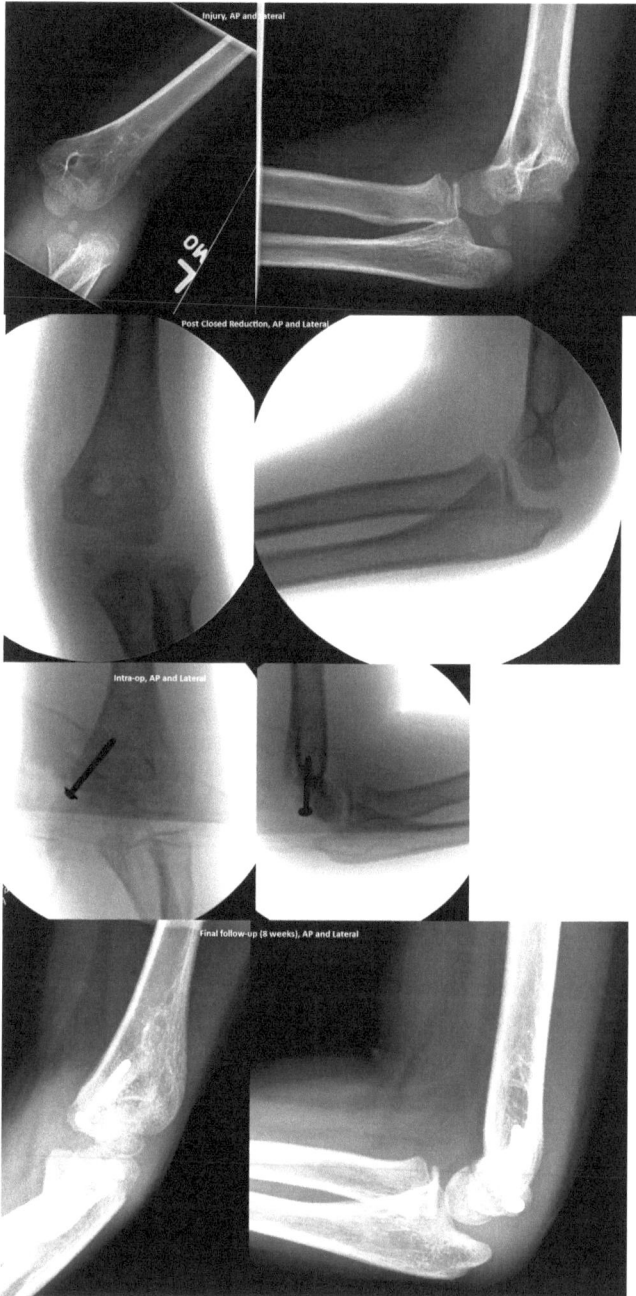

Figure 2. The clinical course of a 9-year-old with a medial epicondyle fracture. Injury (first row from the top, left image—Antero-Posterior (AP); right image—Lateral); Post Closed Reduction (second row from the top, left image—AP scan; right image—Lateral); Intra-operative (third row from the top, left image—AP; right image—Lateral); Final follow up at 8 weeks (fourth from the top/Bottom row, left image—AP; right image—Lateral).

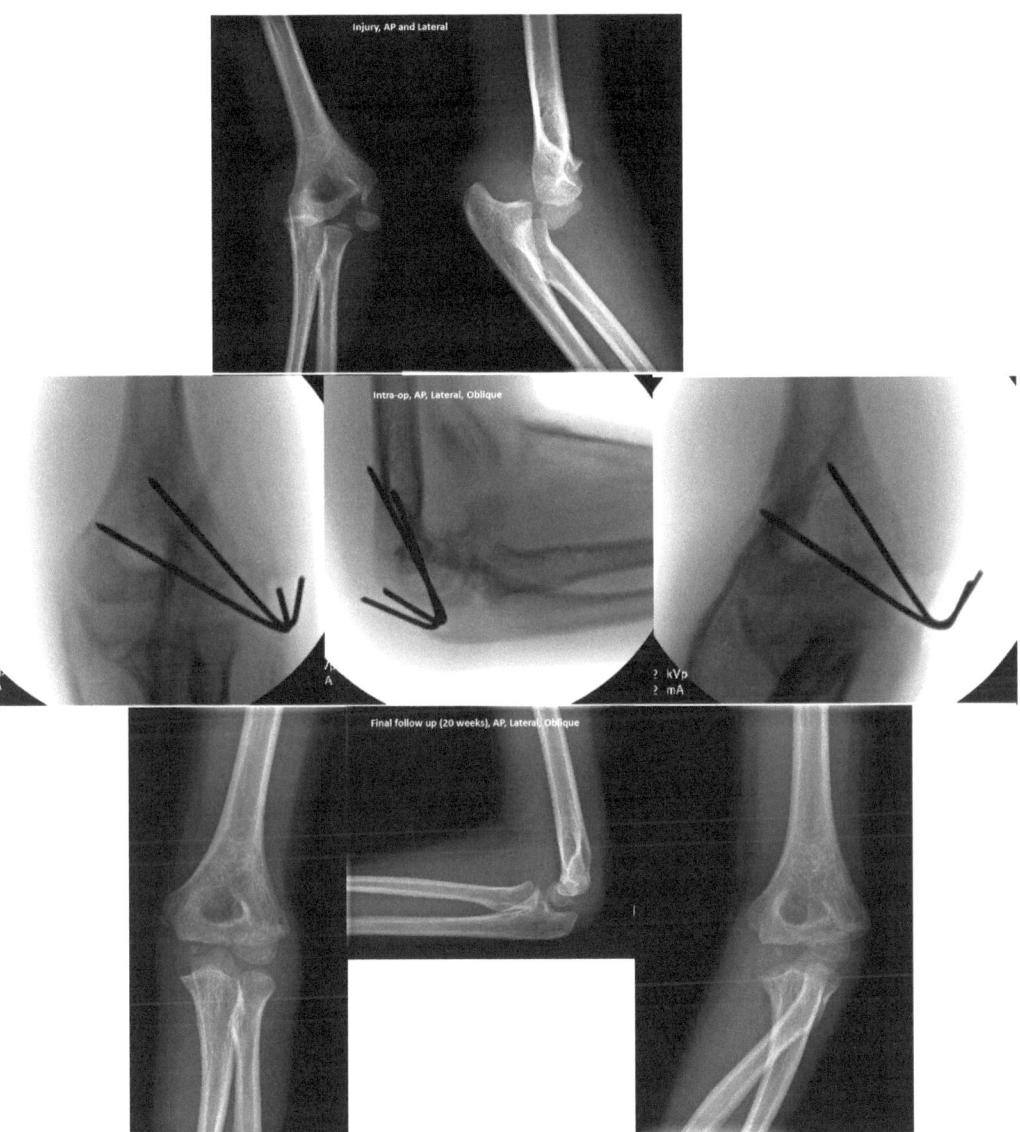

Figure 3. The clinical course of a 7-year-old male with a lateral condyle fracture. Injury (1st row from the top, left image—Antero-Posterior (AP); right image—Lateral); Intra-Operative (2nd row from the top, left image—AP; middle image—Lateral; right image—Oblique); Final follow-up at 20 weeks (3rd row from top/bottom row, left image—AP; middle image—Lateral; right image—Oblique.

Of all patients with an associated fracture in which maximum displacement measurements could be made ($n = 51$), there was a significant difference ($p = 0.0004$) between those treated non-operatively (mean displacement = 4.3 mm) and those treated with ORIF (mean displacement = 10.58 mm). For patients with a medial epicondyle fracture, there was also a statistically significant difference ($p = <0.0001$) between those treated non-operatively (mean displacement = 4.30 mm) and those treated with ORIF (mean displacement = 12.85 mm).

The lateral condyle and radial head/neck groups were too small to make comparisons or draw conclusions regarding fracture displacement.

In summary, 37.5% (30/80) of patients with an associated fracture went on to ORIF. Over 40% of patients with an associated medial epicondyle fracture, and over 50% of those with an associated lateral condyle fracture underwent operative management.

All surgeries were performed by fellowship-trained pediatric orthopedic surgeons. The average time from initial treatment (closed reduction) to surgery was 2.8 days (range 0–13 days, median 1 day). Of the 30 patients who were treated with ORIF, 28 had surgery within 7 days of closed reduction. The other two patients were initially managed non-operatively, then found to have a further displacement at the initial follow up visit, prompting the decision for surgical intervention (at 11 days and 13 days, respectively).

The average follow-up in this series was 65 days (range 0–666 days, median 46 days).

4. Discussion

In our series, none of the patients who presented with a simple elbow dislocation required operative intervention. These findings suggest that these injuries may be treated successfully with closed reduction under sedation in the ED.

Elbow dislocations in the pediatric population are a relatively uncommon injury. A recent study by Hyvonen et al. showed the stable incidence of elbow dislocations in the pediatric population in Finland from 1996–2014 [11]. There is consensus regarding the absolute indications for operative intervention, including neurovascular compromise, open injury, incarcerated fracture fragment, or inability to achieve a concentric, stable reduction. However, controversy exists regarding the management of concomitant injuries and the amount of fracture displacement which is amenable to non-operative treatment [7]. The purpose of this study was to evaluate pediatric patients with an acute elbow dislocation, to further characterize which patients were indicated for surgical intervention.

The average age (10.3 years) and gender distribution (63% male) in our cohort were similar to previous reports [2]. Sporting activities and fall from height/playground equipment were the most common mechanisms of injury.

Nearly 70% (80/117) of patients in our study had an associated fracture. Consistent with previous reports [7,8], medial epicondyle fracture was the most commonly associated injury (74%). As previously reported by Silva et al., associated lateral condyle fractures were uncommon [12]. ORIF was performed in nearly 40% of patients with an associated fracture, most commonly medial epicondyle, and lateral condyle fractures.

Murphy et al. recently reported a series of 145 patients with an elbow dislocation and noted concomitant fractures in 80% (114/145) [2]. Medial epicondyle fracture was the most common (60%). In their series, 59% of patients were treated with ORIF of associated fractures. The complication rate was found to be 14% (21/145). The authors identified risk factors for less than excellent functional outcomes including the presence of multiple associated fractures, operative intervention, and prolonged immobilization.

In our series, over 40% of patients with an associated medial epicondyle fracture and over 50% of patients with an associated lateral condyle fracture were treated surgically. Based on our findings, approximately half of the patients will be going on to surgery within the following day (median time to surgery was 1 day). With the assumption that the patient is neurovascularly intact, with a palpable pulse, and comfortably splinted, it may be reasonable to postpone closed reduction under sedation in the ED and proceed with operative intervention in a timely manner rather than subjecting the child to two anesthetics within 24 h. While both moderate sedation as well as general anesthesia in pediatric patients continues to improve in safety, there is evidence in laboratory animals that early exposure to anesthesia is associated with long-term brain changes [13,14], and that in children under the age of 4 years old, multiple, or prolonged exposures to anesthesia may have adverse effects on behavior, learning, and memory [15–17]. In addition, adverse events are a known risk of sedation and anesthesia, which may range from mild, such as a failed sedation [18,19], to a more serious adverse effect such as cardiac arrest [20]. While there is still no direct evidence linking anesthesia to negative central nervous system effects in children, exposure to anesthetic agents should be minimized, when possible, in the pediatric age group.

On the other hand, acute reduction in the ED is the standard of care for all joint dislocations. Urgent reduction results in improved patient comfort, decreased swelling and tension on the soft tissues, and therefore decreased risk of developing neurovascular complications. It is reasonable to conclude from our findings, that reduction IS indicated in the acute setting given the high likelihood of success and the possibility that surgery may not be necessary. A decision for surgery may then be made electively. This also makes the timing of surgery less urgent, in the event of OR delays and other scheduling hurdles.

Limitations of this study include its retrospective nature and lack of long-term follow-up, as is common in many studies looking at orthopedic trauma injuries. The study was performed in a single institution and is therefore limited in its generalizability. The main weakness of the study is that the indication for operative intervention for the medial epicondyle fracture varied by surgeon, as the indications for fixation of closed, non-incarcerated medial epicondyle fractures are controversial. Some surgeons in our practice feel strongly that any medial epicondyle fracture with an associated dislocation should be surgically fixed to prevent valgus instability, while others feel the non-operative treatment is appropriate with a displacement of the fragment up to 1 cm, consistent with prior published studies [9].

Future studies assessing other methods of evaluating fracture morphology may be worthwhile for these types of injuries. Computed tomography (CT) scans are used with caution in the pediatric population, but may have a role in some cases.

5. Conclusions

In conclusion, patients with a simple elbow dislocation (no associated fracture) can be successfully treated with a closed reduction in the ED. However, nearly half of patients with an elbow dislocation and associated medial epicondyle fracture or lateral condyle fracture go on to secondary operative management. This is important to consider when counseling patients and families regarding the initial management of these injuries, likelihood of surgery, and the possibility of the child having multiple anesthetics. Based on these findings, we recommend urgent reduction in the ED for patients with an associated fracture, with plans for surgery in a timely fashion as indicated.

Author Contributions: Conceptualization, L.L., M.E.E., A.M. and C.A.H.; Data curation, L.L., M.E.E., A.M. and C.A.H.; Formal analysis, L.L., M.E.E., A.M. and C.A.H.; Investigation, L.L., M.E.E., A.M. and C.A.H.; Methodology, L.L., M.E.E., A.M. and C.A.H.; Validation, L.L., M.E.E., A.M. and C.A.H.; Visualization, L.L., M.E.E., A.M. and C.A.H.; Writing—original draft preparation, L.L., M.E.E., A.M. and C.A.H.; Writing—review and editing, L.L., M.E.E., A.M. and C.A.H. All authors have read and agreed to the published version of the manuscript.

Funding: This research received no external funding.

Institutional Review Board Statement: Not applicable.

Informed Consent Statement: Not applicable.

Data Availability Statement: The data presented in this study are available on request from the corresponding author. The data are not available publicly due to privacy reasons.

Conflicts of Interest: The authors declare no conflict of interest.

References

1. Sofu, H.; Gursu, S.; Camurcu, Y.; Yildirim, T.; Sahin, V. Pure elbow dislocation in the paediatric age group. *Int. Orthop.* **2016**, *40*, 541–545. [CrossRef] [PubMed]
2. Murphy, R.F.; Vuillermin, C.; Naqvi, M.; Miller, P.E.; Bae, D.S.; Shore, B.J. Early outcomes of pediatric elbow dislocation-risk factors associated with morbidity. *J. Pediatr. Orthop.* **2017**, *37*, 440–446. [CrossRef] [PubMed]

3. Bilgili, F.; Dikmen, G.; Baş, A.; Asma, A.; Batibay, S.G.; Şirikçi, M.; Atalar, A.C. Acute traumatic posterior fracture dislocation of the elbow in pediatric patients: Impact of surgery time and associated fractures on outcome. *J. Pediatr. Orthop. B* **2016**, *25*, 434–438. [CrossRef] [PubMed]
4. Tarallo, L.; Mugnai, R.; Fiacchi, F.; Adani, R.; Zambianchi, F.; Catani, F. Pediatric medial epicondyle fractures with intra-articular elbow incarceration. *J. Orthop. Traumatol.* **2015**, *16*, 117–123. [CrossRef] [PubMed]
5. Magee, L.C.B.; Baghdadi, S.; Gohel, S.B.; Sankar, W.N. Complex Fracture-Dislocations of the Elbow in the Pediatric Population. *J. Pediatr. Orthop.* **2021**, *41*, e470–e474. [CrossRef] [PubMed]
6. Herring, J.A.; Tachdjian, M.O. *Tachdjian's Pediatric Orthopaedics: From the Texas Scottish Rite Hospital for Children*, 5th ed.; Saunders: Philadelphia, PA, USA, 2014.
7. Knapik, D.M.; Fausett, C.L.; Gilmore, A.; Liu, R.W. Outcomes of Nonoperative Pediatric Medial Humeral Epicondyle Fractures with and without Associated Elbow Dislocation. *J. Pediatr. Orthop.* **2017**, *37*, e224–e228. [CrossRef] [PubMed]
8. Vuillermin, C.; Donohue, K.S.; Miller, P.; Bauer, A.S.; Kramer, D.E.; Yen, Y.-M. Incarcerated Medial Epicondyle Fractures with Elbow Dislocation: Risk Factors Associated with Morbidity. *J. Pediatr. Orthop.* **2019**, *39*, e647–e651. [CrossRef] [PubMed]
9. Farsetti, P.; Potenza, V.; Caterini, R.; Ippolito, E. Long-Term Results of Treatment of Fractures of the Medial Humeral Epicondyle in Children. *J. Bone Jt. Surg.* **2001**, *83*, 1299–1305. [CrossRef] [PubMed]
10. Lawrence, J.T.R.; Patel, N.M.; Macknin, J.; Flynn, J.M.; Cameron, D.; Wolfgruber, H.C.; Ganley, T.J. Return to competitive sports after medial epicondyle fractures in adolescent athletes: Results of operative and nonoperative treatment. *Am. J. Sports Med.* **2013**, *41*, 1152–1157. [CrossRef] [PubMed]
11. Hyvönen, H.; Korhonen, L.; Hannonen, J.; Serlo, W.; Sinikumpu, J.-J. Recent trends in children's elbow dislocation with or without a concomitant fracture. *BMC Musculoskelet. Disord.* **2019**, *20*, 294. [CrossRef] [PubMed]
12. Silva, M.; Cooper, S.D.; Cha, A. Elbow dislocation with an associated lateral condyle fracture of the humerus: A rare occurrence in the pediatric population. *J. Pediatr. Orthop.* **2015**, *35*, 329–333. [CrossRef] [PubMed]
13. Jevtovic-Todorovic, V.; Hartman, R.E.; Izumi, Y.; Benshoff, N.D.; Dikranian, K.; Zorumski, C.F.; Olney, J.W.; Wozniak, D.F. Early exposure to common anesthetic agents causes widespread neurodegeneration in the developing rat brain and persistent learning deficits. *J. Neurosci.* **2003**, *23*, 876–882. [CrossRef] [PubMed]
14. Paule, M.; Li, M.; Allen, R.; Liu, F.; Zou, X.; Hotchkiss, C.; Hanig, J.; Patterson, T.; Slikker, W.; Wang, C. Ketamine anesthesia during the first week of life can cause long-lasting cognitive deficits in rhesus monkeys. *Neurotoxicol. Teratol.* **2011**, *33*, 220–230. [CrossRef] [PubMed]
15. Davidson, A.J.; Disma, N.; de Graaff, J.C.; Withington, D.E.; Dorris, L.; Bell, G.; Stargatt, R.; Bellinger, D.C.; Schuster, T.; Arnup, S.J.; et al. Neurodevelopmental outcome at 2 years of age after general anaesthesia and awake-regional anaesthesia in infancy (GAS): An international multicentre, randomised controlled trial. *Lancet* **2016**, *387*, 239–250, Erratum in *Lancet* **2016**, *387*, 228. [CrossRef] [PubMed]
16. McCann, M.E.; de Graaff, J.C.; Dorris, L.; Disma, N.; Withington, D.; Bell, G.; Grobler, A.; Stargatt, R.; Hunt, R.W.; Sheppard, S.J.; et al. Neurodevelopmental outcome at 5 years of age after general anaesthesia or awake-regional anaesthesia in infancy (GAS): An international, multicentre, randomised, controlled equivalence trial. *Lancet* **2019**, *393*, 664–677. [CrossRef] [PubMed]
17. Sun, L.S.; Li, G.; Miller, T.L.K.; Salorio, C.; Byrne, M.W.; Bellinger, D.C.; Ing, C.; Park, R.; Radcliffe, J.; Hays, S.R.; et al. Association Between a Single General Anesthesia Exposure Before Age 36 Months and Neurocognitive Outcomes in Later Childhood. *JAMA* **2016**, *315*, 2312–2320. [CrossRef] [PubMed]
18. Bjur, K.A.; Payne, E.T.; Nemergut, M.E.; Hu, D.; Flick, R.P. Anesthetic-Related Neurotoxicity and Neuroimaging in Children: A Call for Conversation. *J. Child Neurol.* **2017**, *32*, 594–602. [CrossRef] [PubMed]
19. Warner, D.O.; Zaccariello, M.J.; Katusic, S.K.; Schroeder, D.R.; Hanson, A.C.; Schulte, P.J.; Buenvenida, S.L.; Gleich, S.J.; Wilder, R.T.; Sprung, J.; et al. Neuropsychological and Behavioral Outcomes after Exposure of Young Children to Procedures Requiring General Anesthesia: The Mayo Anesthesia Safety in Kids (MASK) Study. *Anethesiology* **2018**, *129*, 89–105. [CrossRef] [PubMed]
20. Bartels, D.D.; McCann, M.E.; Davidson, A.J.; Polaner, D.M.; Whitlock, E.L.; Bateman, B.T. Estimating pediatric general anesthesia exposure: Quantifying duration and risk. *Paediatr. Anaesth.* **2018**, *28*, 520–527. [CrossRef] [PubMed]

Disclaimer/Publisher's Note: The statements, opinions and data contained in all publications are solely those of the individual author(s) and contributor(s) and not of MDPI and/or the editor(s). MDPI and/or the editor(s) disclaim responsibility for any injury to people or property resulting from any ideas, methods, instructions or products referred to in the content.

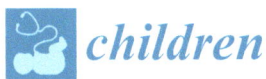

Article

Extra Lateral Pin or Less Radiation? A Comparison of Two Different Pin Configurations in the Treatment of Supracondylar Humerus Fracture

Özgür Kaya [1,*], Batuhan Gencer [2], Ahmet Çulcu [3] and Özgür Doğan [2]

1. Department of Orthopedics and Traumatology, Faculty of Medicine, Lokman Hekim University, Ankara 06000, Turkey
2. Department of Orthopedics and Traumatology, Ankara City Hospital, Ankara 06000, Turkey; gencer.batuhan@gmail.com (B.G.); dr.ozgurdogan@gmail.com (Ö.D.)
3. Department of Orthopedics and Traumatology, Ministry of Health Yüksekova State Hospital, Hakkari 30110, Turkey; dr.ahmetculcu@gmail.com
* Correspondence: ozgur.kaya@lokmanhekim.edu.tr

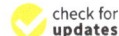

Citation: Kaya, Ö.; Gencer, B.; Çulcu, A.; Doğan, Ö. Extra Lateral Pin or Less Radiation? A Comparison of Two Different Pin Configurations in the Treatment of Supracondylar Humerus Fracture. *Children* **2023**, *10*, 550. https://doi.org/10.3390/children10030550

Academic Editors: Christiaan J. A. van Bergen and Joost W. Colaris

Received: 18 February 2023
Revised: 3 March 2023
Accepted: 13 March 2023
Published: 14 March 2023

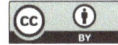

Copyright: © 2023 by the authors. Licensee MDPI, Basel, Switzerland. This article is an open access article distributed under the terms and conditions of the Creative Commons Attribution (CC BY) license (https:// creativecommons.org/licenses/by/ 4.0/).

Abstract: Background: Closed reduction and percutaneous fixation are the most commonly used methods in the surgical treatment of supracondylar humerus fractures. The pin configuration changes stability and is still controversial. The aim of this study was to investigate the relationship between surgical duration and radiation dose/duration for different pinning fixations. Methods: A total of 48 patients with Gartland type 2, 3, and 4 supracondylar fractures of the humerus were randomized into two groups—2 lateral and 1 medial (2L1M) pin fixation ($n = 26$) and 1 lateral 1 medial (1L1M) pin fixation ($n = 22$). A primary assessment was performed regarding surgical duration, radiation duration, and radiation dose. A secondary assessment included clinical outcome, passive range of motion, radiographic measurements, Flynn's criteria, and complications. Results: There were 26 patients in the first group (2L1M) and 22 patients in the second group (1L1M). There was no statistical difference between the groups regarding age, sex, type of fracture, or Flynn's criteria. The overall mean surgical duration with 1L1M fixation (30.59 ± 8.72) was statistically lower ($p = 0.001$) when compared to the 2L1M Kirschner wire K-wire fixation (40.61 ± 8.25). The mean radiation duration was 0.76 ± 0.33 s in the 1L1M K-wire fixation and 1.68 ± 0.55 s in the 2L1M K-wire fixation. The mean radiation dose of the 2L1M K-wire fixation (2.45 ± 1.15 mGy) was higher than that of the 1L1M K-wire fixation (0.55 ± 0.43 mGy) ($p = 0.000$). Conclusions: The current study shows that although there is no difference between the clinical and radiological outcomes, radiation dose exposure is significantly lower for the 1L1M fixation method.

Keywords: supracondylar humeral fracture; pin configuration; radiation dose

1. Introduction

Supracondylar humeral fractures are the most common elbow fractures in children, with incidences reaching a peak at about 5 to 8 years of age [1]. Generally, the fracture occurs due to a fall onto an outstretched hand, causing hyperextension of the elbow joint. The distal fragment is posteriorly displaced in more than 95% of fractures [2,3]. At the same time, these fractures have the potential to cause problems, especially due to elbow varus deformities, neurovascular injuries, stiffness, compartment syndrome, and malunion [4,5]. Therefore, the treatment of supracondylar humerus fractures is important in children because they affect function and elbow appearance.

According to Gartland's criteria, these fractures are classified as nondisplaced fractures (type I), hinged fractures with the posterior cortex intact (type II), and completely displaced fractures (type III) [6], and in 2006, Leitch et al. [7] added type IV, which identifies fractures with multidirectional instability.

The most commonly used treatment for displaced supracondylar humeral fractures is percutaneous pinning after closed or open reduction. Due to the incision scar and long operation time, open surgery has more disadvantages than closed reduction and percutaneous pinning [8]. Although some studies found open reduction superior in terms of more satisfactory results, the general opinion is that supracondylar humerus fractures should be treated with closed reduction and percutaneous pinning [9,10]. The most common pinning configuration for supracondylar humeral fractures is cross-pinning or lateral pinning using two or three pins [4]. Although crossed medial–lateral pin fixation provides more stabilization than the lateral pin fixation method, it poses a greater risk of iatrogenic ulnar nerve damage [10–13]. In many biomechanical studies, the relationship between pin configuration and stability has been evaluated, and it has been shown that lateral pinning is more unstable against torsional forces than cross-pinning [14,15], and a third medial pin must be added whenever there is rotational instability [11,14,16,17].

In supracondylar humeral fracture surgery, the use of fluoroscopy is essential during the fixation phase. Intraoperative fluoroscopy is indispensable to orthopedic surgeons and boosts surgical accuracy. Therefore, both the surgeon and the patient are exposed to ionizing radiation during surgery. This ionizing radiation may increase the risk of developing cancer, which might be higher for pediatric patients [18,19]. Therefore, in supracondylar humeral fracture surgery, the methods that expose patients to less radiation should be chosen.

In our clinic, the surgical treatment of supracondylar humerus fractures generally requires the two lateral and one medial pin (2L1M) configuration, considering that this configuration is more stable, as has been proven in most biomechanical studies [16,17]. However, the prolongation of surgical time and the radiation dose received led us to wonder, "Is the second pin from the lateral side necessary?". This led us to the conception of this study.

The aim of this study was to compare surgical duration, radiation duration, and the radiation dose regarding two different pin configurations (2L1M vs. 1L1M) for supracondylar humeral fracture.

2. Materials and Methods

The study design was a single-center, prospective, randomized clinical trial. Ethics approval was obtained from our institutional review board, and informed consent was provided by all of patients in the study. All study procedures were performed in accordance with the 1964 Declaration of Helsinki and all its subsequent amendments. Patients with Gartland type 2, 3, and 4 supracondylar humeral fractures who were treated (at our clinic) with closed reduction and percutaneous pinning were enrolled from April 2021 to December 2022.

All surgeries were performed by the same surgical team. The inclusion criteria were as follows: age: from 3 to 12 years old and the treatment of a displaced (type 2, 3, or 4) supracondylar fracture of the humerus. The exclusion criteria were as follows: an age of less than 3 years old or greater than 12 years old, an open fracture, a fracture requiring open reduction or neurovascular exploration, a floating elbow injury, and a bilateral upper extremity fracture. A total of 48 patients who met the criteria were included in the study (Figure 1).

All patients underwent general anesthesia, closed reduction, and percutaneous pinning under the supine position [20]. The choice of pin configuration was determined according to the date of the day of surgery. If the date of the surgery fell on an odd day of that month (for example, the 1st, 3rd, or 5th day of the month), the first surgical method was chosen. If the operation date fell on an even day of that month (for example, the 2nd, 4th, or 6th day of the month), the second surgical method was chosen. With this method, patients were randomly differentiated. In the first method, following the closed reduction of the fracture, 2 lateral pins were placed under fluoroscopy in hyperflexion, and then 1 medial pin was placed by extending the elbow (2L1M group) (Figure 2). In the second method, following fracture reduction, 1 lateral pin was placed in hyperflexion under fluoroscopy, and 1 medial pin was placed by extending the elbow (1L1M group) (Figure 3). In both methods, the pins were bent outside the skin, and a bivalved, long-arm cast was applied with approximately 90° of elbow flexion and neutral forearm rotation. The duration of surgery, the duration of fluoroscopy used during surgery, and the amount of dose received were all recorded for both the reduction and fixation phases of the surgery. The radiation dose and duration were obtained through the recording system of the device used (Figure 4).

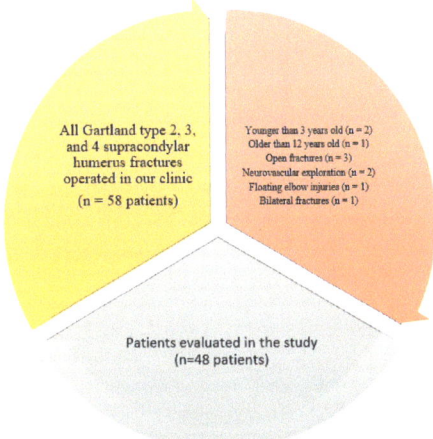

Figure 1. Detailed analysis chart of patients included and excluded from the study.

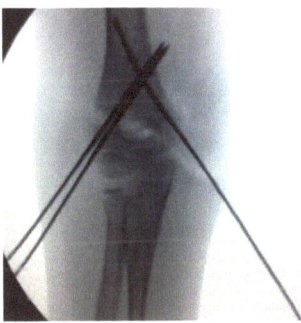

Figure 2. Two lateral and one medial pin configuration for supracondylar humeral fracture.

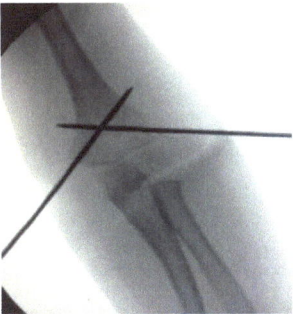

Figure 3. One lateral and one medial pin configuration for supracondylar humeral fracture.

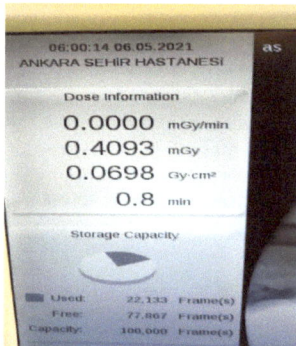

Figure 4. Radiation duration and dose recorded via fluoroscopy.

All of the patients were discharged after 1 or 2 days and were seen in the clinic 1 week after surgery. Radiographs were obtained in both anteroposterior and lateral planes at this follow-up. If these were acceptable, the child was seen again after 3 weeks, the cast was removed, and radiographs were obtained again. When acceptable healing was confirmed, the pins were removed in the clinic, and motion was encouraged. The mean immobilization time with pins in the present study was 5.2 ± 1.24 (4–7) weeks. Only those patients with elbow stiffness were routinely treated with physiotherapy.

Each patient was called for a control assessment every 3 months following pin removal. Clinical evaluation and radiographic evaluation were performed at each control visit. The clinical evaluation included the assessment of the carrying angle, the measurement of the passive range of elbow motion, a neurologic and vascular examination of the extremity, and the determination of any complications, such as superficial infection, deep infection, and the need for reoperation. The clinical results were graded according to the criteria of Flynn et al., which are based on the carrying angle and elbow motion [21]. The radiographic evaluation included an anteroposterior radiograph of the distal part of the humerus and a lateral radiograph of the elbow. A radiological assessment was made by comparing the Baumann angle, the humero-ulnar angle, and the humero-capitaller angle in the initial postoperative and final follow-up radiographs [4,22]. A change in Baumann's angle of more than 12° was defined as a major loss of reduction, a change from 6° to 12° as mild displacement, and a change of less than 6° as no displacement.

The data obtained in the study were analyzed statistically using SPSS v. 22.0 software (IBM Corp., Armonk, NY, USA). Pearson's chi-square and Fisher's exact tests were used to compare the categorical data to independently assess the relationships among sex, age, Flynn's criteria, and type of fracture. The Mann–Whitney U-test was used to compare the mean values between the groups.

3. Results

A total of 48 patients who met the inclusion criteria were operated on for displaced (type 2, 3, and 4) extension supracondylar humeral fracture. The mean age of the patients was 6.54 ± 2.02 (3–11) years. A total of 25 patients (52.1%) were female, with 12 patients (25%) having a Gartland type 2 supracondylar humeral fracture, 25 patients (52.1%) having a Gartland type 3 fracture, and 11 patients (22.9%) having a Gartland type 4 supracondylar humeral fracture.

A total of 26 patients were operated on using the first method (2L1M), and 22 patients were operated on using the second method (1L1M). There were 26 patients in the first group (2L1M), and the mean age of the patients was 6.57 ± 2.01 years. There were 11 (42%) females, and 6 patients (23%) had Gartland type 2 supracondylar humeral fractures, 11 patients (42%) had Gartland type 3 fractures, and 9 patients (35%) had Gartland type 4 supracondylar humeral fractures. According to Flynn's criteria, 24 of the patients had excellent results, and 2 patients had good results.

There were 22 patients in the second group (1L1M), and the mean age of the patients was 6.51 ± 2.08 years. There were 14 (64%) females, and 6 patients (27%) had a Gartland type 2 supracondylar humeral fracture, 14 patients (63%) had a Gartland type 3 fracture, and 2 patients (10%) had a Gartland type 4 supracondylar humeral fracture. According to Flynn's criteria, 17 patients had excellent results, and 7 patients had good results.

There was no statistically significant difference between the groups regarding age, sex, type of fracture, or Flynn's criteria (Table 1).

Table 1. Comparison of clinical results and descriptive features between two groups.

	2L1M	1L1M	p Value
No. of patients	26	22	
Age	6.57 ± 2.01	6.51 ± 2.08	0.925
Sex			0.141
male	15	8	
female	11	14	
Type of Fracture			0.105
Gartland 2	6	6	
Gartland 3	11	14	
Gartland 4	9	2	
Flynn Criteria			0.330
excellent	24	17	
good	2	7	
fair	0	0	
poor	0	0	

Intraoperative radiographs showed that the fracture reductions were acceptable in all cases. A final clinical and radiological assessment confirmed the complete healing of the fractures in all children. There were no complications, such as iatrogenic ulnar nerve injury, a loss of reduction, pin tract infections, nonunions, etc., in either group.

The overall mean surgical duration for the 1L1M fixation (30.59 ± 8.72 min.) was statistically lower ($p = 0.001$) when compared to the 2L1M K-wire fixation (40.61 ± 8.25 min). The mean radiation duration was 0.76 ± 0.33 s. for the 1L1M K-wire fixation and 1.68 ± 0.55 s. for the 2L1M K-wire fixation. The mean radiation dose for the 2L1M K-wire fixation (2.45 ± 1.15 mGy) was higher than the mean radiation dose for the 1L1M K-wire fixation (0.55 ± 0.43 mGy) ($p < 0.001$). A comparison between the two types of fixations showed the mean surgical duration and radiation dose/duration were significantly lower for the 1L1M K-wire fixation compared to the 2L1M K-wire fixation (Table 2).

Table 2. Comparison of surgical time, radiation dose, and duration between pin configurations.

	Pin Configuration	N	Mean Rank	p Value
Surgical duration in min	2L1M	26	40.61 ± 8.25	
	1L1M	22	30.59 ± 8.72	
	Total	48		0.001
Radiation duration in min	2L1M	26	1.68 ± 0.55	
	1L1M	22	0.76 ± 0.33	
	Total	48		<0.001
Radiaton dose in mGy	2L1M	26	2.45 ± 1.15	
	1L1M	22	0.55 ± 0.43	
	Total	48		<0.001

4. Discussion

Although closed reduction and percutaneous pinning are the primarily recommended treatment options in the literature for pediatric supracondylar humeral fractures, discussions continue regarding the superiority of different pin configurations (2L1M vs. 1L1M) to each other [4,9–13]. Although the main focus of these discussions is the absolute necessity of anatomical reduction and stabilization of the fracture, radiation exposure is an important criterion, especially considering that the patient population is in the pediatric age group [14–19]. The number of studies examining the superiority of different pin configurations to each other by including radiation exposure is quite limited in the literature, and this constitutes the main strength of our study. The most important finding of this study was that although there was no difference between the two different pin configuration methods in terms of clinical outcomes ($p > 0.05$ for each), there was a significant difference in terms of surgical duration, radiation dose, and radiation duration ($p < 0.05$ for each). Although the 1L1M pin configuration was clinically and radiologically similar, the radiation dose exposure it required was significantly lower ($p < 0.001$).

While closed reduction and percutaneous fixation are preferred in the surgical treatment of supracondylar humeral fractures in terms of low complication rates and wound healing, the pin configuration is still controversial [8–14]. Biomechanical studies show that cross-pinning is more effective than lateral pinning alone, especially to achieve greater rotational stability. In particular, it has been shown that stability is increased with the cross-pinning of two laterals and one medial [16]. When the literature was reviewed, the relationship between cross-pinning and lateral pinning in the percutaneous treatment of supracondylar humeral fractures was examined and evaluated in terms of stability and function. In particular, cross-pinning is considered to be more advantageous due to its contribution to torsional stability. The treatment of displaced supracondylar humeral fractures using only two lateral pins has been noted to be associated with a higher incidence of loss of reduction [23]. Although the medial pin improves torsional stability, it also introduces the risk of iatrogenic ulnar nerve injury. The reported incidences of postoperative ulnar nerve palsies range from 0% to 12% [24–26]. In a randomized clinical trial in 2007, Kocher et al. showed that both lateral entry pin fixation and medial and lateral entry pin fixation were effective in surgery for supracondylar humeral fractures [4]. They did not observe a functional difference in either group. They did not observe iatrogenic ulnar nerve injury in either group. In their surgical technique, firstly, the lateral pin was placed, the elbow was extended to a position of <90°, and a small incision was made over the medial epicondyle to protect the ulnar nerve. They believed that, with this method, the risk of ulnar nerve injury was reduced. In both groups, we applied medial pins to our patients, similar to the technique of Kocher et al. [4], following lateral pinning with an extension below 90 degrees, and we did not encounter any ulnar nerve injury either. Kocher et al. also suggested that a third pin may need to be administered to lateral entry patients, especially for those who are unstable. We believe that this recommendation is a method of increasing stability in accordance with the literature. In another prospective study conducted by Prashant et al. in 2016, medial–lateral cross-pinning was compared with lateral pinning, and they observed moderate reduction loss in two cases in the lateral pinning group [27]. While achieving similar results in terms of the functional and radiological aspects, they found iatrogenic ulnar nerve injury in two patients in the medial–lateral cross-pinning group. In the systematic review and meta-analysis study conducted by Dekker et al. in 2016 covering the years 1966–2015, it was observed that there was no significant difference between lateral pinning and medial–lateral cross-pinning [28]. Moderate reduction loss was seen in the lateral pinning group, and the medial–lateral cross-pinning group had a three-fold increase in iatrogenic ulnar nerve injury. In our study, we did not observe nerve injury or loss of reduction in any patients. In accordance with our study, it was observed that pin configuration did not have a significant effect on radiological or clinical outcomes ($p < 0.05$). At this point, it is obvious that there are many positive correlations, such as surgical experience and the effective use of fluoroscopy. We believe that having the same surgical team perform all the operations in our study facilitated optimal stability and explains the low complication rates. In addition, the fact that we did not include open fractures, bilateral injuries, or polytraumas may affect our complication rates. Finally, since the study mainly focused on perioperative variables, radiation exposure, and reduction quality, the fact that we did not evaluate our long-term follow-up results and changes in the patient's joint range of motion and bearing angle may have also had an impact on our results. We can optimally compare the stability and functional and radiological results of the 1L1M and 2L1M configurations with further studies that also evaluate the mid-long-term follow-up results.

While the widespread use of radiography and even computed tomography in orthopedic pediatric injuries continues in diagnosis, treatment, and follow-up processes, the concept of limiting radiation exposure after traumatic injuries of pediatric patients has been a controversial issue in the literature for many years. Several studies have reported that with a correct and adequate physical examination of children with elbow injuries, the need for radiographic examination and radiation exposure could be significantly reduced [29–31]. Kraus and Dresing, in their 2023 study, investigated rational imaging in children and emphasized the necessity of protection from radiation [32]. Kocaoglu et al. investigated the necessity of fixation of both bones in children with distal forearm fractures of both bones, considering the surgical time and radiation exposure criteria, and reported that with the fixation of the distal radius fracture alone, optimal functional results could be achieved with less radiation exposure and shorter surgical time [33]. There are a limited number of studies in the literature comparing pin configurations and radiation doses in pediatric supracondylar humeral fractures. Patients with 18 supracondylar humeral fractures fixed by Martus et al. using the same method were shown to experience minimal exposure of radiosensitive organs to radiation doses [34]. Schmucker et al. determined the factors that influence radiation exposure during the fixation of supracondylar fractures [35]. No difference was found when they compared biplanar and uniplanar C-arm use. Both radiation exposure and duration increased with fracture displacement, and the number of pins increased. In the retrospective study conducted by Tzatzairis et al. in 2021, although there was no difference according to Flynn's criteria, a statistically significant decrease in radiation dose was found in the cross-pinning group compared to the lateral pinning group [36]. They believed that the high radiation dose in the lateral pinning group was due to taking more images to assess stability. In our study, although there was no difference between the groups in terms of functional outcome, it was observed that the surgical time was longer and the radiation exposure was higher in the group with three pins (2L1M). We believe that after a safe level of stability of the cross-pin configuration has been achieved, the use of an extra pin may result in increased radiation exposure and prolonged surgical time.

Our study was limited in that only the radiation emitted through the C arm was evaluated, and this does not reflect direct radiation exposure. Although we did not study scatter radiation in our study, it is still an important factor to consider with regard to both the health of the patient and the surgical team. It would be appropriate to investigate this in future studies. Another important limitation was our relatively low number of patients. Finally, although we stated that the extra pin used in the 2L1M configuration did not contribute to stability while extending the surgical time and increasing the radiation exposure, as we mentioned before, our findings are supported by short-term follow-up results. The effect of the extra pin on stability and radiation exposure can be more clearly demonstrated by further studies with a larger patient cohort and including dosimetry analyses in which the mid-long-term follow-up results of the patients are examined.

5. Conclusions

In the surgical treatment of supracondylar humeral fractures, both 2L1M and 1L1M cross-pinning methods are effective. The 2L1M cross-pinning method prolongs the surgical time and causes greater radiation exposure. For this reason, we believe that when cross-pinning is applied in the treatment of supracondylar humeral fractures, the use of one lateral pin and one medial pin provides an effective result by minimizing radiation dose exposure. If persistent instability occurs after the placement of the crossed medial and lateral entry pins, the addition of a third pin is usually recommended in these patients to achieve fracture stability.

Author Contributions: Conceptualization, Ö.K. and B.G.; methodology, Ö.K.; validation, A.Ç. and B.G.; formal analysis, Ö.D.; investigation, Ö.K. and B.G.; resources, B.G.; data curation, A.Ç.; writing—original draft preparation, Ö.K.; writing—review and editing, Ö.D.; visualization, A.Ç.; supervision, Ö.D.; project administration, B.G. and A.Ç.; funding acquisition, Ö.K. All authors have read and agreed to the published version of the manuscript.

Funding: This research received no external funding.

Institutional Review Board Statement: The study was conducted in accordance with the Declaration of Helsinki and was approved by the Institutional Ethics Committee of ANKARA CITY HOSPITAL (protocol code E1-21-1637 and approval date is 17 March 2021).

Informed Consent Statement: Informed consent was obtained from all subjects involved in the study.

Data Availability Statement: The data presented in this study are available on request from the corresponding author. The data are not publicly available due to privacy or ethical restrictions.

Conflicts of Interest: The authors declare no conflict of interest.

References

1. Anjum, R.; Sharma, V.; Jindal, R.; Singh, T.P.; Rathee, N. Epidemiologic pattern of paediatric supracondylar fractures of humerus in a teaching hospital of rural India: A prospective study of 263 cases. *Chin. J. Traumatol.* **2017**, *20*, 158–160. [CrossRef] [PubMed]
2. Mehlman, C.T.; Denning, J.R.; McCarthy, J.J.; Fisher, M.L. Infantile supracondylar humeral fractures (patients less than two years of age): Twice as common in females and a high rate of malunion with lateral column-only fixation. *J. Bone Jt. Surg. Am.* **2019**, *101*, 25–34. [CrossRef]
3. Wilkins, K.E. Supracondylar Fractures. In *Fractures in Children*, 3rd ed.; Rockwood, C.A., Wilkins, K.E., King, R.E., Eds.; Lippincott Williams & Wilkins: Philadelphia, PA, USA, 1991; pp. 526–617.
4. Kocher, M.S.; Kasser, J.R.; Waters, P.M.; Bae, D.; Snyder, B.D.; Hresko, M.T.; Daniel, H.; Lawrence, K.; Kim, Y.J.; Murray, M.M.; et al. Lateral entry compared with medial and lateral entry pin fixation for completely displaced supracondylar humeral fractures in children. A randomized clinical trial. *J. Bone Jt. Surg. Am.* **2007**, *89*, 706–712. [CrossRef]
5. Otsuka, N.Y.; Kasser, J.R. Supracondylar Fractures of the Humerus in Children. *J. Am. Acad. Orthop. Surg.* **1997**, *5*, 19–26. [CrossRef] [PubMed]
6. Gartland, J.J. Management of supracondylar fractures of the humerus in children. *Surg. Gynecol. Obstet.* **1959**, *109*, 145–154. [PubMed]
7. Leitch, K.K.; Kay, R.M.; Femino, J.D.; Tolo, V.T.; Storer, S.K.; Skaggs, D.L. Treatment of multidirectionally unstable supracondylar humeral fractures in children. A modified Gartland type-IV fracture. *J. Bone Jt. Surg. Am.* **2006**, *88*, 980–985. [CrossRef] [PubMed]
8. Keskin, D.; Sen, H. The comparative evaluation of treatment outcomes in pediatric displaced supracondylar humerus fractures managed with either open or closed reduction and percutaneous pinning. *Acta Chir. Orthop. Traumatol. Cech.* **2014**, *81*, 380–386.
9. Rakha, A.; Khan, R.D.A.; Arshad, A.; Khan, Z.A.; Ahmad, S.; Mahmood, S. Comparison of efficacy between open and close reduction in supracondylar fracture of humerus in children using Flynn's criteria. *Ann. Punjab Med. Coll.* **2020**, *14*, 32–36.
10. Maity, A.; Saha, D.; Roy, D.S. A prospective randomised, controlled clinical trial comparing medial and lateral entry pinning with lateral entry pinning for percutaneous fixation of displaced extension type supracondylar fractures of the humerus in children. *J. Orthop. Surg. Res.* **2012**, *7*, 6. [CrossRef]
11. Gordon, J.E.; Patton, C.M.; Luhmann, S.J.; Bassett, G.S.; Schoenecker, P.L. Fracture stability after pinning of displaced supracondylar distal humerus fractures in children. *J. Pediatr. Orthop.* **2001**, *21*, 313–318. [CrossRef]
12. Skaggs, D.L.; Hale, J.M.; Bassett, J.; Kaminsky, C.; Kay, R.M.; Tolo, V.T. Operative treatment of supracondylar fractures of the humerus in children. The consequences of pin placement. *J. Bone Jt. Surg. Am.* **2001**, *83*, 735–740. [CrossRef]
13. Rasool, M.N. Ulnar nerve injury after K-wire fixation of supracondylar humerus fractures in children. *J. Pediatr. Orthop.* **1998**, *18*, 686–690. [CrossRef] [PubMed]
14. Lee, S.S.; Mahar, A.T.; Miesen, D.; Newton, P.O. Displaced pediatric supracondylar humerus fractures: Biomechanical analysis of percutaneous pinning techniques. *J. Pediatr. Orthop.* **2002**, *22*, 440–443. [CrossRef] [PubMed]
15. Feng, C.; Guo, Y.; Zhu, Z.; Zhang, J.; Wang, Y. Biomechanical analysis of supracondylar humerus fracture pinning for fractures with coronal lateral obliquity. *J. Pediatr. Orthop.* **2012**, *32*, 196–200. [CrossRef] [PubMed]
16. Wallace, M.; Johnson, D.B.; Pierce, W.; Iobst, C.; Riccio, A.; Wimberly, R.L. Biomechanical Assessment of Torsional Stiffness in a Supracondylar Humerus Fracture Model. *J. Pediatr. Orthop.* **2019**, *39*, e210–e215. [CrossRef]
17. Larson, L.; Firoozbakhsh, K.; Passarelli, R.; Bosch, P. Biomechanical analysis of pinning techniques for pediatric supracondylar humerus fractures. *J. Pediatr. Orthop.* **2006**, *26*, 573–578. [CrossRef] [PubMed]

18. Richter, P.; Dehner, C.; Scheiderer, B.; Gebhard, F.; Kraus, M. Emission of radiation in the orthopaedic operation room: A comprehensive review. *OA Musculoskelet. Med.* **2013**, *1*, 11. [CrossRef]
19. Ron, E. Ionizing radiation and cancer risk: Evidence from epidemiology. *Pediatr. Radiol.* **2002**, *32*, 232–244. [CrossRef]
20. Sapienza, M.; Testa, G.; Vescio, A.; Panvini, F.M.C.; Caldaci, A.; Parisi, S.C.; Pavone, V.; Canavese, F. The Role of Patient Position in the Surgical Treatment of Supracondylar Fractures of the Humerus: Comparison of Prone and Supine Position. *Medicina* **2023**, *59*, 374. [CrossRef]
21. Flynn, J.C.; Matthews, J.G.; Benoit, R.L. Blind pinning of displaced supracondylar fractures of the humerus in children. Sixteen years' experience with long-term follow-up. *J. Bone Jt. Surg. Am.* **1974**, *56*, 263–272. [CrossRef]
22. Topping, R.E.; Blanco, J.S.; Davis, T.J. Clinical evaluation of crossed-pin versus lateral-pin fixation in displaced supracondylar humerus fractures. *J. Pediatr. Orthop.* **1995**, *15*, 435–439. [CrossRef] [PubMed]
23. Sankar, W.N.; Hebela, N.M.; Skaggs, D.L.; Flynn, J.M. Loss of pin fixation in displaced supracondylar humeral fractures in children: Causes and prevention. *J. Bone Jt. Surg. Am.* **2007**, *89*, 713–717.
24. Lyons, J.P.; Ashley, E.; Hoffer, M.M. Ulnar nerve palsies after percutaneous cross-pinning of supracondylar fractures in children's elbows. *J. Pediatr. Orthop.* **1998**, *18*, 43–45. [CrossRef]
25. Özçelik, A.; Tekcan, A.; Ömeroglu, H. Correlation between iatrogenic ulnar nerve injury and angular insertion of the medial pin in supracondylar humerus fractures. *J. Pediatr. Orthop.* **2006**, *15*, 58–61. [CrossRef] [PubMed]
26. Royce, R.O.; Dutkowsky, J.P.; Kasser, J.R.; Rand, F.R. Neurologic complications after K-wire fixation of supracondylar humerus fractures in children. *J. Pediatr. Orthop.* **1991**, *11*, 191–194. [CrossRef] [PubMed]
27. Prashant, K.; Lakhotia, D.; Bhattacharyya, T.D.; Mahanta, A.K.; Ravoof, A. A comparative study of two percutaneous pinning techniques (lateral vs medial-lateral) for Gartland type III pediatric supracondylar fracture of the humerus. *J. Orthop. Traumatol.* **2016**, *17*, 223–229. [CrossRef] [PubMed]
28. Dekker, A.E.; Krijnen, P.; Schipper, I.B. Results of crossed versus lateral entry K-wire fixation of displaced pediatric supracondylar humeral fractures: A systematic review and meta-analysis. *Injury* **2016**, *47*, 2391–2398. [CrossRef]
29. Appelboam, A.; Reuben, A.D.; Benger, J.R.; Beech, F.; Dutson, J.; Haig, S.; Higginson, I.; Klein, J.A.; Le Roux, S.; Saranga, S.S.; et al. Elbow extension test to rule out elbow fracture: Multicentre, prospective validation and observational study of diagnostic accuracy in adults and children. *BMJ* **2008**, *337*, a2428. [CrossRef]
30. Lennon, R.I.; Riyat, M.S.; Hilliam, R.; Anathkrishnan, G.; Alderson, G. Can a normal range of elbow movement predict a normal elbow X-ray? *Emerg. Med. J. EMJ* **2007**, *24*, 86–88. [CrossRef]
31. Darracq, M.A.; Vinson, D.R.; Panacek, E.A. Preservation of active range of motion after acute elbow trauma predicts absence of elbow fracture. *Am. J. Emerg. Med.* **2008**, *26*, 779–782. [CrossRef]
32. Kraus, R.; Dresing, K. Rational Usage of Fracture Imaging in Children and Adolescents. *Diagnostics* **2023**, *13*, 538. [CrossRef] [PubMed]
33. Kocaoğlu, H.; Kalem, M.; Kavak, M.; Şahin, E.; Başarır, K.; Kınık, H. Comparison of operating time, fluoroscopy exposure time, and functional and radiological results of two surgical methods for distal forearm fractures of both-bones in pediatric patients: Is it necessary to fix both bones? *Acta Orthop. Traumatol. Turc.* **2020**, *54*, 155–160. [CrossRef] [PubMed]
34. Martus, J.E.; Hilmes, M.A.; Grice, J.V.; Stutz, C.M.; Schoenecker, J.G.; Lovejoy, S.A.; Mencio, G.A. Radiation Exposure During Operative Fixation of Pediatric Supracondylar Humerus Fractures: Is Lead Shielding Necessary? *J. Pediatr. Orthop.* **2018**, *38*, 249–253. [CrossRef]
35. Schmucker, A.; Chen, R.; Vachhrajani, S.; Martinek, M.; Albert, M. Radiation exposure in the treatment of pediatric supracondylar humerus fractures. *Arch. Orthop. Trauma Surg.* **2020**, *140*, 449–455. [CrossRef] [PubMed]
36. Tzatzairis, T.; Firth, G.; Bijlsma, P.; Manoukian, D.; Maizen, C.; Ramachandran, M. Radiation Exposure in The Treatment of Pediatric Supracondylar Humerus Fractures: Comparison of Two Fixation Methods. *Open Orthop. J.* **2021**, *15*, 22–26. [CrossRef]

Disclaimer/Publisher's Note: The statements, opinions and data contained in all publications are solely those of the individual author(s) and contributor(s) and not of MDPI and/or the editor(s). MDPI and/or the editor(s) disclaim responsibility for any injury to people or property resulting from any ideas, methods, instructions or products referred to in the content.

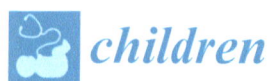

Systematic Review

Management of Traumatic Nerve Palsies in Paediatric Supracondylar Humerus Fractures: A Systematic Review

Christy Graff [1,2,3,*], George Dennis Dounas [1,2,3], Maya Rani Louise Chandra Todd [2,3], Jonghoo Sung [1] and Medhir Kumawat [2]

1 The Women's and Children's Hospital, North Adelaide, SA 5006, Australia; jonghoo.sung@sa.gov.au (J.S.)
2 Faculty of Health and Medical Sciences, University of Adelaide, Adelaide, SA 5005, Australia; medhir.kumawat@student.adelaide.edu.au (M.K.)
3 The Royal Adelaide Hospital, Adelaide, SA 5000, Australia
* Correspondence: christy.graff@sa.gov.au

Abstract: Purpose: Up to 12% of paediatric supracondylar humerus fractures (SCHFs) have an associated traumatic nerve injury. This review aims to summarize the evidence and guide clinicians regarding the timing of investigations and/or surgical interventions for traumatic nerve palsies after this injury. **Methods:** A formal systematic review was undertaken in accordance with the Joanna Briggs Institute (JBI) methodology for systematic reviews and PRISMA guidelines. Manuscripts were reviewed by independent reviewers against the inclusion and exclusion criteria, and data extraction, synthesis, and assessment for methodological quality were undertaken. **Results:** A total of 51 manuscripts were included in the final evaluation, reporting on a total of 510 traumatic nerve palsies in paediatric SCHFs. In this study, 376 nerve palsies recovered without any investigation or intervention over an average time of 19.5 weeks. Comparatively, 37 went back to theatre for exploration beyond the initial treatment due to persistent deficits, at an average time of 4 months. The most common finding at the time of exploration was entrapment of the nerve requiring neurolysis. A total of 27 cases did not achieve full recovery regardless of management. Of the 15 reports of nerve laceration secondary to paediatric SCHFs, 13 were the radial nerve. **Conclusions:** Most paediatric patients who sustain a SCHF with associated traumatic nerve injury will have full recovery. Delayed or no recovery of the nerve palsy should be considered for exploration within four months of the injury; earlier exploration should be considered for radial nerve palsies.

Keywords: fracture; humerus; nerve injury/palsy/palsies; pediatric/paediatric; supracondylar

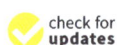

Citation: Graff, C.; Dounas, G.D.; Todd, M.R.L.C.; Sung, J.; Kumawat, M. Management of Traumatic Nerve Palsies in Paediatric Supracondylar Humerus Fractures: A Systematic Review. *Children* **2023**, *10*, 1862. https://doi.org/10.3390/children10121862

Academic Editors: Christiaan J. A. van Bergen and Joost W. Colaris

Received: 17 October 2023
Revised: 20 November 2023
Accepted: 22 November 2023
Published: 27 November 2023

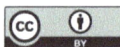

Copyright: © 2023 by the authors. Licensee MDPI, Basel, Switzerland. This article is an open access article distributed under the terms and conditions of the Creative Commons Attribution (CC BY) license (https://creativecommons.org/licenses/by/4.0/).

1. Introduction

Nerve palsy is a common complication of paediatric supracondylar humerus fractures (SCHFs), affecting approximately 12% of patients [1,2]. The median nerve proper, or its branching anterior interosseous nerve, is the most commonly impaired nerve from extension-type fractures, while the ulnar nerve is the most at risk of injury in flexion-type fractures [1–3]. Over 70% of cases of nerve palsies are present pre-operatively [1].

From the literature and clinical opinion, most reported nerve injuries are managed with a 'watch and wait' approach, based on the assumption that the nerve injury is a transient neuropraxia, although the exact resolution details are often unclear [4–6]. There is currently no clear evidence regarding the timing of investigation, intervention, and recovery.

This systematic review aims to summarize the current evidence and guide clinicians regarding the timing of investigation and/or surgical intervention for traumatic nerve palsies sustained at the time of injury in paediatric SCHFs and compare the outcomes of nerve palsy in this population with surgical intervention compared with expectant management.

2. Methods

The review has been conducted in accordance with the Joanna Briggs Institute (JBI) methodology for systematic reviews of effectiveness with reference to the a priori protocol published in the same journal [7,8]. The review has been registered with the International Prospective Register of Systematic Reviews PROSPERO (CRD42019121581).

A comprehensive search strategy was conducted on 7 June 2021 (Supplementary S1). Randomised controlled trials, cohort studies, case series, and case studies published after 1950 were included. The databases searched were Ovid Medline, Embase, and Cochrane Central, as well as a grey literature search using Google Scholar with the first 200 results returned also reviewed. The bibliographies of the accepted manuscripts were reviewed to identify other relevant published research. The search was re-executed on 23 May 2022, due to the longevity of data curation.

The aim of the study was to compare the effectiveness of operative versus expectant management on the recovery of nerve palsies in paediatric supracondylar fractures. The inclusion criteria were papers that included:

- A paediatric patient with;
- An ipsilateral traumatic upper limb nerve palsy after a SCHF;
- With no pre-existing neurological impairment.

Studies were excluded if:

- They did not provide details regarding follow up or the outcome of the traumatic nerve palsy;
- It was not possible from the reporting to separate individual outcomes from large groups of nerve palsies.

Sequential screening of the manuscripts by title, abstract, and full text were performed by two independent reviewers to determine suitability based on the inclusion and exclusion criteria. The results of the final search were reported in accordance with the preferred reporting items for the systematic reviews and meta-analysis (PRISMA) guidelines [9] (Supplementary S2).

Data extraction was performed by two independent reviewers using a prescribed extraction form. Each eligible manuscript underwent critical appraisal and assessment of methodological quality by two independent reviewers using standardized critical appraisal instruments from the Joanna Briggs Institute (JBI) for Systematic Reviews and Research Synthesis (Supplementary S3–S6) [8]. Cohort studies with complete follow up were scored out of eleven, case series out of ten, and case reports out of eight. Cohort studies without confounding factors or incomplete follow up were scored out of ten, and cohort studies without confounding factors and without incomplete follow up were scored out of nine.

Discrepancies between reviewers at all stages were resolved by a senior reviewer. The primary outcome was nerve palsy recovery, ranging from "full recovery" to "no recovery" as a descriptive measure. Secondary outcomes include time to recovery, modality of treatment, use and timing of investigations, findings at operation, and duration of follow up. Data were synthesised in narrative and tabular format. Due to considerable clinical heterogeneity, a meta-analysis was not performed. Where appropriate, frequencies, percentages, and summaries of data were included for analysis.

3. Results

A total of 7919 results were identified on initial search. All of the results were collated and uploaded into EndNote version X.9 (Clarivate Analytics, Philadelphia, PA, USA) and de-duplication occurred, with a final number of 2744 articles retrieved [10]. After title and abstract screening, there were 218 manuscripts reviewed in full including bibliography reviews, of which 51 met the inclusion criteria and were included in this systematic review as demonstrated in the PRISMA flow diagram (Figure 1) [9]. From the final 51 manuscripts, 16 were case reports/series with the remainder being cohort studies. There were 509 nerve palsies described, with the median nerve most commonly affected and the most common fracture type reported as Gartland type 3. No studies were excluded due to bias (Table 1).

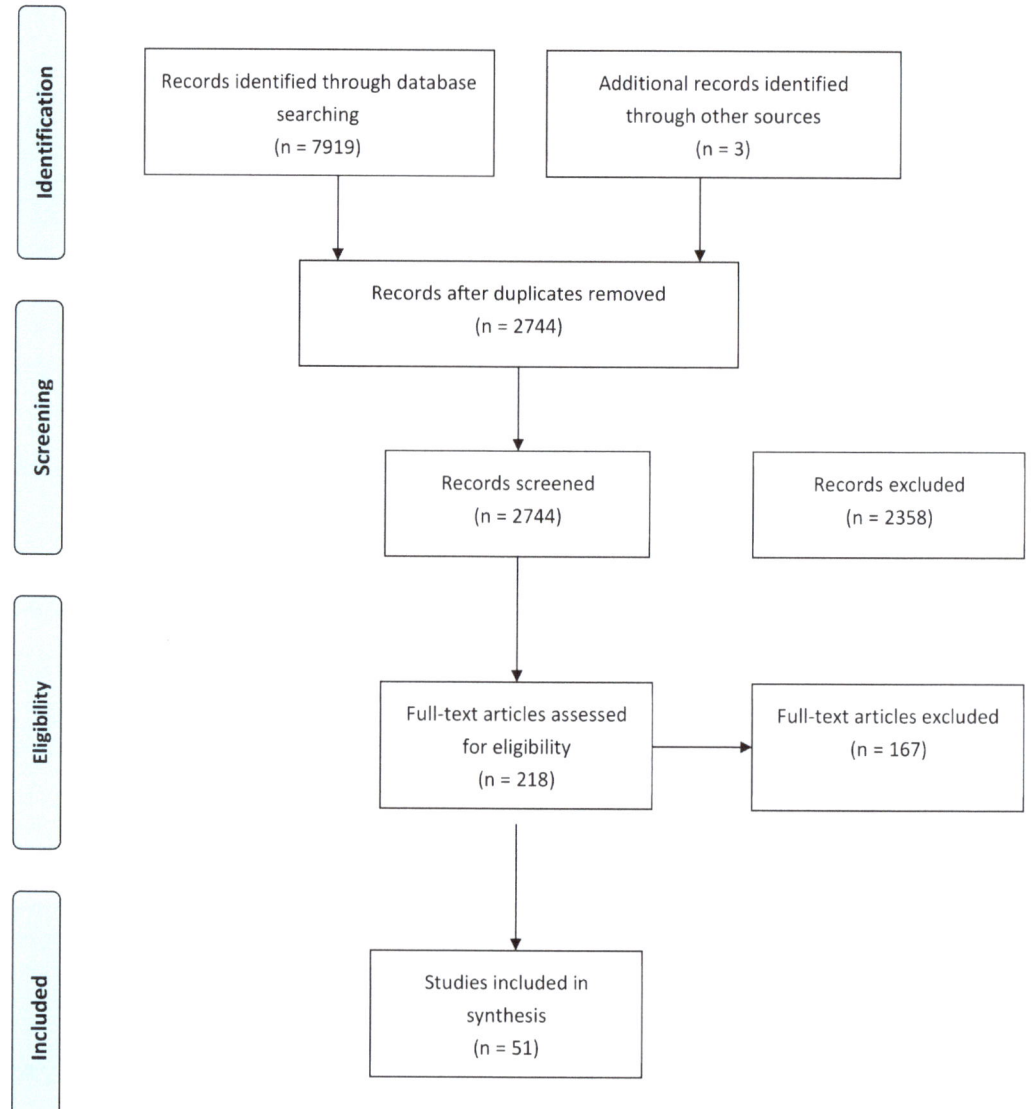

Figure 1. PRISMA flow diagram of the final search.

Table 1. Main characteristics of studies included in analysis.

Paper	Study Type	Risk of Bias	No. of Nerve Palsies	Surgical Exploration at ORIF			Delayed Surgical Exploration			Time to Final Follow up in Months
				No	Reason	Findings	No	Timing in Months	Findings	
Ababneh M et al. [11]	RCS	8/10	7	0	n/a	n/a	0	n/a	n/a	6
Aronson DC et al. [12]	RCS	9/11	1	0	n/a	n/a	0	n/a	n/a	12
Ay S et al. [13]	RCS	7/10	9	9	Describing open surgical technique	Median in fracture site ×3, radial kinked ×6	0	0	0	3
Barrett KK et al. [14]	RCS	8/8	35	0	n/a	n/a	0	n/a	n/a	7.4
Bertelli JS & Ghizoni MF [15]	RCS	9/11	6	0	n/a	n/a	6	6–9	Entrapment ×2, laceration ×4	16–24
Boyd DW & Aronson DD [16]	RCS	8/10	3	0	n/a	n/a	0	n/a	n/a	12
Brown IC et al. [5]	RCS	8/9	14	0	n/a	n/a	0	n/a	n/a	6
Campbell CC et al. [17]	RCS	7/9	25	4	3 = VE 1 = FCR	In continuity	0	n/a	n/a	10
Chakrabarti AJ et al. [18]	RCS	7/10	1	1	NE	Complete division	0	n/a	n/a	36
Cheng JC et al. [19]	RCS	7/9	19	1	VE	In continuity	0	n/a	n/a	4–13
Culp RW et al. [20]	RCS	8/9	18	0	n/a	n/a	9	7.5 (mean)	Fibrous scarring ×6, entrapment ×2, laceration ×2	25
Davis RT et al. [21]	RCS	7/9	10	0	n/a	n/a	0	0	0	48
Devkota P et al. [22]	RCS	10/10	6	0	n/a	n/a	0	0	0	3
Dormans JP et al. [23]	CS	5/5	7	0	n/a	n/a	0	0	0	27
Garg B et al. [24]	CS	8/11	1	1	NE	In continuity	0	n/a	n/a	14–36
Gosens T et al. [25]	RCS	9/11	34	10	VE and FCR	In continuity	0	n/a	n/a	6
Horst M et al. [26]	RCS	8/9	2	0	n/a	n/a	0	n/a	n/a	17 (mean)
Ippolito E et al. [27]	RCS	6/9	14	0	n/a	n/a	1	8	Entrapment in scar tissue	132 (longest)
Jones ET et al. [28]	CS	8/8	6	0	n/a	n/a	0	n/a	n/a	24
Karlsson J et al. [29]	CS	8/8	4	4	VE and FCR	Interposed between bone fragments	0	n/a	n/a	72–108
Khademolhosseini M et al. [30]	RCS	7/9	9	4	FCR	In continuity ×2, entrapment in fracture ×1, contusion ×1	0	n/a	n/a	8
Khan AQ et al. [31]	RCS	8/10	8	0	n/a	n/a	0	n/a	n/a	3
Khan MY et al. [32]	PCaS	8/10	25	2	VE	Entrapment at fracture site	0	n/a	n/a	3
Kirz PH and Marsh HO [33]	CS	8/10	11	0	n/a	n/a	1	4	Lacerated	65
Kiyoshige Y et al. [34]	RCS	7/10	6	0	n/a	n/a	0	n/a	n/a	5–120
Krusche-Mandl I et al. [35]	RCS	8/11	8	0	n/a	n/a	1	2	Compressive scar tissue	12
Kuoppala E et al. [36]	CS	10/10	1	0	n/a	n/a	0	n/a	n/a	12
Lalanandham T et al. [37]	CR	7/8	1	0	n/a	n/a	1	2	Encased in callus; unable to be retrieved	14
Larson AN et al. [38]	RCS	9/11	2	0	n/a	n/a	0	n/a	n/a	10
Leonardi LL et al. [39]	CS	8/10	3	0	n/a	n/a	1	3	Encased at fracture site	12
Li YA et al. [40]	RCS	7/11	7	0	n/a	n/a	0	n/a	n/a	34

Table 1. Cont.

Paper	Study Type	Risk of Bias	No. of Nerve Palsies	Surgical Exploration at ORIF			Delayed Surgical Exploration			Time to Final Follow up in Months
				No	Reason	Findings	No	Timing in Months	Findings	
Louahem DM et al. [41]	RCS	8/11	66	11	FCR	10 in continuity; 1 radial nerve complete laceration	4	3	Severe compression ×3, laceration and retraction ×1 (lacerated radial nerve failed suture repair)	18
Mangat et al. [42]	CS	10/10	9	5	VE	Entrapment at fracture site	4	1× at 48 h, 2× at 2 weeks, 1× at 3 weeks	Tethered or entrapped	12
Marck KW et al. [43]	CR	8/8	2	2	VE	Laceration ×1, traction ×1	0	n/a	n/a	18–48
Martin DF et al. [44]	CR	8/8	1	0	n/a	n/a	1	6	Laceration	18
McGraw J. et al. [45]	RCS	8/10	17	2	FCR and VE	In continuity	1	6	Laceration	14
Oh CW et al. [46]	RCS	7/10	4	1	VE	Entrapment in fracture	0	n/a	n/a	3
Post M. et al. [47]	CR	8/8	1	0	n/a	n/a	1	6	Encased in callous	30
Rasool MN et al. [48]	CS	8/10	27	27	VE	Kinked ×21, intact ×6	0	n/a	n/a	6
Reigstad O et al. [49]	CS	8/10	2	2	VE	Entrapped in fracture site	0	n/a	n/a	10
Sairyo K et al. [50]	CR	8/8	1	0	n/a	n/a	1	3	Laceration	8
Silva M et al. [51]	RCS	8/11	11	0	n/a	n/a	0	n/a	n/a	6
Solak S et al. [52]	RCS	7/9	6	0	n/a	n/a	0	n/a	n/a	36
Steinman et al. [53]	RCS	8/9	1	1	FCR	Entrapment in fracture site	0	n/a	n/a	1–9
Thorleifsson R et al. [54]	CR	8/8	1	0	n/a	n/a	1	2.5	Entrapment in the fracture site	120
Tokutake et al. [55]	CR	8/8	2	1	NE	Entrapment at the fracture site	1	3	Entrapment at the fracture site	4–6
Tomaszewski et al. [56]	RCS	7/10	22	0	n/a	n/a	2	2	Entrapment at the fracture site	10
Tunku-Naziha TZ et al. [57]	RCS	7/9	2	2	VE	Contused but in continuity	0	n/a	n/a	1.5
van Vugt AB et al. [58]	RCS	7/9	23	1	VE	Complete laceration	0	n/a	n/a	'Good result'
Yano K et al. [59]	CR	8/8	1	0	n/a	n/a	1	11	Entrapment in callus	36
Yaokreh JB et al. [60]	RCS	7/9	8	0	n/a	n/a	0	n/a	n/a	5–6

RCS = retrospective cohort study; CS = case series; PcaS = prospective case series; CR = case report. VE = vascular exploration; FCR – failed closed reduction; NE = nerve exploration; n/a = Not Applicable.

There were 372 traumatic nerve palsies which had full recovery with no intervention (such as nerve exploration) or investigation (such as imaging or nerve conduction studies) undertaken (73.9%) (see Table S1 Supplementary S7). The mean duration of time to full recovery at final follow up in these patients was 19.5 weeks (approximately 5 months) (ranging from 3 days to 1 year). Eight nerve palsies had no intervention (such as nerve exploration) or investigation (such as imaging or nerve conduction studies) and were not fully recovered at last follow up. Davis et al. [21] described an ulnar nerve palsy with sensory disturbance at the 4-year follow up, and two radial nerve palsies with wrist extension weakness at the 4-year follow up. Van Vught et al. [58] reported one patient with ulnar, median, and radial sensory loss after a patient presented to them after 5 days with

Volkmann's ischaemic contracture. Yaokreh et al. [60] reported on two nerves that 'required electrophysiological studies' at final follow up but no other detail was given.

There were 26 traumatic nerve palsies which did not document full recovery by the final follow up (5.3%) (see Table S2 Supplementary S7).

There were 92 (18%) nerve palsies which underwent exploration at the time of initial operation (see Table S3 Supplementary S7) of which 89 were described as a secondary intention whilst exploring the brachial artery or an open fracture or converting to open reduction. Three were explored due to surgeon preference of treatment of nerve palsies at presentation [1,19,54]. Eighty-eight which were explored at the time of the initial operation had full recovery by the final follow up, one incomplete recovery, and three were lost to follow up. The findings at exploration in forty-six out of ninety-two nerves were tethered or entrapped in the fracture site, thirty-seven were in continuity, three lacerated, and four contused.

A total of 37 nerves (7.3%) underwent delayed exploration with an average time of 4.4 months (0.5 to 11 months) (see Table S4 Supplementary S7). It was found that 27 were recorded as entrapped in the fracture site/callous/scarring and 10 were found to be completely transected. The radial nerve was involved in sixteen cases, while the median in twelve, and the ulnar in nine. Full recovery at final follow up was reported in 26 nerves. One radial nerve was lacerated, explored, and repaired primarily, but then did not recover, and went on to have a delayed exploration [41]. The primary repair was found to have failed, and was then managed with a nerve graft, and ultimately, tendon transfers.

A total of 13 nerves were found to be completely lacerated on exploration (see Table S5 Supplementary S7). Interestingly, 10 of these were radial nerves. Most of these occurred at the time of the injury, prior to reduction (see Table S5 Supplementary S7).

4. Discussion

Our systematic review focused on traumatic nerve palsies in paediatric supracondylar humerus fractures. Iatrogenic or K-wire-associated nerve palsies represent a different spectrum of nerve trauma and have been described elsewhere [30,61]. This review represents the most current comprehensive description of outcomes after traumatic nerve palsies in paediatric supracondylar humerus fractures in the literature, with a total of 510 nerve injuries identified. The characteristics of a Gartland type 3 fracture were consistent with previously reported papers, supporting the opinion that neurological injury is more prevalent amongst more severely displaced fractures [2,24,62]. A total of 18 of the 51 papers did not report the Gartland type, and therefore we did not think a percentage of Gartland type would be accurate to report.

The previous literature reports that 86–100% of nerve injuries will recover spontaneously by 6 months, with a mean time of approximately 3 months [41,63]. Most nerves in the current series were managed expectantly, and had full spontaneous recovery, in keeping with this 'watch and wait' policy which is consistently advocated in the literature for patients with anatomical reduction [17,58]. However, an adequate reduction does not rule out the possibility of entrapment and does not account for lacerations [42,55].

A comparison of time frame to full recovery between no exploration, exploration at initial operation, and delayed exploration was unable to be calculated in this review as the majority of papers reported recovery 'at time of final follow up' or provided a broad range, such as 1 day to 10 months or 1 to 4 years [17,43]. It is important to recognize that the 'time to full recovery' for nerve palsies is the time of final follow up. The literature is not robust enough to determine how long it took for the nerve palsies to fully recover.

It was found that 7.4% of nerve palsies required delayed exploration due to persistent deficits or stagnated recovery at an average of 4 months. Exploration has been advocated for if there is no clinical recovery from 6 weeks to 3 months [30,41,64]. If the nerve is found in continuity at 3 months and is neurolysed, there is a trend to complete recovery [20,58]. Incomplete recovery was more common after complete nerve transection, or if exploration occurred after 4 months. There were 13 reports of nerve laceration secondary to paediatric SCHFs, of which 10 were the radial nerve, and had poorer outcomes.

Nerve exploration is recommended to be undertaken when there is no evidence of clinical or electrophysiological improvement by 8 weeks to 6 months after injury [19,20,45,50,63,65]. Ultrasound has been advocated as useful to evaluate the continuity of the nerve in a small percentage of series pre-operatively, intraoperatively, and post-operatively; ultrasound, however, is highly user dependent [55]. Only three of the papers that met the inclusion criteria reported the use of ultrasound [39,47,55]. Nerve conduction studies and EMG can be poorly tolerated in children, which may explain why most series did not use these in their management of nerve palsies. Magnetic resonance imaging (MRI) can sometimes require a general anaesthetic in this age group but can often be useful in older children to investigate nerve injuries. No study reported on the use of MRI. Additionally, newer surgical techniques such as nerve transfer have not been documented at all in the current literature. From this systematic review, our recommendation would be nerve exploration if there is no or little clinical recovery at 3 months, and exploration within 4 months, except in the case to the radial nerve, which is discussed below. For the consideration of exploration in this time frame, investigations such as ultrasound, MRI, and/or nerve conduction studies should be considered at 6–12 weeks (Figure 2). Liaison with the local nerve injury unit is imperative regarding the timing of referral for the consideration of nerve exploration, repair, nerve grafting, nerve transfer, and/or tendon transfer.

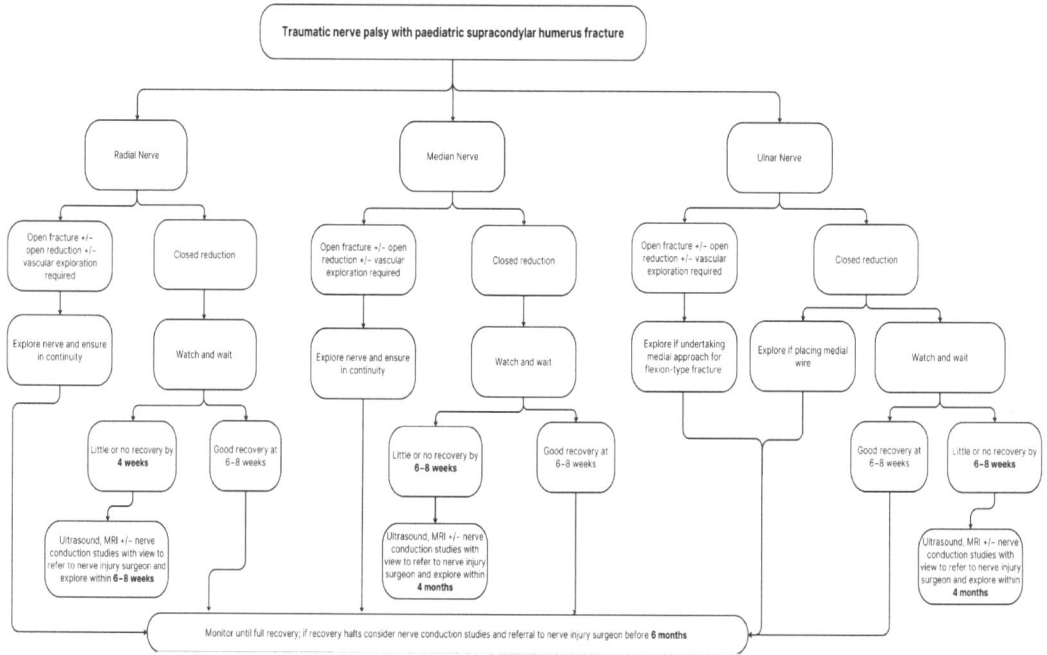

Figure 2. Algorithm for the management of traumatic nerve palsies after paediatric supracondylar humerus fractures.

The majority of included papers did not have a primary objective of nerve palsy outcomes; they were commonly reported on only as a complication in part of a wider review of SCHF management techniques. Those that described nerve palsy in detail were often case studies and thus have impacts of selection bias confounding the results. The 5% of nerves that did not fully recover in this series is likely overinflated due to the selection bias of persistent deficits being reported in case series. Our review included eight case reports, focusing only on nerves that were lacerated or entrapped, and so were not typical of the normal pathway of nerve palsies after paediatric supracondylar humerus fractures.

There is unfortunately very limited literature dedicated to the management of these injuries from injury to full recovery, which is surprising considering the importance of the topic. Retrospective or prospective data from large centres or multicentre trials on the recovery of nerve palsies in this population is required for improved confidence in recommendations for management.

Another limitation is that two of the largest series describing 425 nerve palsies were excluded by full text; a report of the interventions and outcomes was unclear for the purposes of this review. The authors were contacted for further details which were not able to be obtained at the time of submission [63,66].

The incidence of complete lacerations of nerves after paediatric SCHFs has never been reported before. This systematic review suggests that the radial nerve is more often lacerated than other nerves, which is a new finding to our knowledge. This needs further investigation, and a radial nerve that is not recovering after a paediatric SCHF may need earlier investigation or exploration.

5. Conclusions and Recommendations

This is the largest systematic review to report outcomes of investigations and interventions on the recovery of traumatic nerve palsies in paediatric patients after sustaining a supracondylar humerus fracture. From the findings, the authors recommend the below to be included in discussions with parents of these patients:

i. Almost all nerves will fully recover without intervention or investigation within the first 4–5 months;
ii. In nerves with little or no recovery at 3 months, a return to theatre before 4 months is recommended, as full recovery was more likely than those that were not explored, unless the nerve was lacerated;
iii. Although rare, complete transection was reported more commonly in the radial nerve; no recovery of the radial nerve at 6 weeks should alert earlier exploration;
iv. A small percentage (<5%) of traumatic nerve palsies will not fully recover regardless of investigation or surgical exploration; it is likely that permanent damage to the nerve has occurred at the time of fracture, or a failure of the nerve graft or repair.

We encourage centres to report on their outcomes of traumatic nerve palsies after paediatric SCHFs to clarify these recommendations and further guide clinicians.

Supplementary Materials: The following supporting information can be downloaded at: https://www.mdpi.com/article/10.3390/children10121862/s1, Supplementary S1: Search Strategies. Supplementary S2: PRISMA 2020 Checklist. Supplementary S3: JBI Critical Appraisal Checklist for Case Control studies. Supplementary S4: JBI Critical Appraisal Checklist for Cohort Studies. Supplementary S5: JBI Critical Appraisal Checklist for Case Series. Supplementary S6: JBI Critical Appraisal Checklist for Case Reports. Supplementary S7: Tables S1–S5. References [67–74] are cited in the supplementary materials.

Author Contributions: C.G.: writing of protocol, data collection, data extraction, results interpretation, writing of paper, supervision of authors. M.R.L.C.T.: writing of protocol, data collection, data extraction, results interpretation, writing of paper. G.D.D.: writing of protocol, data collection, data extraction, results interpretation, writing of paper. J.S.: data extraction, assessment of papers. M.K.: data extraction, assessment of papers. All authors have read and agreed to the published version of the manuscript.

Funding: This research received no external funding.

Institutional Review Board Statement: Not applicable due to the nature of the study.

Informed Consent Statement: Not applicable due to the nature of the study.

Data Availability Statement: Raw data is available on request to the primary author.

Conflicts of Interest: The authors declare no conflict of interest.

References

1. Garg, S.; Weller, A.; Larson, A.N.; Fletcher, N.D.; Kwon, M.; Schiller, J.; Browne, R.; Copley, L.; Ho, C. Clinical characteristics of severe supracondylar humerus fractures in children. *J. Pediatr. Orthop.* **2014**, *34*, 34–39. [CrossRef] [PubMed]
2. Babal, C.J.; Mehlman, T.C.; Klein, T.G. Nerve Injuries Associated with Pediatric Supracondylar Humeral Fractures: A Meta-analysis. *J. Pediatr. Orthop.* **2010**, *30*, 253–263. [CrossRef] [PubMed]
3. Dekker, A.E.; Krijnen, P.; Schipper, I.B. Results of crossed versus lateral entry K-wire fixation of displaced pediatric supracondylar humeral fractures: A systematic review and meta-analysis. *Injury* **2016**, *47*, 2391–2398. [CrossRef] [PubMed]
4. Cramer, E.K.; Green, E.N.; Devito, P.D. Incidence of Anterior Interosseous Nerve Palsy in Supracondylar Humerus Fractures in Children. *J. Pediatr. Orthop.* **1993**, *13*, 502–505. [CrossRef] [PubMed]
5. Brown, I.C.; Zinar, D.M. Traumatic and iatrogenic neurological complications after supracondylar humerus fractures in children. *J. Pediatr. Orthop.* **1995**, *15*, 440–443. [CrossRef]
6. Tomaszewski, R.; Gap, A.; Wozowicz, A.; Wysocka, P. Analysis of early vascular and neurological complications of supracondylar humerus fractures in children. *Pol. Orthop. Traumatol.* **2012**, *77*, 101–104.
7. Todd, M.; Dounas, G.; Chataway, J.; Salih, S.; Graff, C. Effectiveness of operative versus expectant management on recovery of nerve palsies in pediatric supracondylar fractures: A systematic review protocol. *JBI Evid. Synth.* **2020**, *18*, 1788–1793. [CrossRef]
8. Tufanaru, C.; Munn, Z.; Aromataris, E.; Campbell, J.; Hopp, L. Chapter 3: Systematic reviews of effectiveness. In *Joanna Briggs Institute Reviewer's Manual*; Aromataris, E., Munn, Z., Eds.; Joanna Briggs Institute: Adelaide, SA, Australia, 2017.
9. Moher, D.; Liberati, A.; Tetzlaff, J.; Altman, D.G. Preferred reporting items for systematic reviews and meta-analyses: The PRISMA statement. *Int. J. Surg.* **2010**, *8*, 336–341. [CrossRef]
10. Bramer, W.M.; Giustini, D.; de Jonge, G.B.; Holland, L.; Bekhuis, T. De-duplication of database search results for systematic reviews in EndNote. *J. Med. Libr. Assoc.* **2016**, *104*, 240–243. [CrossRef]
11. Ababneh, M.; Shannak, A.; Agabi, S.; Hadidi, S. The treatment of displaced supracondylar fractures of the humerus in children. A comparison of three methods. *Int. Orthop.* **1998**, *22*, 263–265. [CrossRef]
12. Aronson, D.C.; van Vollenhoven, E.; Meeuwis, J.D. K-wire fixation of supracondylar humeral fractures in children: Results of open reduction via a ventral approach in comparison with closed treatment. *Injury* **1993**, *24*, 179–181. [CrossRef] [PubMed]
13. Ay, S.; Akinci, M.; Kamiloglu, S.; Ercetin, O. Open reduction of displaced paediatric supracondylar humeral fractures through the anterior cubital approach. *J. Pediatr. Orthop.* **2005**, *25*, 149–153. [CrossRef] [PubMed]
14. Barrett, K.K.; Skaggs, D.L.; Sawyer, J.R.; Andras, L.; Moisan, A.; Goodbody, C.; Flynn, J.M. Supracondylar humeral fractures with isolated anterior interosseous nerve injuries: Is urgent treatment necessary? *J. Bone Jt. Surg. Am.* **2014**, *96*, 1793–1797. [CrossRef] [PubMed]
15. Bertelli, J.; Soldado, F.; Ghizoni, M.F. Outcomes of Radial Nerve Grafting In Children After Distal Humerus Fracture. *J. Hand Surg. Am.* **2018**, *43*, 1140.e1141–1140.e1146. [CrossRef] [PubMed]
16. Boyd, D.W.; Aronson, D.D. Supracondylar fractures of the humerus: A prospective study of percutaneous pinning. *J. Pediatr. Orthop.* **1992**, *12*, 789–794. [CrossRef] [PubMed]
17. Campbell, C.C.; Waters, P.M.; Emans, J.B.; Kasser, J.R.; Millis, M.B. Neurovascular injury and displacement in type III supracondylar humerus fractures. *J. Pediatr. Orthop.* **1995**, *15*, 47–52. [CrossRef]
18. Chakrabarti, A.J.; Kunzru, K.M. Complete ulnar nerve division in a displaced supracondylar fracture: A case report. *J. Bone Jt. Surg. Br.* **1995**, *77*, 977–978. [CrossRef]
19. Cheng, J.C.; Lam, T.P.; Shen, W.Y. Closed reduction and percutaneous pinning for type III displaced supracondylar fractures of the humerus in children. *J. Orthop. Trauma* **1995**, *9*, 511–515. [CrossRef]
20. Culp, R.W.; Osterman, A.L.; Davidson, R.S.; Skirven, T.; Bora, F.W. Neural injuries associated with supracondylar fractures of the humerus in children. *J. Bone Jt. Surg. Am.* **1990**, *72*, 1211–1215. [CrossRef]
21. Davis, R.T.; Gorczyca, J.T.; Pugh, K. Supracondylar humerus fractures in children. Comparison of operative treatment methods. *Clin. Orthop. Relat. Res.* **2000**, *376*, 49–55. [CrossRef]
22. Devkota, P.; Khan, J.A.; Acharya, B.M.; Pradhan, N.M.; Mainali, L.P.; Singh, M.; Shrestha, S.K.; Rajbhandari, A.P. Outcome of supracondylar fractures of the humerus in children treated by closed reduction and percutaneous pinning. *JNMA J. Nepal Med. Assoc.* **2008**, *47*, 66–70. [CrossRef] [PubMed]
23. Dormans, J.P.; Squillante, R.; Sharf, H. Acute neurovascular complications with supracondylar humerus fractures in children. *J. Hand Surg. Am.* **1995**, *20*, 1–4. [CrossRef] [PubMed]
24. Garg, B.; Pankaj, A.; Malhotra, R.; Bhan, S. Treatment of flexion-type supracondylar humeral fracture in children. *J. Orthop. Surg.* **2007**, *15*, 174–176. [CrossRef] [PubMed]
25. Gosens, T.; Bongers, K.J. Neurovascular complications and functional outcome in displaced supracondylar fractures of the humerus in children. *Injury* **2003**, *34*, 267–273. [CrossRef] [PubMed]
26. Horst, M.; Altermatt, S.; Weber, D.M.; Weil, R.; Ramseier, L.E. Pitfalls of lateral external fixation for supracondylar humeral fractures in children. *Eur. J. Trauma Emerg. Surg.* **2011**, *37*, 405–410. [CrossRef]
27. Ippolito, E.; Caterini, R.; Scola, E. Supracondylar fractures of the humerus in children. Analysis at maturity of fifty-three patients treated conservatively. *J. Bone Jt. Surg. Am.* **1986**, *68*, 333–344. [CrossRef]
28. Jones, E.T.; Louis, D.S. Median nerve injuries associated with supracondylar fractures of the humerus in children. *Clin. Orthop. Relat. Res.* **1980**, *150*, 181–186. [CrossRef]

29. Karlsson, J.; Thorsteinsson, T.; Thorleifsson, R.; Arnason, H. Entrapment of the median nerve and brachial artery after supracondylar fractures of the humerus in children. *Arch. Orthop. Trauma Surg.* **1986**, *104*, 389–391. [CrossRef]
30. Khademolhosseini, M.; Abd Rashid, A.H.; Ibrahim, S. Nerve injuries in supracondylar fractures of the humerus in children: Is nerve exploration indicated? *J. Pediatr. Orthop. B* **2013**, *22*, 123–126. [CrossRef]
31. Khan, A.Q.; Goel, S.; Abbas, M.; Sherwani, M.K. Percutaneous K-wiring for Gartland type III supracondylar humerus fractures in children. *Saudi Med. J.* **2007**, *28*, 603–606.
32. Khan, A.A.; Younas, M.; Mehmood, A.; Laraib, B. Compare the functional outcomes of closed reduction and percutaneous cross pinning versus lateral pinning in supracondylar fracture of humerus in children. *Pak. J. Med Health Sci.* **2021**, *15*, 2154–2156. [CrossRef]
33. Kirz, P.; Marsh, H. Supracondylar Fractures of the Humerus in Children. *J. Pediatr. Orthop.* **1982**, *2*, 338. [CrossRef]
34. Kiyoshige, Y. Critical displacement of neural injuries in supracondylar humeral fractures in children. *J. Pediatr. Orthop.* **1999**, *19*, 816–817. [CrossRef] [PubMed]
35. Krusche-Mandl, I.; Aldrian, S.; Kottstorfer, J.; Seis, A.; Thalhammer, G.; Egkher, A. Crossed pinning in paediatric supracondylar humerus fractures: A retrospective cohort analysis. *Int. Orthop.* **2012**, *36*, 1893–1898. [CrossRef] [PubMed]
36. Kuoppala, E.; Parviainen, R.; Pokka, T.; Sirvio, M.; Serlo, W.; Sinikumpu, J.J. Low incidence of flexion-type supracondylar humerus fractures but high rate of complications. *Acta Orthop.* **2016**, *87*, 406–411. [CrossRef] [PubMed]
37. Lalanandham, T.; Laurence, W.N. Entrapment of the ulnar nerve in the callus of a supracondylar fracture of the humerus. *Injury* **1984**, *16*, 129–130. [CrossRef] [PubMed]
38. Larson, A.N.; Garg, S.; Weller, A.; Fletcher, N.D.; Schiller, J.R.; Kwon, M.; Browne, R.; Copley, L.A.; Ho, C.A. Operative treatment of type II supracondylar humerus fractures: Does time to surgery affect complications? *J. Pediatr. Orthop.* **2014**, *34*, 382–387. [CrossRef] [PubMed]
39. Leonardi, L.; Loreti, S.; Di Pasquale, A.; Morino, S.; Fionda, L.; Vanoli, F.; Garibaldi, M.; Antonini, G. Nerve high-resolution ultrasonography in peripheral nerve injuries associated with supracondylar humeral fractures in children. *J. Clin. Neurosci.* **2020**, *71*, 119–123. [CrossRef]
40. Li, Y.A.; Lee, P.C.; Chia, W.T.; Lin, H.J.; Chiu, F.Y.; Chen, T.H.; Feng, C.K. Prospective analysis of a new minimally invasive technique for paediatric Gartland type III supracondylar fracture of the humerus. *Injury* **2009**, *40*, 1302–1307. [CrossRef]
41. Louahem, D.M.; Nebunescu, A.; Canavese, F.; Dimeglio, A. Neurovascular complications and severe displacement in supracondylar humerus fractures in children: Defensive or offensive strategy? *J. Pediatr. Orthop. B* **2006**, *15*, 51–57. [CrossRef]
42. Mangat, K.S.; Martin, A.G.; Bache, C.E. The 'pulseless pink' hand after supracondylar fracture of the humerus in children: The predictive value of nerve palsy. *J. Bone Jt. Surg. Br.* **2009**, *91*, 1521–1525. [CrossRef] [PubMed]
43. Marck, K.W.; Kooiman, A.M.; Binnendijk, B. Brachial artery rupture following supracondylar fracture of the humerus. *Neth. J. Surg.* **1986**, *38*, 81–84. [PubMed]
44. Martin, D.F.; Tolo, V.T.; Sellers, D.S.; Weiland, A.J. Radial nerve laceration and retraction associated with a supracondylar fracture of the humerus. *J. Hand Surg.* **1989**, *14*, 542–545. [CrossRef] [PubMed]
45. McGraw, J.J.; Akbarnia, B.A.; Hanel, D.P.; Keppler, L.; Burdge, R.E. Neurological complications resulting from supracondylar fractures of the humerus in children. *J. Pediatr. Orthop.* **1986**, *6*, 647–650. [CrossRef]
46. Oh, C.W.; Park, B.C.; Kim, P.T.; Park, I.H.; Kyung, H.S.; Ihn, J.C. Completely displaced supracondylar humerus fractures in children: Results of open reduction versus closed reduction. *J. Orthop. Sci.* **2003**, *8*, 137–141. [CrossRef]
47. Post, M.; Haskell, S.S. Reconstruction of the median nerve following entrapment in supracondylar fracture of the humerus: A case report. *J. Trauma* **1974**, *14*, 252–264. [CrossRef]
48. Rasool, M.N.; Naidoo, K.S. Supracondylar fractures: Posterolateral type with brachialis muscle penetration and neurovascular injury. *J. Pediatr. Orthop.* **1999**, *19*, 518–522. [CrossRef]
49. Reigstad, O.; Thorkildsen, R.; Grimsgaard, C.; Reigstad, A.; Røkkum, M. Supracondylar fractures with circulatory failure after reduction, pinning, and entrapment of the brachial artery: Excellent results more than 1 year after open exploration and revascularization. *J. Orthop. Trauma* **2011**, *25*, 26–30. [CrossRef]
50. Sairyo, K.; Henmi, T.; Kanematsu, Y.; Nakano, S.; Kajikawa, T. Radial nerve palsy associated with slightly angulated pediatric supracondylar humerus fracture. *J. Orthop. Trauma* **1997**, *11*, 227–229. [CrossRef]
51. Silva, M.; Cooper, S.D.; Cha, A. The Outcome of Surgical Treatment of Multidirectionally unstable (Type IV) Pediatric Supracondylar Humerus Fractures. *J. Pediatr. Orthop.* **2015**, *35*, 600–605. [CrossRef]
52. Solak, S.; Aydin, E. Comparison of two percutaneous pinning methods for the treatment of the pediatric type III supracondylar humerus fractures. *J. Pediatr. Orthop. B* **2003**, *12*, 346–349. [CrossRef] [PubMed]
53. Steinman, S.; Bastrom, T.P.; Newton, P.O.; Mubarak, S.J. Beware of ulnar nerve entrapment in flexion-type supracondylar humerus fractures. *J. Child. Orthop.* **2007**, *1*, 177–180. [CrossRef] [PubMed]
54. Thorleifsson, R.; Karlsson, J.; Thorsteinsson, T. Median nerve entrapment in bone after supracondylar fracture of the humerus. Case report. *Arch. Orthop. Trauma Surg.* **1988**, *107*, 183–185. [CrossRef]
55. Tokutake, K.; Okui, N.; Hirata, H. Primary Radial Nerve Exploration Determined by Ultrasound in Paediatric Supracondylar Humerus Fracture: A Report of Two Cases. *J. Hand Surg. Asian-Pac. Vol.* **2021**, *26*, 284–289. [CrossRef] [PubMed]
56. Tomaszewski, R.; Wozowicz, A.; Wysocka-Wojakiewicz, P. Analysis of Early Neurovascular Complications of Paediatric Supracondylar Humerus Fractures: A Long-Term Observation. *Biomed. Res. Int.* **2017**, *2017*, 2803790. [CrossRef] [PubMed]

57. Tunku-Naziha, T.Z.; Wan-Yuhana, W.; Hadizie, D.; Muhammad, P.; Abdul-Nawfar, S.; Wan-Azman, W.S.; Arman, Z.M.; Abdul-Razak, S.; Rhendra-Hardy, M.Z.; Wan-Faisham, W.I. Early Vessels Exploration of Pink Pulseless Hand in Gartland III Supracondylar Fracture Humerus in Children: Facts and Controversies. *Malays. Orthop. J.* **2017**, *11*, 12–17. [CrossRef] [PubMed]
58. van Vugt, A.B.; Severijnen, R.V.; Festen, C. Neurovascular complications in supracondylar humeral fractures in children. *Arch. Orthop. Trauma Surg.* **1988**, *107*, 203–205. [CrossRef] [PubMed]
59. Yano, K.; Ishiko, M.; Iida, K.; Sasaki, K.; Kojima, T.; Kaneshiro, Y.; Sakanaka, H. High Median Nerve Entrapment by Fracture Callus in Surgically Treated Paediatric Supracondylar Humeral Fracture: A Case Report. *JBJS Case Connect.* **2022**, *12*, 737. [CrossRef]
60. Yaokreh, J.B.; Gicquel, P.; Schneider, L.; Stanchina, C.; Karger, C.; Saliba, E.; Ossenou, O.; Clavert, J.M. Compared outcomes after percutaneous pinning versus open reduction in paediatric supracondylar elbow fractures. *Orthop. Traumatol. Surg. Res.* **2012**, *98*, 645–651. [CrossRef]
61. Graff, C.; Dounas, G.D.; Sung, J.; Kumawat, M.; Huang, Y.; Todd, M. Management of iatrogenic ulnar nerve palsies after cross pinning of pediatric supracondylar humerus fractures: A systematic review. *J. Child. Orthop.* **2022**, *16*, 366–373. [CrossRef]
62. Reitman, R.D.; Waters, P.; Millis, M. Open Reduction and Internal Fixation for Supracondylar Humerus Fractures in Children. *J. Pediatr. Orthop.* **2001**, *21*, 157–161. [CrossRef] [PubMed]
63. Shore, B.J.; Gillespie, B.T.; Miller, P.E.; Bae, D.S.; Waters, P.M. Recovery of Motor Nerve Injuries Associated with Displaced, Extension-type Pediatric Supracondylar Humerus Fractures. *J. Pediatr. Orthop.* **2019**, *39*, e652–e656. [CrossRef] [PubMed]
64. Ramachandran, M.; Birch, R.; Eastwood, D.M. Clinical outcome of nerve injuries associated with supracondylar fractures of the humerus in children: The experience of a specialist referral centre. *J. Bone Jt. Surg. Br.* **2006**, *88*, 90. [CrossRef] [PubMed]
65. Galbraith, K.A.; McCullough, C.J. Acute nerve injury as a complication of closed fractures or dislocations of the elbow. *Injury* **1979**, *11*, 159–164. [CrossRef]
66. Kwok, I.H.Y.; Silk, Z.M.; Quick, T.J.; Sinisi, M.; Macquillan, A.; Fox, M. Nerve injuries associated with supracondylar fractures of the humerus in children: Our experience in a specialist peripheral nerve injury unit. *Bone Jt. J.* **2016**, *98-B*, 851. [CrossRef]
67. Gagnier, J.J.; Kienle, G.; Altman, D.G.; Moher, D.; Sox, H.; Riley, D.; CARE Group. The CARE Guidelines: Consensus-Based Clinical Case Reporting Guideline Development. *Headache J. Head Face Pain* **2013**, *53*, 1541–1547. [CrossRef]
68. Dekkers, O.M.; Egger, M.; Altman, D.G.; Vandenbroucke, J.P. Distinguishing case series from cohort studies. *Ann. Intern. Med.* **2012**, *156*, 37–40. [CrossRef]
69. Esene, I.N.; Ngu, J.; El Zoghby, M.; Solaroglu, I.; Sikod, A.M.; Kotb, A.; Dechambenoit, G.; El Husseiny, H. Case series and descriptive cohort studies in neurosurgery: The confusion and solution. *Child's Nerv. Syst.* **2014**, *30*, 1321–1332. [CrossRef]
70. Abu-Zidan, F.M.; Abbas, A.K.; Hefny, A.F. Clinical "case series": A concept analysis. *Afr. Health Sci.* **2012**, *12*, 557–562. [CrossRef]
71. Straus, S.E.; Richardson, W.S.; Glasziou, P.; Haynes, R.B. *Evidence-Based Medicine: How to Practice and Teach EBM*, 3rd ed.; Elsevier: Amsterdam, The Netherlands, 2005.
72. Moola, S.; Munn, Z.; Tufanaru, C.; Aromataris, E.; Sears, K.; Sfetcu, R.; Currie, M.; Qureshi, R.; Mattis, P.; Lisy, K.; et al. Chapter 7: Systematic reviews of etiology and risk. In *JBI Manual for Evidence Synthesis*; Aromataris, E., Munn, Z., Eds.; JBI: Adelaide, Australia, 2020; Available online: https://synthesismanual.jbi.global (accessed on 20 July 2022).
73. Page, M.J.; McKenzie, J.E.; Bossuyt, P.M.; Boutron, I.; Hoffmann, T.C.; Mulrow, C.D.; Shamseer, L.; Tetzlaff, J.M.; Akl, E.A.; Brennan, S.E.; et al. The PRISMA 2020 statement: An updated guideline for reporting systematic reviews. *BMJ* **2021**, *37*, n71. [CrossRef]
74. Law, K.; Howick, J. OCEBM Table of Evidence Glossary. 2013. Available online: http://www.cebm.net/index.aspx?o=1116 (accessed on 10 January 2014).

Disclaimer/Publisher's Note: The statements, opinions and data contained in all publications are solely those of the individual author(s) and contributor(s) and not of MDPI and/or the editor(s). MDPI and/or the editor(s) disclaim responsibility for any injury to people or property resulting from any ideas, methods, instructions or products referred to in the content.

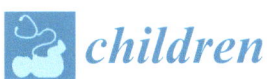

Review

Indications and Timing of Guided Growth Techniques for Pediatric Upper Extremity Deformities: A Literature Review

Mark F. Siemensma [1], Christiaan J.A. van Bergen [1,2], Eline M. van Es [1], Joost W. Colaris [1] and Denise Eygendaal [1,*]

1 Department of Orthopedics and Sports Medicine, Erasmus University Medical Center—Sophia Children's Hospital, 3000 CA Rotterdam, The Netherlands
2 Department of Orthopaedic Surgery, Amphia Hospital, 4800 RK Breda, The Netherlands
* Correspondence: d.eygendaal@erasmusmc.nl

Abstract: Osseous deformities in children arise due to progressive angular growth or complete physeal arrest. Clinical and radiological alignment measurements help to provide an impression of the deformity, which can be corrected using guided growth techniques. However, little is known about timing and techniques for the upper extremity. Treatment options for deformity correction include monitoring of the deformity, (hemi-)epiphysiodesis, physeal bar resection, and correction osteotomy. Treatment is dependent on the extent and location of the deformity, physeal involvement, presence of a physeal bar, patient age, and predicted length inequality at skeletal maturity. An accurate estimation of the projected limb or bone length inequality is crucial for optimal timing of the intervention. The Paley multiplier method remains the most accurate and simple method for calculating limb growth. While the multiplier method is accurate for calculating growth prior to the growth spurt, measuring peak height velocity (PHV) is superior to chronological age after the onset of the growth spurt. PHV is closely related to skeletal age in children. The Sauvegrain method of skeletal age assessment using elbow radiographs is possibly a simpler and more reliable method than the method by Greulich and Pyle using hand radiographs. PHV-derived multipliers need to be developed for the Sauvegrain method for a more accurate calculation of limb growth during the growth spurt. This paper provides a review of the current literature on the clinical and radiological evaluation of normal upper extremity alignment and aims to provide state-of-the-art directions on deformity evaluation, treatment options, and optimal timing of these options during growth.

Keywords: limb length discrepancy; alignment; growth correction; children; timing

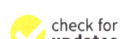

Citation: Siemensma, M.F.; van Bergen, C.J.A.; van Es, E.M.; Colaris, J.W.; Eygendaal, D. Indications and Timing of Guided Growth Techniques for Pediatric Upper Extremity Deformities: A Literature Review. *Children* **2023**, *10*, 195. https://doi.org/10.3390/children10020195

Academic Editor: Vito Pavone

Received: 30 December 2022
Revised: 13 January 2023
Accepted: 18 January 2023
Published: 20 January 2023

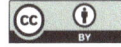

Copyright: © 2023 by the authors. Licensee MDPI, Basel, Switzerland. This article is an open access article distributed under the terms and conditions of the Creative Commons Attribution (CC BY) license (https:// creativecommons.org/licenses/by/ 4.0/).

1. Introduction

In contrast with adults, children have the unique capability to correct bone deformities by growth. Most deformities have a traumatic origin. Traumatic injury can occur at the level of the epiphysis, the physis, the metaphysis, or diaphysis [1]. Most correction can be expected in younger children in deformities near the most active growth plate and in the direction of the dominant movement. Most often, growth behaves like a friend, allowing the deformity to correct itself naturally during extensive follow-up. Natural correction follows two principles. The first principle is formed by the Hueter–Volkmann law, in which a degree of pressure on the convex side increases periosteal bone formation and relatively inhibits longitudinal growth [2]. Conversely, bone formation on the concave side is stimulated, increasing bone formation and resulting in a relative increase of longitudinal growth. In the second principle, Wolff's Law addresses the ability of the bone and joint surfaces to remodel according to local mechanical loads [3].

Sometimes growth behaves less favorably, leading to severe malunions, joint instability, joint incongruence, impairment of movement, and eventually to early posttraumatic arthritis. Especially fractures through or nearby the physis are renowned for problems during growth, such as premature closure caused by bone bars, resulting in asymmetrical growth or even growth arrest. It is, therefore, of great importance to closely monitor these cases and, if needed, intervene surgically to correct the deformity.

While in the lower extremity, guided growth by epiphysiodesis or hemi-epiphysiodesis is described extensively, little is known about the techniques, timing, and principles in the upper extremity. The purpose of this paper is to provide a review of the current literature concerning the clinical and radiological evaluation of normal upper extremity alignment and the causes and assessment of deformities in the upper extremity. Moreover, it aims to provide state-of-the-art directions on deformity evaluation and monitoring, different treatment options, and the timing of these options during growth.

2. Methods

For this narrative review, the Medline Ovid and Embase databases were searched for peer-reviewed studies in English until 30 November 2022. The search was divided into subcategories regarding each section using the following keywords and synonyms. Clinical and radiological evaluation: alignment, carrying angle, Baumann angle, Hafner method, cubitus varus, physical examination, radiograph. Causes of deformity: epiphyseal plate, (Salter–Harris) fracture, ischemia, repetitive stress, physeal plate, Madelung deformity. Treatment options: eight-plate, tension band, transphyseal screw, physeal bar resection Timing of intervention: skeletal age, growth chart, multiplier method, guided growth. A total of 716 articles were screened by title and abstract for relevance, twenty-two articles were additionally included by snowballing, and 83 articles were included in the final synthesis. All articles were screened by two independent reviewers. Single case reports and studies based on expert opinions were excluded from the synthesis. Because symptomatic deformities of the upper extremity occur primarily at the distal parts of the humerus and forearm with relation to the elbow and wrist, other upper extremity parts are deemed outside of the scope of this review. All patients and parents gave written informed consent for the publication of the anonymized images used in this review.

3. Clinical Evaluation

Standard physical examination is a quick and reliable method for the assessment of gross deformities of the upper limb [4]. Comparison to the uninjured side is mandatory in posttraumatic deformities. The examination should include the assessment of alignment in three directions, joint effusion, active and passive range of motion, evaluation of stability and points of tenderness, and finally, neurovascular assessment.

Because symptomatic deformities of the upper extremity occur primarily at the distal part of the humerus and in the forearm, range of motion (ROM) of the elbow and wrist is important to assess. Pediatric ROM of both the elbow and the wrist is slightly increased compared to adults, caused by hyperlaxity of the joints in childhood (Table 1). Despite the slight differences, a separate set of normal values is not defined for children in most hospitals, and the adult ROM-values are often used during clinical evaluation.

Table 1. Normal range of motion (ROM) of the elbow and wrist in degrees for both adults [4] and children [5].

Elbow	Adult ROM (Degrees)	Pediatric ROM (Degrees, SD)	Wrist	Adult ROM (Degrees)	Pediatric ROM (Degrees, SD)
Flexion	140	145 ± 5	Flexion	60	78 ± 6
Extension	0	1 ± 4	Extension	60	76 ± 6
Pronation	80	77 ± 5	Radial deviation	20	22 ± 4
Supination	80	83 ± 3	Ulnar deviation	30	37 ± 4

3.1. Elbow

During visual inspection, the patient is placed in front of the examiner, standing in the anatomical position with both elbows fully extended (Figure 1). The carrying angle is measured best in a standing patient with arms in the anatomical position, with arms fully extended and wrists fully supinated. The carrying angle is the angle deviated from the line parallel to the humerus and the forearm. The carrying angle is usually greater in women, with an average of 15–20 degrees. In men, the carrying angle is, on average, 10–15 degrees [5–7]. Therefore, the carrying angle is compared best with the contralateral side. A physiological change in the carrying angle from valgus to varus can be observed as the patient flexes the elbow and supinates the forearm [8]. Assessment of the carrying angle is therefore performed in the same amount of flexion and rotation of both arms to optimize adequate comparison. In most female patients and children, a slight hyperextension of the elbow of 0 to 10 degrees is physiological [9]. Deformities in the sagittal plane are measured with the humerus in 90 degrees anteflexion and by flexing and extending the elbow with the forearm in a supinated position.

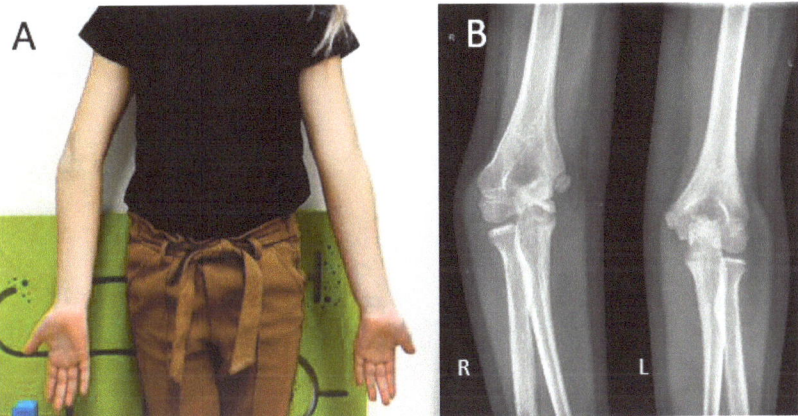

Figure 1. (**A**) Visual inspection of the carrying angle of the elbow in a 10-year-old girl showing a unilateral cubitus varus on the right side. (**B**) Anteroposterior radiographic views of the elbow with the unaffected contralateral side for comparison.

Forearm rotation is measured by having the patient place the arms parallel to the side of the patient with the elbows in 90 degrees flexion. A pen in the child's fist improves rotatory measurements.

3.2. Wrist

There are multiple ways of measuring wrist dorsal flexion. One quick way to assess for gross deformities is to have the patient put their palms together with their fingers pointing upwards and their elbows kept horizontally. Wrist palmar flexion can be performed similarly by putting both dorsal sides of the hand together with the fingers pointing downwards. Angular deviation in the coronal plane is measured by the radial and ulnar deviation of the wrist. It is measured best by having the patient place the supinated forearm on a flat surface with the palm of the hand lying flat. A small reference line is then drawn on the dorsum of the hand along the third metacarpus.

4. Radiological Evaluation
4.1. Humerus

Different radiographic angles have been described for the assessment of humeral alignment. The Baumann's angle is measured on an anteroposterior (AP) radiograph with the elbow in extension. It is formed by the angle between the long axis of the humeral shaft and a straight line through the epiphyseal plate of the capitellum or the lateral condylar physis (Figure 2A). There is a considerable variation in individuals, ranging from 64 to 82 degrees [10,11]. Therefore, the Baumann's angle is best compared to the contralateral side, where a difference >5 degrees is deemed abnormal.

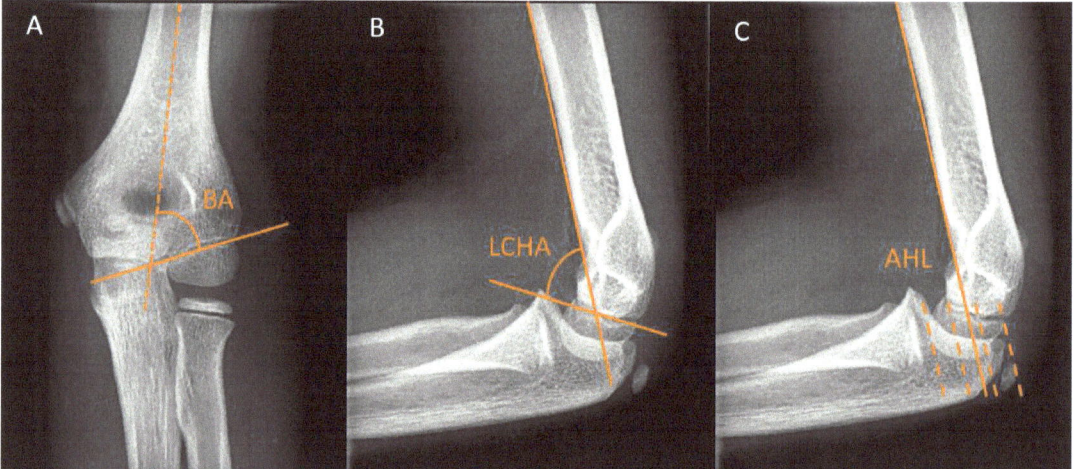

Figure 2. Distal humerus radiographic reference lines. (**A**) Baumann angle (BA) on an anteroposterior elbow view. (**B**) The lateral capitellohumeral angle (LCHA) on a lateral elbow view. (**C**) Anterior humeral line (AHL) on a lateral view. This line should pass between the two dotted lines in the middle.

The lateral capitellohumeral angle (LCHA) is measured on a lateral radiograph as the angle between the line along the anterior surface of the humerus and a line along the open capitellar physis (Figure 2B). The LCHA has a smaller normal range from 45 to 57 degrees and does not vary by age, side, or sex [12] (Figure 2B).

The lateral anterior humeral line (AHL) or capitellohumeral line is a line drawn along the anterior surface of the humerus, which should pass through the middle third of the capitellum on a lateral view (Figure 2C).

4.2. Radius

Radial height is measured on posteroanterior (PA) views as the distance between two parallel lines: one perpendicular to the long axis of the radius along the ulnar aspect of the articular surface and the other one at the tip of the radial styloid (Figure 3A). A normal adult radial height is 8 to 14 mm [13]; however, the values range in the literature, and those for children are unknown.

Volar tilt is measured on the lateral view as the angle between a line drawn perpendicular to the long axis of the radius and a tangent line along the slope of the articular surface of the radius (Figure 3B). A normal volar tilt ranges between 10 and 25 degrees [14,15].

Radial inclination is measured on the PA view as the angle between a line perpendicular to the long axis of the radius at the level of the radial styloid tip and a line along the articular surface of the distal radius (Figure 3C). A normal radial inclination ranges between 15 and 25 degrees [14,16].

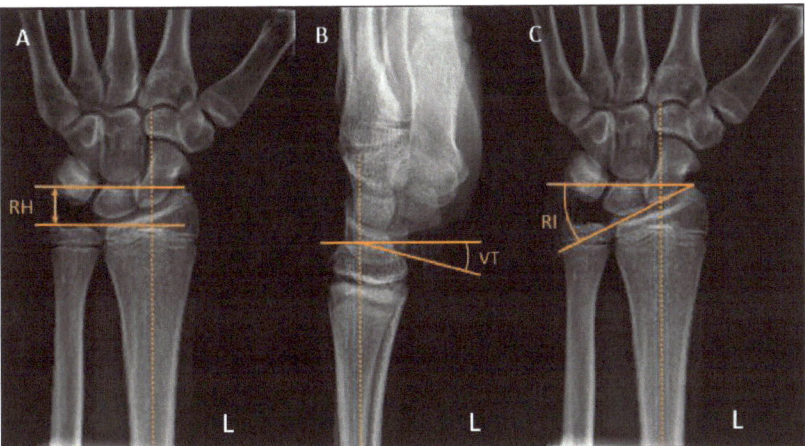

Figure 3. Distal radius radiographic reference lines. (**A**) Radial height (RH). (**B**) Volar tilt (VT). (**C**) Radial inclination (RI).

4.3. Ulna

Ulnar variance, or Hulten variance, can be positive, negative, or neutral. In positive ulnar variance, the ulna is longer than the radius. Conversely, in negative ulnar variance, the radius is longer than the ulna. In neutral ulnar variance, both the articular surfaces of the radius and the ulna are at the same height. Ulnar variance is independent of the length of the ulnar styloid process, which may also vary.

There are multiple ways of measuring the ulnar variance. In the method of perpendiculars, a line is drawn perpendicular to the longitudinal axis of the radius and through the most distal ulnar part of the radius. The distance between the adjacent distal cortical rim of the ulna relative to this line is then measured as the variance [17] (Figure 4A). In the method as described by Hafner et al. [18], a line is drawn perpendicular to the longitudinal axis of the ulna, touching the most proximal prominent point of the ulnar metaphysis on the radial side. Secondly, a line is drawn on the radius perpendicular to its longitudinal axis touching the most proximal point of the radial metaphysis on the ulnar side. Ulnar variance is then defined as the distance between these lines. In the literature, these distances are referred to as "Proximal–PRoximal distance [17]. Conversely, the variance can be measured using the distance of the most distal points of the radial and ulnar metaphysis. This method is referred to as "Distal–DIstal" distance. (Figure 4B).

Kox et al. investigated the difference between the above-stated methods for measuring ulnar variance in a group of 350 healthy children and adolescents. It was found that the Hafner method was the preferred method for children with unfused growth plates or those younger than 13 years, and the adapted perpendicular method was recommended in children with fused growth plates or those 14 years and older [17].

Ulnar variance changes with wrist position and during clenching of the wrist. It is more positive during pronation and becomes more negative during supination. In addition, a clenched fist results in a relatively more ulna plus compared with a neutral grip. Therefore, obtaining only a PA-view with a neutral grip may underestimate maximal variance, and obtaining clenched fist view radiographs can be a useful addition [15].

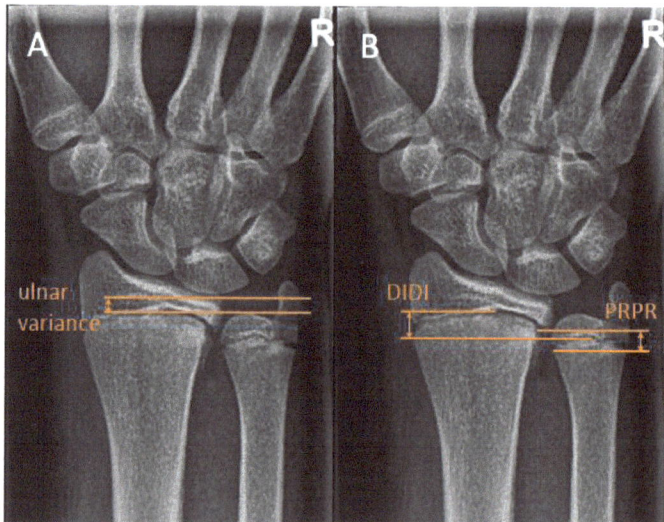

Figure 4. Distal ulna radiographic reference lines. (**A**) The Hafner method for measuring ulnar variance. (**B**) The method of perpendiculars for measuring ulnar variance, with 'PRPR termed as the two most proximal points of the physis and 'DIDI' termed as the two most distal points of the physis.

5. Causes of Upper Extremity Deformity

Osseous deformities can arise at different levels of the bone, dependent on the pathophysiology. Deformities occurring at the level of the diaphysis and the metaphysis are often the result of a malunited fracture [1]. Deformities at the level of the physis have a broader spectrum of causes. They can be congenital, developmental, or acquired as the result of an infection, arthritis, compartment syndrome, avascular necrosis, or trauma, with the latter being the most common cause [18,19].

In up to 10% of physeal fractures, some form of growth disturbance occurs [20–22]. The main traumatic factors contributing to the growth arrest of the physeal plate are crush fractures from high-energy injury or repetitive stress (i.e., Salter–Harris type V) and physeal injuries crossing the germinal layer (i.e., Salter–Harris type III and IV) [21]. Traumatic growth disturbance may cause slower, asymmetrical, or arrested growth. These growth disturbances are often the result of an incorrect or overstimulated fracture repair. During fracture healing, when blood vessels reach the hypertrophic zone of the physis, ossification is stimulated, and a physiologic bridge of sclerotic bone forms eccentrically between the epiphyseal ossification center and the metaphyseal bone [20]. This effectively replaces a segment of the physis and the zone of Ranvier [23]. The effects of this bony bridge vary with its location and size but will result in either a complete or a partial growth disturbance. A large central bar will slow down or completely arrest the growth of the entire physis, creating a short bone, which in term may lead to limb length inequality or joint congruity if the bone of a pair is affected in the case of the radius and ulna. When the bar is eccentrically formed within the physis, growth stops at that point but continues in the rest of the physis. This results in a progressive angular deformity [24].

5.1. Humerus

Cubitus varus is most often seen as late sequela after a distal humerus fracture (Figure 1B). The current stance in the literature is that it is caused by malunion of a humeral fracture rather than a growth arrest. The most common type of distal humerus fracture in children is the supracondylar fracture [25]. They are classified using the Gartland type classification, ranging from type I to type III, depending on the amount of posterior displacement of the capitellum and the intactness of the posterior humeral cortex [26]. Cubitus varus, however, results from displacement or comminution in the coronal plane. These injuries are often overlooked or difficult to judge on standard radiographs. Therefore, in type II and type III fractures, an oblique view may be helpful in identifying minimally displaced fractures [27]. Rotational malalignment can be difficult to assess radiographically. A high index of suspicion for rotational malalignment is required in cases of posteromedial displacement. These cases may also lead to a higher Baumann angle and hence combined cubitus varus deformity [28]. If missed or left untreated, the malunion leads to a progressive angular deformity in the coronal plane. The result at patient presentation is often a painless varus deformity evident at visual inspection that may not always be accompanied by limitations in ROM [25]. Although diagnosis is usually based on clinical evaluation alone, measuring the radiological Baumann angle compared to the contralateral side may give a more accurate measure of the extent of the deformity.

5.2. Radius

Proximal radial fractures represent up to 10% of all pediatric elbow fractures [29,30]. The mechanism of injury is usually a fall on an outstretched hand, combined with a compressive valgus force across the elbow joint. Despite the occurrence of these fractures around the growth plate, premature physeal closure occurs in about 1.5% of patients [30]. Growth has more impact, however, in congenital radial head dislocations (Figure 5). Although rare in absolute numbers, it is the most common congenital elbow abnormality, accounting for up to 10% [31]. Dislocations occur bilaterally in most cases. Around 70% of dislocations occur posteriorly, followed by anterior and lateral dislocations, occurring around 15% each [31]. With frequent dislocations, the normal anatomical relation of the radial head with the capitellum and the proximal radioulnar joint (PRUJ) during growth may be lost. Without the pressure of the radial head onto the capitellum during growth, a malformation of the radial head with loss of concavity occurs, making reduction in longstanding cases impossible [31]. Patients are generally presented with a painless mass at visual inspection or palpation. Elbow flexion may be slightly decreased in the case of an anterior dislocation, and extension may be slightly decreased in the case of a posterior dislocation. Additionally, DRUJ alignment may be lost, resulting in decreased ROM during pronation and supination [31]. A lateral elbow radiograph is often sufficient to diagnose this condition. Herein, the extent of radial head deformation is a reliable guideline in the decision of whether to operate on a patient [32]. If the radial head is more dome-shaped and has lost all its concavity, surgery tends to be unsuccessful.

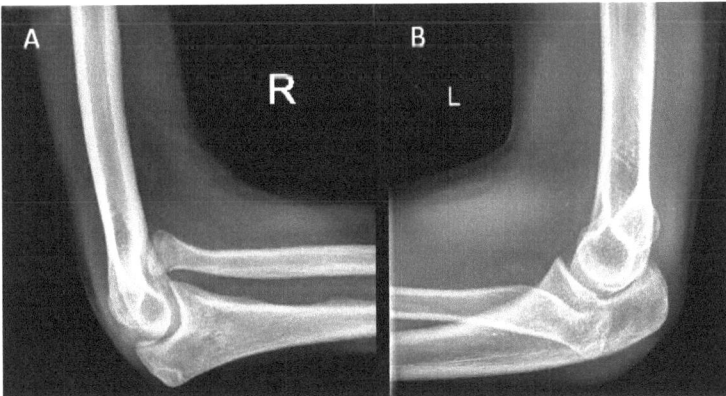

Figure 5. (**A**) A 17-year-old boy with congenital anterior radial head dislocations of the right arm. (**B**) A 16-year-old girl with congenital posterior radial head dislocations of the left arm, accompanied by a symptomatic elbow contracture. The girl was treated conservatively with a static progressive elbow flexion brace.

The distal radius is the most common site of physeal injury of the upper extremity, accounting for 30% to 39% of all physeal injuries [33]. The incidence of growth disturbances in the forearm caused by distal physeal injuries has been reported at a rate of up to 28% [18]. Despite the generally good outcomes of distal radius fractures, the incidence of a premature complete distal radius growth arrest is up to 7% [34–36]. Risk factors for developing premature physeal arrest are repeated forceful manipulation during reduction, multiple reduction attempts, and late reduction [34]. A posttraumatic radial physeal arrest can result in ulnar overgrowth, otherwise known as positive ulnar variance or ulna-plus. This occurs when the level of the ulna is >2.5 mm beyond the radius margin of the distal radioulnar joint (DRUJ). Gross deformity develops if the discrepancy between the radial and the ulnar length is more than 4 mm [34]. Despite the presence of gross deformity, functional problems do not always occur, and therefore, clinical presentation can be variable [18]. However, the majority of patients report significant impairment, most commonly by activity-related pain and loss of pronation–supination. Some asymptomatic patients in which radiographic signs of physeal arrest and positive ulnar variance are seen may opt for early surgery to prevent progressive deformity [36].

Chronic repetitive stress injuries of the distal wrist are increasingly being mentioned as a distinct diagnosis. This type of injury has a high incidence in competitive gymnasts. It is, therefore, also known as the 'gymnast wrist'. As the result of repetitive axial loading with microtraumata of both the distal radial and ulnar physis, premature closure of the physis can occur, mimicking a Salter–Harris type V injury [33]. In a study by DiFiori et al. in which fifty-nine gymnasts were examined, 51% had radiological findings of stress injury to the distal radial physis, and 7% had distinct widening of the growth plate. In addition, wrist pain was significantly related to the grade of radiographic injury. Prolonged repetitive stress on the distal radial physis can even lead to complete physeal arrest [37]. Radiologic criteria for the diagnosis of stress injuries in the physis of the distal radius include widening of the growth plate, especially on the volar and radial side, cystic changes of the metaphyseal aspect of the growth plate, a beaked distal volar and radial physis, and haziness within the growth plate [38]. These criteria are named in multiple reports; however, a comprehensive guideline for the classification of these injuries is lacking [38,39].

Madelung deformity is a rare congenital arm condition that affects the growth plate of the distal radius. The lagging growth of the distal radius results in a radioulnar and radiocarpal misalignment. The progressive growth disturbance may eventually lead to a three-dimensional wrist deformity [40]. Madelung deformity is usually diagnosed between the ages of 6 and 13 years [41]. In children with Madelung deformity, additional ulnar radiological measurements are indicated. Farr et al. [40] stated that in addition to ulnar variance, a lunate subsidence (LS) >4 mm and a palmar carpal displacement (PCD) >20 mm were radiographic criteria for undergoing an ulnar shortening osteotomy. They measured PCD on a lateral radiograph as the distance between the longitudinal ulna axis and the most volar aspect of the lunate (Figure 6A). LS was measured on a PA radiograph as the distance between a perpendicular line to the longitudinal ulna axis and the most proximal point of the lunate. (Figure 6B). Symptoms of Madelung deformity can range from wrist pain to decreased function. Most commonly, patients experience a limited range of motion in the wrist and continuous or post-activity wrist pain.

5.3. Ulna

In the proximal part of the ulna, physeal fractures of the olecranon account for 4% of all pediatric elbow fractures [42]. They usually occur as a result of a fall onto an outstretched hand with the elbow in flexion. Nondisplaced fractures respond well to conservative treatment, and growth disturbances are rare. Growth disturbances in the distal ulna, caused by physeal injuries, however, have been reported at a rate of up to 50% [18]. The higher percentage may be explained by the higher force required to overcome the cushioning effect of the cartilage between the ulna and the proximal carpal row and the dissipation of impact forces through the triangulate fibrocartilage complex [43]. A shortened distal ulna results more commonly from any of the surgical procedures that involve resection of the distal ulna secondary to prior wrist trauma or correction of Madelung deformity.

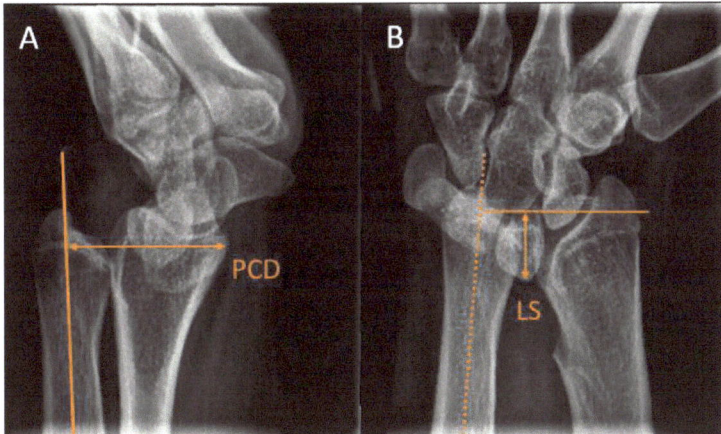

Figure 6. Radiographic wrist measurements used for the assessment of Madelung deformity. (**A**) Palmar carpal displacement (PCD) on a lateral wrist view, measured as the distance between the longitudinal ulna axis and the most volar lunate aspect. (**B**) Lunate subsidence (LS) on a posteroanterior view, measured as the distance between a perpendicular line to the longitudinal ulna axis and the most proximal lunate point.

5.4. Combined Radioulnar

During forearm rotation, the relation in the distance between the radius and ulna changes dynamically. Angular deformities in either bone can further increase or decrease the distance between both bones during rotation [44–46]. During pronation, the radius crosses the ulna, and their respective distance decreases. Radial bowing and radius malunions with the deformity pointed towards the ulnar side may cause a pronation deficit by a collision of the radius and ulna [45,46]. Conversely, during supination, an increase in distance between both bones is seen. The radius and ulna are interconnected by the central band. This ligament allows for the dissipation of forces from one bone to the other but can also pose problems in the case of osseous deformity. In radius malunions directed away from the ulna, the rigid central band length can impair further rotation and cause a supination deficit [15,16].

6. Treatment Options

In contrast to the lower extremity, where even minor limb length differences can lead to symptoms, minor differences in length in the upper extremity pose a lesser problem. In general, expected length differences of less than 5 cm in the humerus are generally treated conservatively. If the bones of the distal radius and ulna are affected, the margins are smaller. Radioulnar variance greater than 4 mm is considered a gross deformity [34]. Any physeal arrest in either the radius or the ulna can therefore be a good indication for surgical intervention. In general, treatment options for physeal arrest include observation, (temporary-) epiphysiodesis or hemiepiphysiodesis, physeal bar resection, and corrective osteotomy.

6.1. Observation

Growth arrest, angular deformities, and consequentially altered joint mechanics may develop up to 2 years post-injury [47]. Secondary to the injury, damaged cartilage tissue within the physis is often replaced by unwanted bony tissue, forming a bony bar or bony bridge. If the fracture is aligned correctly with or without reduction, physicians may choose for casting to ensure anatomic alignment and to prevent displacement accompanied by close radiological follow-up for observation of bony bar formation [48]. If a bar appears to involve the entire physis and the predicted length inequality or angular deformity at skeletal maturity is acceptable, observation may be the best option. Because growth often naturally corrects the deformity, another consideration can be to initially observe the deformity until skeletal maturity and to plan a correction osteotomy to correct the deformity if needed.

6.2. Hemiepiphysiodesis

In (progressive) angular deformities, hemiepiphysiodesis can be performed by tethering the proximal and distal physeal parts together. This results in a temporary halt of the growth at one side while the other side can catch up, correcting the deformity by growth. Growth plates can be tethered together using metal clips over the physis, by drilling screws through the physis, or by connecting the proximal and distal part of the physis together by non-resorbable filament, Kirschner wires, or a nonlocking plate that acts as a tension band. Due to its reversibility, this technique is safer and more predictable than a classic permanent epiphysiodesis. In addition, the exact timing of the intervention is of lesser importance because the implant is removed when the desired correction is achieved. The required second surgery to remove the implant, however, is a considerable disadvantage compared to permanent epiphysiodesis [49].

In the lower limb, modulation of growth by tethering part of the growth plate using tension-band plates (TBPs) or eight-plates is an established technique. The literature shows high efficacy and low complications with success rates for correction up to 93% [50,51]. Despite the high efficacy of the technique, no cohort studies of sufficient size have been published using TBPs in the upper extremity. A rebound phenomenon after using tension band hemiepiphysiodesis is known to occur. This happens when the growth of the inhibited side of the physis exceeds that of the contralateral side due to transient overstimulation after tension band removal [52]. To compensate for this, a slight overcorrection can be aimed for. A high correction rate is a significant risk factor for developing overcorrection. This is found to be a direct indicator of physeal activity, wherein a higher rate of correction is indicative of a larger residual growth plate activity [52]. Younger age at initial surgery and implant removal may also pose a risk factor [53,54]. The younger the patient is at the initial procedure, the higher the growth plate activity, leading to a more rapid correction and concomitant longer time between plate removal and skeletal maturity. Most studies advocate delaying temporary hemiepiphysiodesis until 8–10 years for the lower extremities due to the occurrence of rebound or concerns about causing permanent physeal damage [55]. Despite the lower growth rates of the upper extremity compared to the lower extremity, clinicians should monitor patients closely after tension band hemiepiphysiodesis for rebound phenomena, especially in younger patients.

An alternative technique to tether the growth plate is to use transphyseal screws (Figure 7). This technique has a faster correction rate than the tension band principle [56,57]. Hence, this technique may better serve patients that are near skeletal maturity. Soldado et al. [58] used transphyseal crossed cannulated screws (Metaizeau technique) to correct cubitus varus deformities in five very young children. The children had a mean age of 3 years and 7 months and were followed over a mean period of 3 years and 10 months. No correction was observed in all cases. The authors postulated that the ineffectiveness may be explained by the modest growth capacity of the distal humeral physis and because most growth occurs during the pubertal growth spurt, while their follow-up finished before any of their patients reached that stage. Dai et al. [59] studied temporary hemiepiphysiodesis in a total of 135 physes in 66 children with a mean age of 4.69 years old (ranging from 1 to 10 years). In a mean deformity correction period of 13.26 months, 94.06% of the angular deformities were corrected. Thus, posing temporary hemiepiphysiodesis using the Metaizeau technique is an effective method for correcting angular deformities in younger children. A probable reason why the deformity correction for young children in the lower extremity is more successful than in the distal humerus is the difference in axial growth speeds and the percentage of contribution of the physes with regard to the total limb growth. Only 20% of growth takes place in the distal humerus, accounting for a mean of 0.26 cm per year. Conversely, in the distal femur and proximal tibia these percentages are 70% and 60%, respectively, which corresponds to 1.2 cm and 0.9 cm per year [60–62].

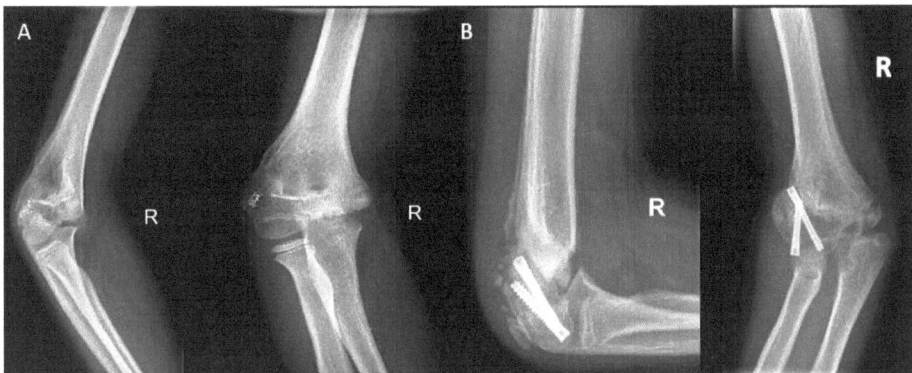

Figure 7. (**A**) Elbow radiographs of a 9-year-old girl with a posttraumatic cubitus varus, a flexion deficit of 60 degrees, and avascular necrosis of the medial condyle after a fall from height. (**B**) An epiphysiodesis using transphyseal screws was performed in addition to an arthrolysis with reduction of the coronoid fossa and release of the ulnar nerve.

6.3. Complete Epiphysiodesis

In complete epiphysiodesis, the physis is completely removed or temporarily tethered across the entire width. This procedure is performed to prevent overgrowth. Surgical options range from percutaneous techniques using drills and curettes to more invasive open techniques. For example, premature closure of the distal radial physis can be associated with ulnar overgrowth, leading to altered wrist mechanics and pain. An epiphysiodesis of the ulna can prevent worsening of the deformity (Figure 8).

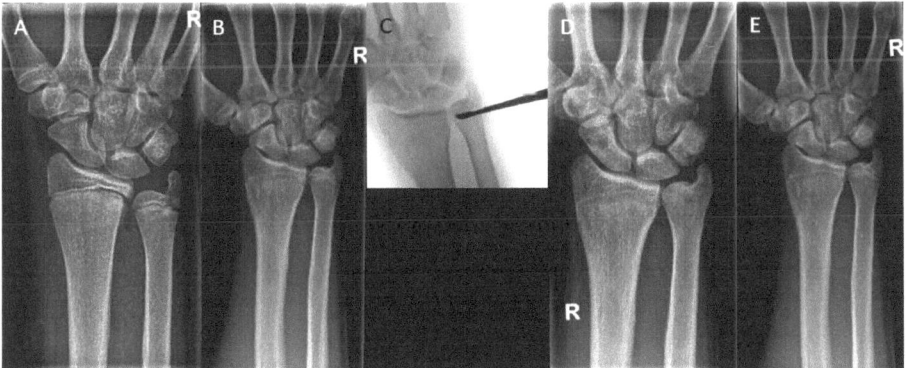

Figure 8. (**A**) A 15-year-old boy with premature closure of the distal radial physis after a Salter–Harris type 2/4 fracture. Initially, the boy had an ulna minus wrist. (**B**) A closed radial physis, accompanied by an impending ulna plus. (**C**) Intraoperative radiographs during epiphysiodesis of the ulna. (**D**) Postoperative radiographs show a closed physis of both the radius and the ulna. Note that the ulna had been growing until the epiphysiodesis, leading to an ulna zero. (**E**) Radiographs after 1-year follow-up. Note the unaltered ulnar variance.

Scheider et al. [49] reported seven cases with the diagnosis of a painful ulnar positive variance in four individuals who underwent a temporary epiphysiodesis. This was done using a customized shortened 1.0 mm thick nonlocking two- or three-hole plate with 2.3 mm wide screw holes and screw lengths between 10 and 14 mm. The average age at implantation was 12.4 years and 14.7 years at explantation. The mean ulnar variance of +3.9 mm preoperatively was reduced to +0.1 mm, which led to satisfactory results in six out of seven cases. One case needed a secondary ulnar shortening osteotomy, which can be explained by having too little residual growth of the physis remaining at the beginning of therapy.

Campbell et al. [63] followed 31 wrists in 30 patients with premature distal radius physeal closure. Patients had an average age of 13.8 years [SD 1.6] at the time of surgery and were followed for a median of 163 days (ICR 101-419). The success rate of the procedure for the total group was 93.5%. However, because there were additional procedures performed at the time of epiphysiodesis in 67.7% of patients, including ulnar shortening osteotomies and distal radius osteotomies, the exact contribution of isolated epiphysiodeses could not be extracted from these results.

Waters et al. [36] followed thirty adolescents who underwent surgery after posttraumatic distal radial growth arrest at the average age of 14.8 years. Patients underwent ulnar epiphysiodesis in 11 cases and a combined radial and ulnar epiphysiodesis in three cases. Average ulnar variance among all patients improved from 4 mm positive (range −9 mm to +13 mm) before the procedure to 0 mm (range −6 mm to +4 mm) at the most recent follow-up radiographic evaluation ($p < 0.01$).

In a study by Farr et al. [40], performed on children with Madelung deformity, a series of 10 wrists out of 41 received an ulnar epiphysiodesis. Of these ten wrists, none of them required another intervention in correcting the deformity. The mean age of performed procedures was 13.4 ± 1.5 years. The authors postulate that ulnar epiphysiodesis may be considered in skeletally immature children older than 10 years of age with Madelung deformity.

6.4. Physeal Bar Resection

Resection of a physeal bar can be indicated in young children with a partial physeal closure, with the aim of restoring growth. The procedure for the removal of a physeal bar was first introduced by Langenskiöld [64] and is currently still being used in modified approaches. Success rates range from 15% to 38%, depending on the size and location of the bar [65]. Patients should have at least 50% of a healthy physeal surface in addition to 2 years of skeletal growth remaining [65,66]. Peterson et al. [67] classified the type and locations of a physeal bar into three subtypes: central, peripheral, and linear. A peripheral bar can be approached directly. Herein, excision of the overlying periosteum and removal of abnormal bone is carried out until the normal physeal cartilage is exposed completely. The remaining cavity is often interposed using fat or wax. Central and linear bars are more difficult to locate and visualize accurately. Preoperatively, the physeal bar must be identified correctly, preferably by computed tomography (CT) [65,68]. Fluoroscopy can be used to visualize the bar intraoperatively, but this may sometimes be difficult. In recent years, the use of a CT-guided navigation system helped identify the location, while an endoscope enables direct visualization of the physeal bar [66]. During follow-up, early magnetic resonance imaging (MRI) within four weeks has shown signs of incomplete resection [65].

6.5. Osteotomy

In severe deformities or in cases with too little growth remaining, a corrective osteotomy can be performed in addition to or without epiphysiodesis to correct the length and restore the anatomical alignment (Figure 9). In the forearm, performing a dome or wedge osteotomy allows for an accurate correction of alignment and restoration of the axial length, but it is an invasive procedure with a longer recovery time than epiphysiodesis. Patients with a cubitus varus may need a rotational correction in addition to angular correction. In these cases, either a dome osteotomy or a closed lateral wedge osteotomy is a reliable and powerful method to achieve correction [25]. In isolated growth arrest of the radius, an ulnar shortening osteotomy may be needed to correct the ulnar overgrowth [63].

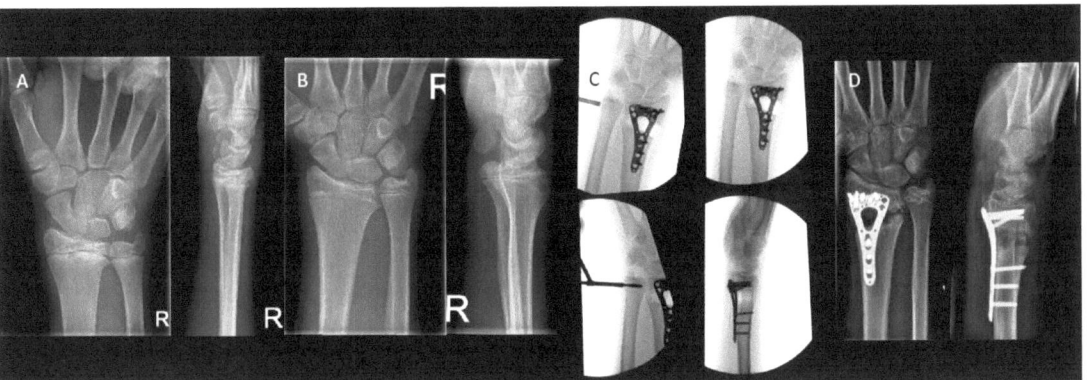

Figure 9. (**A**) A 17-year-old boy with a traumatic premature closure of the distal radial physis. (**B**) A closed radial physis, accompanied by an ulna plus. (**C**) Intraoperative radiographs during correction osteotomy of the radius combined with an epiphysiodesis of the ulna. (**D**) Radiographs six weeks postoperatively.

7. Timing of Intervention

The timing of epiphysiodesis is crucial when planning guided correction of a limb or bone-length inequality, e.g., in the forearm. Estimating limb-length inequality starts with an estimation of the length of the unaffected limb at skeletal maturity. This is followed by determining the growth rate of the affected limb compared to the rate of the unaffected limb. The difference in rates can then be used to estimate the final limb-length inequality [69]. It is important to realize that not all length discrepancies increase continuously over time. Shapiro et al. described five different patterns of growth in lower-extremity length discrepancies [70]. A Type-I proportionate progression pattern was seen in children with destroyed physes. In this type, the length discrepancy develops and increases continually with time at the same proportionate rate. This allows for the estimation of the ultimate limb length or growth remaining.

A multitude of methods to accurately determine final limb length or remaining growth have been developed over the course of the years. Anderson and Green first introduced growth-remaining charts using skeletal age [60]. This method was later simplified by the introduction of the Moseley straight-line graphs in which only skeletal maturity is used [61]. The Rotterdam straight-line graph can be seen as an improvement of the Moseley straight-line graphs by means of a further expansion of that database [71]. The White–Menelaus formula uses chronological age and is based on a simple calculation with the assumption of a fixed mean annual growth and the assumption of physeal closure at a specific age for boys and girls [72]. The Paley multiplier method (MM) also uses chronological age and is based on an age-based multiplier specific for each age to calculate the final limb growth and remaining growth [73].

Each method has its pitfalls and potential advantages, but none of them is universally accepted as the gold standard in determining the timing of epiphysiodesis. For the upper limb, only the Anderson and Green-based growth charts of Stahl et al. and the Paley multiplier have been developed [74,75]. Birch and Makarov compared different methods of limb length prediction and found skeletal age to be superior to chronological age for prediction [76,77]. Sanders et al. [69] compared both the MM and skeletal age measurements and found that chronological age was superior to skeletal age for predicting ultimate limb length in children prior to their adolescent growth spurt. In contrast, after the start of the growth spurt, predicting limb length using skeletal age proved superior. This observation is consistent with other studies [60,78].

This raises further questions as to why chronological age is a better predictor prior to the adolescent growth spurt but worse after it. The Paley multiplier was based on the assumption of a Shapiro type-I linear growth pattern that remains the same during maturity and the multipliers remaining the same regardless of the growth phase the child is in. Differences in accuracy between the MM and the other methods might be due to each method having its own way of taking the growth spurt into account. Sanders et al. suggested that using peak height velocity (PHV) was the best marker for maturity during the transition into adolescence [69]. Growth measurements can then easily be calculated using PHV-derived multipliers. These multipliers are currently made using skeletal age, which is closely related to PHV during adolescence.

Different methods of measuring skeletal maturity are currently used. Historically, the Greulich and Pyle atlas for hand bone age is the most widely known and used [79]. The Sauvegrain method assesses skeletal age from elbow radiographs based on a 27-point scoring system [80]. This method uses four ossification centers of the elbow: the lateral condyle, trochlea, olecranon apophysis, and proximal radial epiphysis as landmarks. The scores of these structures are summed, and a graph is then used to determine the skeletal age. In contrast to the GP atlas, this method allows for the assessment of skeletal age in 6-month intervals during the phase of accelerating growth velocity, which makes it markedly suitable for the period of growth spurt.

When compared to the Greulich and Pyle atlas, the Sauvegrain method has been proven to be a more accurate method for the assessment of skeletal age during puberty, with the addition of having a high inter- and intra-observer reliability [81,82]. Furthermore, it is shown that the Sauvegrain score is a reliable marker for measuring PHV in children [83]. It should therefore prove suitable for predicting PHV-derived multipliers used for a more accurate prediction of growth in children during their growth spurt.

8. Conclusions and Recommendations

Because of the ability of children to correct osseous deformities during longitudinal growth, often, the deformity is corrected naturally. Their frequent relation with joints, however, may potentially have harmful consequences if discovered late or left untreated. Therefore, early clinical evaluation is often helpful in giving a quick indication, followed by additional radiologic evaluation for a more concise measure of the deformity. Current methods of measuring humeral and radial alignment prove sufficient for children, regardless of their age. However, in measuring ulnar variance, the use of age-specific methods such as the Hafner method and the method of perpendiculars may additionally improve accuracy.

If surgical intervention is necessary, deformity correction by means of guided growth poses an elegant and low-invasive option. Surgical treatment options include (hemi-) epiphysiodesis, physeal bar resection, and osteotomy, as well as combinations of techniques. The preferred treatment option is dependent on the location of the deformity, involvement of the physis, presence of a physeal bar, and predicted length inequality at skeletal maturity.

An accurate estimation of the limb or bone length at skeletal maturity is crucial for the correct timing of intervention. To date, the Paley multiplier method based on chronological age remains the most accurate method for calculating final and remaining limb growth in the upper extremity. Multiple studies found that the calculation of growth using chronological age is superior prior to the growth spurt. Skeletal age is found to be more accurate during the growth spurt. These calculations are generally performed using peak-height velocity. The Sauvegrain method of skeletal age assessment using elbow radiographs proves to be a more simple and more reliable method than the current widespread method of assessment using hand radiographs by Greulich and Pyle. The Sauvegrain method also proves to be a reliable marker for measuring peak-height velocity in children.

For children prior to their growth spurt, the Paley multiplier method remains the most accurate and simple method. In the absence of other validated methods, the Paley method can additionally be used for predicting growth during the growth spurt. However, because the Sauvegrain method has been proven suitable for measuring the peak-height velocity, further research should be carried out on calculating and validating specific PHV-based multipliers. Furthermore, the Paley multiplier still needs validation in the upper extremity. When both validation studies have been performed, a subsequent algorithm can be developed using the MM prior to the growth spurt and PHV-based multipliers based on the Sauvegrain method during the growth spurt. This combines the current two best methods and allows for a more accurate calculation of limb growth in the upper extremity. Because growth is not a two-dimensional progress, deformities often do not conform to a single plane during further growth. Therefore, apart from calculating the projected upper limb growth, an accurate assessment of which direction the deformity grows in should be carried out. Therefore, more research is needed for a better assessment and growth prediction of osseous deformities in 3D.

Author Contributions: Conceptualization, M.F.S., C.J.A.v.B., J.W.C. and D.E.; methodology, M.F.S. and E.M.v.E.; investigation, M.F.S.; resources, M.F.S.; data curation, M.F.S.; writing—original draft preparation, M.F.S.; writing—review and editing, M.F.S., C.J.A.v.B., E.M.v.E., J.W.C. and D.E.; visualization, M.F.S.; supervision, C.J.A.v.B., J.W.C. and D.E.; project administration, M.F.S. All authors have read and agreed to the published version of the manuscript.

Funding: This research received no external funding.

Institutional Review Board Statement: Not applicable.

Informed Consent Statement: Informed consent was obtained from all subjects involved in the study.

Data Availability Statement: Not applicable.

Acknowledgments: The authors wish to thank Wichor Bramer from the Erasmus MC Medical Library for developing and updating the search strategies.

Conflicts of Interest: The authors declare no conflict of interest.

References

1. Gupta, P.; Gupta, V.; Patil, B.; Verma, V. Angular deformities of lower limb in children: Correction for whom, when and how? *J. Clin. Orthop. Trauma* **2020**, *11*, 196–201. [CrossRef] [PubMed]
2. Mehlman, C.; Araghi, A.; Roy, D. Hyphenated history: The Hueter-Volkmann law. *Am. J. Orthop.* **1997**, *26*, 798–800. [PubMed]
3. Teichtahl, A.J.; Wluka, A.E.; Wijethilake, P.; Wang, Y.; Ghasem-Zadeh, A.; Cicuttini, F.M. Wolff's law in action: A mechanism for early knee osteoarthritis. *Arthritis Res. Ther.* **2015**, *17*, 207. [CrossRef] [PubMed]
4. Armstrong, A.D.; MacDermid, J.C.; Chinchalkar, S.; Stevens, R.S.; King, G.J. Reliability of range-of-motion measurement in the elbow and forearm. *J. Shoulder Elbow Surg.* **1998**, *7*, 573–580. [CrossRef]
5. Amis, A.A.; Dowson, D.; Unsworth, A.; Miller, J.H.; Wright, V. An Examination of the Elbow Articulation with Particular Reference to Variation of the Carrying Angle. *Eng. Med.* **1977**, *6*, 76–80. [CrossRef]
6. Beals, R.K. The normal carrying angle of the elbow. A radiographic study of 422 patients. *Clin. Orthop. Relat. Res.* **1976**, *119*, 194–196. [CrossRef]
7. Keats, T.E.; Teeslink, R.; Diamond, A.E.; Williams, J.H. Normal axial relationships of the major joints. *Radiology* **1966**, *87*, 904–907. [CrossRef]
8. Morrey, B.F.; Chao, E.Y. Passive motion of the elbow joint. *J. Bone Joint Surg. Am.* **1976**, *58*, 501–508. [CrossRef]
9. Soucie, J.M.; Wang, C.; Forsyth, A.; Funk, S.; Denny, M.; Roach, K.E.; Boone, D. Range of motion measurements: Reference values and a database for comparison studies. *Haemophilia* **2011**, *17*, 500–507. [CrossRef]
10. Keenan, W.N.; Clegg, J. Variation of Baumann's angle with age, sex, and side: Implications for its use in radiological monitoring of supracondylar fracture of the humerus in children. *J. Pediatr. Orthop.* **1996**, *16*, 97–98. [CrossRef]
11. Williamson, D.M.; Coates, C.J.; Miller, R.K.; Cole, W.G. Normal characteristics of the Baumann (humerocapitellar) angle: An aid in assessment of supracondylar fractures. *J. Pediatr. Orthop.* **1992**, *12*, 636–639. [CrossRef]
12. Shank, C.F.; Wiater, B.P.; Pace, J.L.; Jinguji, T.M.; Schmale, G.A.; Bittner, R.C.; Bompadre, V.; Stults, J.; Krenger, W.F. The lateral capitellohumeral angle in normal children: Mean, variation, and reliability in comparison to Baumann's angle. *J. Pediatr. Orthop.* **2011**, *31*, 266–271. [CrossRef] [PubMed]

13. Dario, P.; Matteo, G.; Carolina, C.; Marco, G.; Cristina, D.; Daniele, F.; Ferretti, A. Is it really necessary to restore radial anatomic parameters after distal radius fractures? *Injury* **2014**, *45*, S21–S26. [PubMed]
14. Greenspan, A. *Orthopedic Radiology*; VCH Verlagsges Edition Medizin: Weinheim, Germany, 1990.
15. Hanel, D.P.; Jones, M.D.; Trumble, T.E. Wrist fractures. *Orthop. Clin. N. Am.* **2002**, *33*, 35–57. [CrossRef] [PubMed]
16. Wood, M.B.; Berquist, T.H. *The Hand and Wrist*; WB Saunders Co.: Philadelphia, PA, USA, 1985.
17. Kox, L.S.; Jens, S.; Lauf, K.; Smithuis, F.F.; van Rijn, R.R.; Maas, M. Well-founded practice or personal preference: A comparison of established techniques for measuring ulnar variance in healthy children and adolescents. *Eur. Radiol.* **2020**, *30*, 151–162. [CrossRef]
18. Cannata, G.; De Maio, F.; Mancini, F.; Ippolito, E. Physeal Fractures of the Distal Radius and Ulna: Long-Term Prognosis. *J. Orthop. Trauma* **2003**, *17*, 172–179. [CrossRef]
19. Gauger, E.M.; Casnovsky, L.L.; Gauger, E.J.; Bohn, D.C.; Van Heest, A.E. Acquired Upper Extremity Growth Arrest. *Orthopedics* **2017**, *40*, e95–e103. [CrossRef]
20. Eastwood, D.M.; de Gheldere, A.; Bijlsma, P. Physeal injuries in children. *Surgery* **2014**, *32*, 1–8.
21. Mizuta, T.; Benson, W.M.; Foster, B.K.; Morris, L.L. Statistical Analysis of the Incidence of Physeal Injuries. *J. Pediatr. Orthop.* **1987**, *7*, 518–523. [CrossRef]
22. Salter, R.B.; Harris, W.R. Epiphyseal plate injuries. In *Management of Pediatric Fractures*; Churchill Livingstone: New York, NY, USA, 1994; pp. 11–26.
23. Ogden, J.A. The evaluation and treatment of partial physeal arrest. *Jbjs* **1987**, *69*, 1297–1302. [CrossRef]
24. Ecklund, K.; Jaramillo, D. Patterns of Premature Physeal Arrest. *Am. J. Roentgenol.* **2002**, *178*, 967–972. [CrossRef] [PubMed]
25. Vaquero-Picado, A.; González-Morán, G.; Moraleda, L. Management of supracondylar fractures of the humerus in children. *EFORT Open Rev.* **2018**, *3*, 526–540. [CrossRef]
26. Gartland, J.J. Management of supracondylar fractures of the humerus in children. *Surg. Gynecol. Obstet.* **1959**, *109*, 145–154.
27. Abzug, J.M.; Herman, M.J. Management of Supracondylar Humerus Fractures in Children: Current Concepts. *JAAOS J. Am. Acad. Orthop. Surgeons* **2012**, *20*, 69–77. [CrossRef]
28. de Gheldere, A.; Bellan, D. Outcome of Gartland type II and type III supracondylar fractures treated by Blount's technique. *Indian J. Orthop.* **2010**, *44*, 89–94. [CrossRef] [PubMed]
29. Apoorva Khajuria, V.T. *Radial Neck Fracture Repair in a Child*; StatPearls Publishing: Treasure Island, FL, USA, 2022.
30. Kumar, S.; Mishra, A.; Odak, S.; Dwyer, J. Treatment principles, prognostic factors and controversies in radial neck fractures in children: A systematic review. *J. Clin. Orthop. Trauma* **2020**, *11*, S456–S463. [CrossRef]
31. Sachar, K.; Mih, A.D. Congenital radial head dislocations. *Hand Clin.* **1998**, *14*, 39–47. [CrossRef]
32. Langenberg, L.C.; Beumer, A.; The, B.; Koenraadt, K.; Eygendaal, D. Surgical treatment of chronic anterior radial head dislocations in missed Monteggia lesions in children: A rationale for treatment and pearls and pitfalls of surgery. *Shoulder Elb.* **2020**, *12*, 422–431. [CrossRef]
33. Bley, L.; Seitz, W.H. Injuries about the distal ulna in children. *Hand Clin.* **1998**, *14*, 231–237. [CrossRef]
34. Lee, B.S.; Esterhai, J.L., Jr.; Das, M. Fracture of the Distal Radial Epiphysis: Characteristics and Surgical Treatment of Premature, Post-traumatic Epiphyseal Closure. *Clin. Orthop. Relat. Res.* **1984**, *185*, 90–96. [CrossRef]
35. Samora, J.B. Distal Radius Physeal Bar and Ulnar Overgrowth: Indications for Treatment. *J. Pediatr. Orthop.* **2021**, *41*, S6–S13. [CrossRef]
36. Waters, P.M.; Bae, D.S.; Montgomery, K.D. Surgical Management of Posttraumatic Distal Radial Growth Arrest in Adolescents. *J. Pediatr. Orthop.* **2002**, *22*, 717–724. [CrossRef]
37. DiFiori, J.P.; Puffer, J.C.; Aish, B.; Dorey, F. Wrist pain, distal radial physeal injury, and ulnar variance in young gymnasts: Does a relationship exist? *Am. J. Sports Med.* **2002**, *30*, 879–885. [CrossRef]
38. Roy, S.; Caine, D.; Singer, K.M. Stress changes of the distal radial epiphysis in young gymnasts. A report of twenty-one cases and a review of the literature. *Am. J. Sports Med.* **1985**, *13*, 301–308. [CrossRef]
39. Caine, D.; Roy, S.; Singer, K.M.; Broekhoff, J. Stress changes of the distal radial growth plate. A radiographic survey and review of the literature. *Am. J. Sports Med.* **1992**, *20*, 290–298. [CrossRef]
40. Farr, S.; Kalish, L.A.; Bae, D.S.; Waters, P.M. Radiographic Criteria for Undergoing an Ulnar Shortening Osteotomy in Madelung Deformity: A Long-term Experience From a Single Institution. *J. Pediatr. Orthop.* **2016**, *36*, 310–315. [CrossRef]
41. Knutsen, E.J.; Goldfarb, C.A. Madelung's Deformity. *Hand* **2014**, *9*, 289–291. [CrossRef]
42. Holme, T.J.; Karbowiak, M.; Arnander, M.; Gelfer, Y. Paediatric olecranon fractures: A systematic review. *EFORT Open Rev.* **2020**, *5*, 280–288. [CrossRef]
43. Golz, R.J.; Grogan, D.P.; Greene, T.L.; Belsole, R.J.; Ogden, J.A. Distal Ulnar Physeal Injury. *J. Pediatr. Orthop.* **1991**, *11*, 318–326. [CrossRef]
44. Yasutomi, T.; Nakatsuchi, Y.; Koike, H.; Uchiyama, S. Mechanism of limitation of pronation/supination of the forearm in geometric models of deformities of the forearm bones. *Clin. Biomech.* **2002**, *17*, 456–463. [CrossRef]
45. Mania, S.; Zindel, C.; Götschi, T.; Carrillo, F.; Fürnstahl, P.; Schweizer, A. Malunion deformity of the forearm: Three-dimensional length variation of interosseous membrane and bone collision. *J. Orthop. Res.* **2022**, 1–10. [CrossRef] [PubMed]
46. Abe, S.; Murase, T.; Oka, K.; Shigi, A.; Tanaka, H.; Yoshikawa, H. In Vivo Three-Dimensional Analysis of Malunited Forearm Diaphyseal Fractures with Forearm Rotational Restriction. *J. Bone Joint Surg. Am.* **2018**, *100*, e113. [CrossRef] [PubMed]

47. Shaw, N.; Erickson, C.; Bryant, S.J.; Ferguson, V.L.; Krebs, M.D.; Hadley-Miller, N.; Payne, K.A. Regenerative Medicine Approaches for the Treatment of Pediatric Physeal Injuries. *Tissue Eng. Part B Rev.* **2018**, *24*, 85–97. [CrossRef] [PubMed]
48. Larsen, M.C.; Bohm, K.C.; Rizkala, A.R.; Ward, C.M. Outcomes of Nonoperative Treatment of Salter-Harris II Distal Radius Fractures:A Systematic Review. *Hand* **2016**, *11*, 29–35. [CrossRef] [PubMed]
49. Scheider, P.; Ganger, R.; Farr, S. Temporary epiphysiodesis in adolescent patients with ulnocarpal impaction syndrome: A preliminary case series of seven wrists. *J. Pediatr. Orthop. B* **2021**, *30*, 601–604. [CrossRef]
50. Danino, B.; Rödl, R.; Herzenberg, J.E.; Shabtai, L.; Grill, F.; Narayanan, U.; Segev, E.; Wientroub, S. Growth modulation in idiopathic angular knee deformities: Is it predictable? *J. Child Orthop.* **2019**, *13*, 318–323. [CrossRef]
51. Kumar, S.; Sonanis, S.V. Growth modulation for coronal deformity correction by using Eight Plates-Systematic review. *J. Orthop.* **2018**, *15*, 168–172. [CrossRef]
52. Choi, K.J.; Lee, S.; Park, M.S.; Sung, K.H. Rebound phenomenon and its risk factors after hemiepiphysiodesis using tension band plate in children with coronal angular deformity. *BMC Musculoskelet. Disord.* **2022**, *23*, 339. [CrossRef]
53. Leveille, L.A.; Razi, O.; Johnston, C.E. Rebound Deformity After Growth Modulation in Patients With Coronal Plane Angular Deformities About the Knee: Who Gets It and How Much? *J. Pediatr. Orthop.* **2019**, *39*, 353–358. [CrossRef]
54. Ramazanov, R.; Ozdemir, E.; Yilmaz, G.; Caglar, O.; Cemalettin Aksoy, M. Rebound phenomenon after hemiepiphysiodesis: Determination of risk factors after tension band plate removal in coronal plane deformities of lower extremities. *J. Pediatr. Orthop. B* **2021**, *30*, 52–58. [CrossRef]
55. Zajonz, D.; Schumann, E.; Wojan, M.; Kübler, F.B.; Josten, C.; Bühligen, U.; Heyde, C.E. Treatment of genu valgum in children by means of temporary hemiepiphysiodesis using eight-plates: Short-term findings. *BMC Musculoskelet. Disord.* **2017**, *18*, 456. [CrossRef] [PubMed]
56. Park, H.; Park, M.; Kim, S.M.; Kim, H.W.; Lee, D.H. Hemiepiphysiodesis for Idiopathic Genu Valgum: Percutaneous Transphyseal Screw Versus Tension-band Plate. *J. Pediatr. Orthop.* **2018**, *38*, 325–330. [CrossRef] [PubMed]
57. Shapiro, G.; Adato, T.; Paz, S.; Shrabaty, T.; Ron, L.; Simanovsky, N.; Zaidman, M.; Goldman, V. Hemiepiphysiodesis for coronal angular knee deformities: Tension-band plate versus percutaneous transphyseal screw. *Arch. Orthop. Trauma Surg.* **2022**, *142*, 105–113. [CrossRef] [PubMed]
58. Soldado, F.; Diaz-Gallardo, P.; Cherqaoui, A.; Nguyen, T.-Q.; Romero-Larrauri, P.; Knorr, J. Unsuccessful mid-term results for distal humeral hemiepiphysiodesis to treat cubitus varus deformity in young children. *J. Pediatr. Orthop. B* **2022**, *31*, 431–433. [CrossRef] [PubMed]
59. Dai, Z.Z.; Liang, Z.P.; Li, H.; Ding, J.; Wu, Z.K.; Zhang, Z.M.; Li, H. Temporary hemiepiphysiodesis using an eight-plate implant for coronal angular deformity around the knee in children aged less than 10 years: Efficacy, complications, occurrence of rebound and risk factors. *BMC Musculoskelet. Disord.* **2021**, *22*, 53. [CrossRef]
60. Anderson, M.; Green, W.T.; Messner, M.B. Growth and predictions of growth in the lower extremities. *J. Bone Joint Surg. Am.* **1963**, *45*, 1–14. [CrossRef]
61. Moseley, C.F. A straight-line graph for leg-length discrepancies. *J. Bone Joint Surg. Am.* **1977**, *59*, 174–179. [CrossRef]
62. Tupman, G.S. A study of bone growth in normal children and its relationship to skeletal maturation. *J. Bone Joint Surg. Br.* **1962**, *44*, 42–67. [CrossRef]
63. Campbell, T.; Faulk, L.W.; Vossler, K.; Goodrich, E.; Lalka, A.; Sibbel, S.E.; Sinclair, M.K. Ulnar Epiphysiodesis: Success of the Index Procedure. *J. Pediatr. Orthop.* **2022**, *42*, 158–161. [CrossRef]
64. Langenskiöld, A. Traumatic Premature Closure of the Distal Tibial Epiphyseal Plate. *Acta Orthop. Scand.* **1967**, *38*, 520–531. [CrossRef]
65. Hasler, C.C.; Foster, B.K. Secondary tethers after physeal bar resection: A common source of failure? *Clin. Orthop. Relat. Res.* **2002**, *405*, 242–249. [CrossRef] [PubMed]
66. Marsh, J.S.; Polzhofer, G.K. Arthroscopically Assisted Central Physeal Bar Resection. *J. Pediatr. Orthop.* **2006**, *26*, 255–259. [CrossRef] [PubMed]
67. Peterson, H.A. Partial Growth Plate Arrest and Its Treatment. *J. Pediatr. Orthop.* **1984**, *4*, 246–258. [CrossRef] [PubMed]
68. Wang, D.C.; Deeney, V.; Roach, J.W.; Shah, A.J. Imaging of physeal bars in children. *Pediatr. Radiol.* **2015**, *45*, 1403–1412. [CrossRef]
69. Sanders, J.O.; Howell, J.; Qiu, X. Comparison of the Paley Method Using Chronological Age with Use of Skeletal Maturity for Predicting Mature Limb Length in Children. *Jbjs* **2011**, *93*, 1051–1056. [CrossRef]
70. Shapiro, F. Developmental patterns in lower-extremity length discrepancies. *J. Bone Joint Surg. Am.* **1982**, *64*, 639–651. [CrossRef]
71. Beumer, A.; Lampe, H.I.H.; Swierstra, B.A.; Diepstraten, A.F.M.; Mulder, P.G.H. The straight line graph in limb length inequality a new design based on 182 Dutch children. *Acta Orthop. Scand.* **1997**, *68*, 355–360. [CrossRef]
72. Menelaus, M.B. Correction of leg length discrepancy by epiphysial arrest. *J. Bone Joint Surg. Br.* **1966**, *48*, 336–339. [CrossRef]
73. Paley, D.; Bhave, A.; Herzenberg, J.E.; Bowen, J.R. Multiplier Method for Predicting Limb-Length Discrepancy. *Jbjs* **2000**, *82*, 1432. [CrossRef]
74. Paley, D.; Gelman, A.; Shualy, M.B.; Herzenberg, J.E. Multiplier method for limb-length prediction in the upper extremity. *J. Hand Surg. Am.* **2008**, *33*, 385–391. [CrossRef]
75. Stahl, E.J.; Karpman, R. Normal growth and growth predictions in the upper extremity. *J. Hand Surg. Am.* **1986**, *11*, 593–596.

76. Birch, J.G.; Makarov, M.A.; Jackson, T.J.; Jo, C.-H. Comparison of Anderson-Green Growth-Remaining Graphs and White-Menelaus Predictions of Growth Remaining in the Distal Femoral and Proximal Tibial Physes. *Jbjs* **2019**, *101*, 1016–1022. [CrossRef] [PubMed]
77. Birch, J.G.; Makarov, M.R.; Sanders, J.O.; Podeszwa, D.A.; Honcharuk, E.M.; Esparza, M.; Tran, E.Y.; Joo, C.H.; Rodgers, J.A. Lower-Extremity Segment-Length Prediction Accuracy of the Sanders Multiplier, Paley Multiplier, and White-Menelaus Formula. *J. Bone Joint Surg. Am.* **2021**, *103*, 1713–1717. [CrossRef]
78. Kasser, J.R.; Jenkins, R. Accuracy of leg length prediction in children younger than 10 years of age. *Clin. Orthop. Relat. Res.* **1997**, 9–13. [CrossRef]
79. Greulich, W.W. *Radiograph Atlas of Skeletal Development of the Hand and Wrist*, 2nd ed.; Stanford University Press: Stanford, CA, USA, 1959.
80. Sauvegrain, J.; Nahum, H.; Carle, F. Bone maturation. Importance of the determination of the bone age. Methods of evaluation. *Ann. Radiol.* **1962**, *5*, 535–541. [PubMed]
81. Breen, A.B.; Steen, H.; Pripp, A.; Gunderson, R.; Mentzoni, H.K.S.; Merckoll, E.; Zaidi, W.; Lambert, M.; Hvid, I.; Horn, J. A comparison of 3 different methods for assessment of skeletal age when treating leg-length discrepancies: An inter- and intra-observer study. *Acta Orthop.* **2022**, *93*, 222–228. [CrossRef] [PubMed]
82. Jang, W.Y.; Ahn, K.S.; Oh, S.; Lee, J.E.; Choi, J.; Kang, C.H.; Kang, W.E.; Hong, S.-J.; Shim, E.; Kim, B.H.; et al. Difference between bone age at the hand and elbow at the onset of puberty. *Medicine* **2022**, *101*, e28516. [CrossRef]
83. Hans, S.D.; Sanders, J.O.; Cooperman, D.R. Using the Sauvegrain method to predict peak height velocity in boys and girls. *J. Pediatr. Orthop.* **2008**, *28*, 836–839.

Disclaimer/Publisher's Note: The statements, opinions and data contained in all publications are solely those of the individual author(s) and contributor(s) and not of MDPI and/or the editor(s). MDPI and/or the editor(s) disclaim responsibility for any injury to people or property resulting from any ideas, methods, instructions or products referred to in the content.

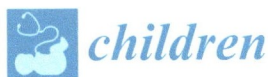

Article

Accuracy of 3D Corrective Osteotomy for Pediatric Malunited Both-Bone Forearm Fractures

Kasper Roth [1], Eline van Es [1], Gerald Kraan [2], Denise Eygendaal [1], Joost Colaris [1] and Filip Stockmans [3,*]

1. Department of Orthopedics and Sports Medicine, Erasmus University Medical Centre, Dr. Molewaterplein 40, 3015 GD Rotterdam, The Netherlands
2. Department of Orthopedics, Reinier HAGA Orthopedic Centre, Toneellaan 2, 2725 NA Zoetermeer, The Netherlands
3. Department of Development and Regeneration, Faculty of Medicine, University of Leuven Campus Kortrijk, Etienne Sabbelaan 53, 8500 Kortrijk, Belgium
* Correspondence: filip.stockmans@kuleuven.be

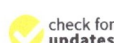

Citation: Roth, K.; van Es, E.; Kraan, G.; Eygendaal, D.; Colaris, J.; Stockmans, F. Accuracy of 3D Corrective Osteotomy for Pediatric Malunited Both-Bone Forearm Fractures. *Children* 2023, 10, 21. https://doi.org/10.3390/children10010021

Academic Editor: Johannes Mayr

Received: 30 November 2022
Revised: 8 December 2022
Accepted: 20 December 2022
Published: 23 December 2022

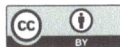

Copyright: © 2022 by the authors. Licensee MDPI, Basel, Switzerland. This article is an open access article distributed under the terms and conditions of the Creative Commons Attribution (CC BY) license (https:// creativecommons.org/licenses/by/ 4.0/).

Abstract: Re-displacement of a pediatric diaphyseal forearm fracture can lead to a malunion with symptomatic impairment in forearm rotation, which may require a corrective osteotomy. Corrective osteotomy with two-dimensional (2D) radiographic planning for malunited pediatric forearm fractures can be a complex procedure due to multiplanar deformities. Three-dimensional (3D) corrective osteotomy can aid the surgeon in planning and obtaining a more accurate correction and better forearm rotation. This prospective study aimed to assess the accuracy of correction after 3D corrective osteotomy for pediatric forearm malunion and if anatomic correction influences the functional outcome. Our primary outcome measures were the residual maximum deformity angle (MDA) and malrotation after 3D corrective osteotomy. Post-operative MDA > 5° or residual malrotation > 15° were defined as non-anatomic corrections. Our secondary outcome measure was the gain in pro-supination. Between 2016–2018, fifteen patients underwent 3D corrective osteotomies for pediatric malunited diaphyseal both-bone fractures. Three-dimensional corrective osteotomies provided anatomic correction in 10 out of 15 patients. Anatomic corrections resulted in a greater gain in pro-supination than non-anatomic corrections: 70° versus 46° (p = 0.04, ANOVA). Residual malrotation of the radius was associated with inferior gain in pro-supination (p = 0.03, multi-variate linear regression). Three-dimensional corrective osteotomy for pediatric forearm malunion reliably provided an accurate correction, which led to a close-to-normal forearm rotation. Non-anatomic correction, especially residual malrotation of the radius, leads to inferior functional outcomes.

Keywords: corrective osteotomy; three-dimensional; malunion; fracture; forearm; radius; pediatric

1. Introduction

In midshaft forearm fractures, growth will not remodel angular deformity as it does in distal fractures [1]. Impairment in forearm rotation is a critical problem associated with malunions of the forearm bones [2]. Malunited diaphyseal forearm fractures in children leading to a severe restriction in pro-supination may require corrective osteotomies [3]. A conventional corrective osteotomy can be technically demanding due to the multiplanar deformity of both forearm bones [4]. In a series by Miyake et al., one patient even had a rotational malunion of the radius of 136°, which is difficult to assess precisely using two-dimensional (2D) radiographic planning. Recent advancements in three-dimensional (3D) planning and 3D printing of patient-specific instruments (PSIs) can aid the surgeon in achieving a more accurate correction. Non-anatomic correction of the bony anatomy in malunions, especially of the upper extremity, may lead to inferior functional outcomes. Several authors have stated anatomically accurate correction during 3D corrective osteotomy is highly desirable to achieve a good outcome [5,6]. Few studies have tested this assumption nor have examined the effectiveness of 3D corrective osteotomy for pediatric malunited forearm fractures concerning the radiographic accuracy of the correction [3,7]. This prospective study aimed to assess the accuracy of correction after 3D corrective osteotomy for pediatric forearm malunion and if anatomic correction influences the functional outcome.

2. Materials and Methods

This study represents an additional analysis of the radiographic outcomes of a prospective cohort of patients whose clinical outcomes have been published previously [8]. Patients were eligible for enrollment if they met the following inclusion criteria: having a symptomatic forearm malunion after a diaphyseal both-bone forearm fracture sustained during childhood (<18 years), resulting in a limitation in pro-supination (pronation or supination of <50°), with unsatisfactory improvement after physiotherapy and a minimum age of 10 years at 3D corrective osteotomy. In addition, patients were excluded if they had an osseous deformity of the contralateral forearm. The pre-operative planning, surgical technique, and post-operative management of our 3D corrective osteotomies are described in our previous publication [8]. Planning of 3D corrective osteotomy and 3D printing of PSIs were performed at Materialise N.V., Leuven, Belgium in collaboration with our surgeons. An example of pre- and post-operative radiographs is provided in Figure 1.

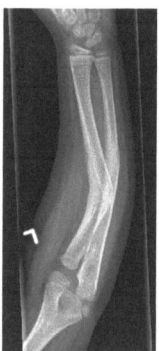 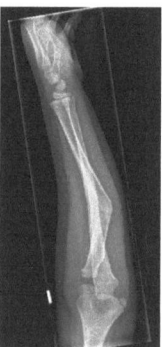 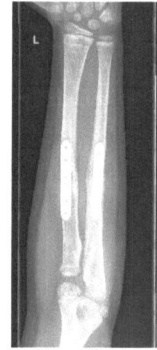 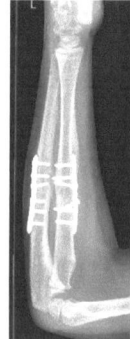

Figure 1. Example of pre- and post-operative radiographs.

2.1. Outcome Measures

Our primary outcome measure was the radiographic accuracy of the achieved correction after 3D corrective osteotomy. To assess the accuracy of correction, we compared the 3D pre-operative plan with the one-year post-operative computed tomography (CT). The residual maximum deformity angle (MDA) and malrotation after 3D corrective osteotomy were used to describe the accuracy of correction. The MDA is calculated by combining the angular deformity on both the coronal and sagittal plane derived from CT, as described by Nagy et al., illustrated in Figure 2 [3,9]. Similar to the study by Byrne et al., we assessed how often angular deformities could be corrected to within 5° of contralateral by 3D corrective osteotomy. Residual MDA $\geq 5°$ was defined as a non-anatomic correction. Unlike for the lower extremity, which most authors recommend to correct a torsional deformity of $\geq 15°$ [10], there are still no uniform cut-off values as to when a correction is indicated in post-traumatic rotational deformity of the forearm [11]. In the current study, malrotation of the radius or ulna $\geq 15°$ was defined as a non-anatomic correction.

Our secondary outcome measures were: functional gain in pro-supination and patient-reported outcome measures (PROMs): the QuickDASH questionnaire (11 items, range 0–100), numerical rating scale (NRS) scores for pain and appearance (range 0–10), and maximal grip strength using a JAMAR hand dynamometer (J.A. Preston Corporation, New York, NY, USA). Pro-supination was measured with a universal goniometer utilizing the method of the American Society of Hand Therapists [12]. Functional outcome was measured by two authors independently (E.E. and J.C.).

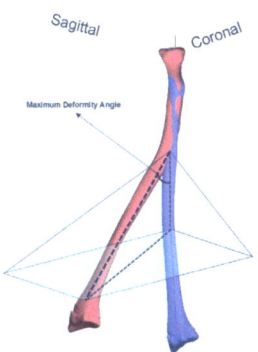

Figure 2. The maximal deformity angle (MDA) was calculated by combining the measurements of angular deformity in the coronal and sagittal plane according to the following formula:

$$MDA = \sqrt{tan^2(Coronal) + tan^2(Sagittal)}$$

2.2. 3D Radiographic Assessment

Radiographic evaluation of the accuracy of the performed correction was performed by analyzing the 3D models of the pre- and post-operative forearm bones according to the following steps: using Mimics software (Mimics Research 25.0), segmentation is performed using a threshold-connected region growing algorithm that collects voxels that belong to the affected bone. Then, the forearm bones are extracted as separate 3D objects.

Next, 3-Matic software (3-Matic Research 17.0) was used to compare 3D models of the pre-operative situation, planned correction, and post-operative result. First, analytic cylinders of the proximal and distal shafts of the radius and ulna are created to establish the axis of the proximal and distal parts of both bones in all three situations. Next, using a closest fit algorithm, the proximal ends of the radius and ulna of all three situations are aligned proximally. The axes of the proximal shaft proximal to the planned correction were used for the coordinate system, as this axis was alike in all three situations. Finally, the deviation between the distal segments in all three situations was measured to assess the degree of angular and rotational malalignment in the coronal, sagittal, and axial planes. The coordinate system of the radius was established as described by the International Society of Biomechanics (ISB) 2005 recommendations [13]. The maximum deformity angle (MDA) was calculated by combining the measurements of angular deformity in the coronal and sagittal planes, according to the Pythagorean theorem. MDA was calculated from the coronal and sagittal planes derived from CT instead of plain radiographs to increase the accuracy of the measurement because the reliability of measurements from 2D images is hampered by over-projection [14]. Two authors measured radiographic outcomes independently (K.R. and E.E). Mean values of both assessors are presented.

2.3. Statistical Analysis

p-values < 0.05 were considered statistically significant. The intraclass correlation coefficient (ICC) was measured to assess the inter-observer reliability of the radiographic measurements. One-way analysis of variance (ANOVA) was performed to study the relationship between an anatomic correction and functional outcomes (gain in pro-supination and PROMs). Subsequently, multi-variate linear regression analysis was performed to investigate the relationship between the accuracy of correction (residual MDA and malrotation of radius and ulna) and gain in pro-supination, both on a continuous scale.

3. Results

Between October 2016 and July 2018, 3D corrective osteotomies of both the radius and ulna were performed in fifteen patients due to pediatric malunited both-bone diaphyseal forearm fractures. Patients had a mean age at trauma of 9.6 years, a mean time until 3D corrective osteotomy of 5.9 years, and a mean age at osteotomy of 15.5 years. There was a mean operating time of 138 min (SD 35) for the 3D corrective osteotomies of the radius and ulna. In addition, four out of fifteen patients underwent an additional soft-tissue release. There were three minor complications: ulnar plate removal, delayed union, and transient neuropraxia of the superficial radial nerve. There were three minor complications: ulnar plate removal, delayed union, and transient neuropraxia of the superficial radial nerve.

3.1. Primary Outcomes

The pre- and post-operative malalignments of the radius and ulna are provided in Table 1. Anatomic correction was achieved in 10 out of 15 patients (25 out of 30 forearm bones) after 3D corrective osteotomy. Examples of an anatomic and a non-anatomic correction of the radius are supplied in Figures 3 and 4 (Case 1 and 4). Likewise, an example of residual malrotation of the radius is provided in Figure 5 (Case 13).

Table 1. Radiographic outcomes: pre- and post-operative malalignment (°).

		Radius							Ulna						
		Pre-Operative			Final Follow-Up					Pre-Operative			Final Follow-Up			
Pt	Cor	Sag	MDA	Ax	Cor	Sag	MDA	RM	Cor	Sag	MDA	Ax	Cor	Sag	MDA	RM
1	3	14	14	−6	0	0	0	6	−5	7	32	−5	5	7	−12
2	9	22	23	24	0	0	1	−2	16	1	16	−1	1	0	1	15
3	−4	8	8	−11	−3	0	3	−9	8	−6	11	−4	1	0	1	−16
4	0	17	17	−26	11	7	13	−6	8	−20	21	11	1	−1	2	2
5	−2	22	23	−8	−1	0	1	14	9	−7	11	0	0	0	0	4
6	7	27	27	−31	0	−3	3	−3	8	−18	19	6	1	0	1	3
7	−11	0	11	−13	1	−1	1	−4	−7	19	20	3	0	1	1	−5
8	5	18	19	18	−1	−1	1	−8	11	2	11	−1	−1	0	1	3
9	0	16	16	1	−1	−1	2	10	6	−5	8	−7	0	−1	1	0
10	17	24	29	−4	0	−2	2	−5	1	−13	13	13	−1	−1	2	9
11	6	19	20	−12	3	3	5	0	3	−15	15	−4	0	0	0	0
12	1	11	11	49	−1	0	1	−1	5	−3	6	−3	−1	−4	4	5
13	9	4	10	15	−2	4	5	17	7	2	7	−20	0	2	2	0
14	−2	6	6	−5	1	1	1	−10	13	−1	13	−7	0	1	1	−1
15	−7	3	7	−17	2	0	2	−3	4	3	5	5	−2	−1	3	−6
Mean	8.1	14.0	16.1	15.9	1.8	1.7	2.6	6.6	7.4	8.0	12.2	7.7	1.0	1.2	1.7	5.5
SD	9.4	8.4	7.2	12.4	2.7	2.0	3.1	4.8	3.7	6.9	5.2	8.7	1.2	1.4	1.7	5.3

Cor = coronal plane; Sag = sagittal plane; Ax = axial plane. MDA = maximum deformity angle; RM = residual malrotation. Dorsal angulation = positive; volar = negative; radial = positive; ulnar = negative; axial malrotation in pronation = positive; axial malrotation in supination = negative. Means are calculated based on absolute values.

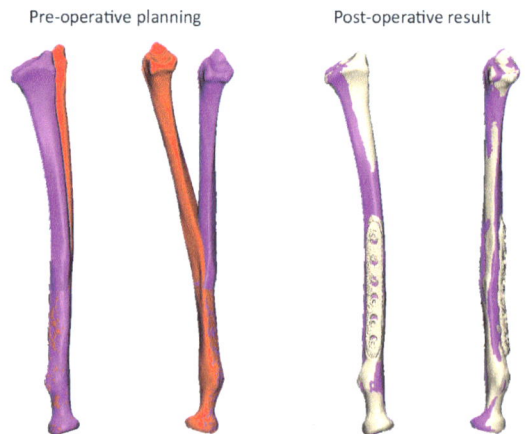

Red = Pre-operative situation; Purple = Planned correction, White = Achieved correction

Figure 3. Example of an anatomic correction of the radius.

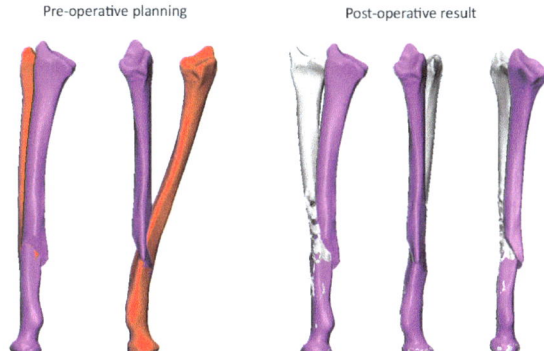

Residual Malalignment of 11° radially and 7° dorsally: a Maximum Deformity Angle (MDA) of 13°

Figure 4. Example of a non-anatomic correction of the radius.

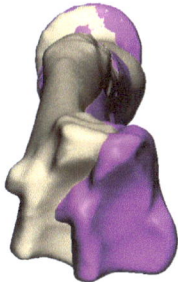

Residual rotational deformity of the radius of 17°

Figure 5. Example of residual malrotation of the radius.

3.2. Is Anatomic Correction Associated with Greater Functional Outcomes?

Three dimensional corrective osteotomy provided a mean gain in pro-supination from 67° (44% of contralateral) pre-operatively to 128° (85% of contralateral), thus a mean total gain of 62°. The results of ANOVA are presented in Table 2. ANOVA revealed ten patients who achieved anatomic correction after 3D corrective osteotomies had significantly greater gains in pro-supination than those with non-anatomic corrections: 70° (95% CI: 55–85°) versus 46° (95% CI: 28–64°). Patient-reported outcome measures or grip strength measurements between anatomic and non-anatomic corrections showed no significant differences. Multi-variate linear regression analysis revealed residual malrotation of the radius was associated with inferior pro-supination ($p = 0.026$); the model is provided in Table 3.

Table 2. ANOVA.

	Anatomic Correction (n = 10)	Non-Anatomic Correction (n = 5)	$p =$
Pre-op pro-supination	67° (53–80°)	66° (36–97°)	0.97
Pro-supination at FU	136° (125–148°)	112° (95–129°)	0.01
Gain in pro-supination	70° (55–85°)	46° (28–85°)	0.04
Pre-op QUICKDASH	22 (13–30)	31 (19–43)	0.16
QUICKDASH at FU	13 (10–16)	17 (14–20)	0.07
Δ QUICKDASH	8 (0–17)	14 (2–26)	0.38
NRS pain score	1.1 (−0.5–2.7)	3.0 (−0.4–6.4)	0.18
NRS cosmetics	2.3 (0.5–4.2)	4.6 (1.3–8.0)	0.13
Grip strength (%)	94 (88–98)	90 (78–102)	0.41

Confidence interval of 95% presented as: (95% CI); FU: follow-up; NRS: numeric rating scale.

Table 3. Multi-variate linear regression.

Model	Unstandardized Coefficients		
	B	Std. Error	Significance
(Constant)	79.0	8.4	<0.001
Residual malrotation Radius	−2.6	1.1	0.026

Dependent variable: gain in pro-supination.

In our radiographic assessment, the interrater reproducibility showed intra-class correlations of 0.996 (95% CI: 0.991–0.998) and 0.992 (0.984–0.996) for measurement of the MDA of the radius and ulna; 0.990 (0.979–0.995) and 0.971 (0.938–0.986) for rotational assessment of the radius and ulna.

4. Discussion

This prospective study aimed to assess the accuracy of correction after 3D corrective osteotomy for pediatric forearm malunion and if anatomic correction influences the functional outcome. In this study, 3D-planned corrective osteotomies for pediatric malunited both-bone forearm fractures resulted in anatomic corrections in 10 out of 15 patients (25 out of 30 operated forearm bones). Patients with anatomic corrections had statistically significantly greater gains in pro-supination after 3D corrective osteotomies than non-anatomic corrections (70° versus 46°). Residual malrotation of the radius after 3D corrective osteotomy was associated with an inferior gain in forearm rotation.

Understanding the complex 3D deformities of both forearm bones in a malunited forearm fracture remains challenging. Therefore, a 3D corrective osteotomy is a promising technique. Recurrent patterns in forearm malunion are often seen. The supinator, pronator teres, and pronator quadratus muscles exert a pulling force upon fracture fragments, which can lead to angular deformity, malrotation, or narrowing of the interosseous space. In fractures located proximal to the pronator teres insertion, the proximal fragment supinates and flexes due to unopposed forces of the supinator and biceps brachii, whereas the distal fragment pronates due to the pronator quadratus and pronator teres. In contrast, in fractures located distal to the pronator teres insertion, the proximal fragment will not rotate as the supinator opposes the forces of the pronator teres and biceps brachii. The distal fragment will pronate and deviate towards the ulna due to the pronator quadratus [4]. Angular deformities of the radius and ulna lead to bony impingement or increased interosseous membrane (IOM) tension, which causes impairment in forearm rotation [15]. In a cadaveric study, a dorsal angular deformity of 20° caused a limitation in pronation. Correspondingly, a volar angular deformity of 20° led to supination limitation. Lastly, angular deformity narrowing the interosseous space limited both pro- and supination [16]. In 2018, Abe et al. stated a pronation limitation was found if there was bony impingement due to dorsal angulation of the radius (>8°) because the interosseous space is encroached during pronation [17]. A supination limitation was found if there was a tightness of the transverse central band (CB) due to valgus deformity of the ulna (>6°), which increases the interosseous space during supination.

Unfortunately, there is no published literature with CT-based accuracy assessment of conventional 2D planned corrective osteotomies with which to compare.

In 2008, Murase and colleagues reported the accuracy of 3D corrective osteotomy for malunited forearm fractures in 10 patients. The mean angle of deformity improved from 16° pre-operatively to 1° after surgery. The mean pro-supination improved from 79° to 155° post-operatively.

In 2012, Miyake et al. published the outcomes of 3D corrective osteotomies for malunited forearm fractures in 20 patients. The average radiographic deformity improved from 21° pre-operatively to 1° post-operatively. In addition, their forearm motion improved from 76° pre-operatively to 152° post-operatively.

In 2013, Kataoka et al. published the results of 3D corrective osteotomies with PSIs for malunited forearm fractures in four patients. They used standard plates, which were pre-bent to fit around 3D-printed, real-sized plastic bone models of the radius and ulna. They achieved an accuracy of correction with a mean error in all directions of <2° for both the radius and the ulna. Mean errors were greater in growing children, as longitudinal forearm growth was not considered. They achieved a mean gain in pro-supination from 106° pre-operatively to 158° post-operatively [18].

In 2015, Bauer et al. performed 19 3D corrective osteotomies due to forearm deformity in children of which 15 were post-traumatic. In their study, maximum deformity angulation of the radius and ulna improved from 23° and 23° to 9° and 8°, respectively. Ten patients were operated on due to limited pro-supination, and a gain in pro-supination was seen from 85° to 138°.

In 2017, Byrne et al. published the outcomes of five patients who underwent 3D corrective osteotomies for malunited diaphyseal forearm fractures. Besides 3D-printed PSIs, they also used patient-specific plates. They found a mean error in the correction of 1.4° for the radius and 1.8° for the ulna. They aimed to correct angular deformities within 5° of the contralateral side and succeeded in 80% of cases. In addition, 3D corrective osteotomy improved mean pro-supination from 115° to 176°.

In 2019, Oka et al. performed 16 3D corrective osteotomies for malunited fractures of the upper extremity. They also used patient-matched plates. They achieved a correction to within 5° of contralateral in 15 of 16 patients after 3D corrective osteotomies. In their study, the mean difference between the planned correction and the achieved result was <1° in all three planes. In patients who were operated on due to limited pro-supination, a gain in pro-supination was seen from 115° to 162°.

In our series, the 3D osteotomy to correct a pediatric forearm malunion provided a highly accurate correction comparable to the studies mentioned above. Anatomic corrections were associated with greater gains in pro-supination. Thus, a lesser gain in forearm rotation was seen if a greater residual angular or rotational deformity persisted after 3D corrective osteotomy. Besides the highly accurate correction and excellent functional outcomes, another potential advantage of 3D modeling and 3D printing is to improve the patient–doctor relationship by giving them insights into the deformity's complexity and the surgical procedure's goal [19].

In our study, residual malrotation of the radius was associated with inferior pro-supination. Not restoring the natural radial bow may lead to bony impingement or too tight soft-tissue, which hinders the radius from swiveling around the ulna. In 1984, Tarr et al. claimed any torsional deformity of the radius leads to a loss of forearm rotation equal to the magnitude of the rotational malalignment but in the opposite direction [16]. However, in a cadaveric study by Kasten et al., a rotational malalignment of the radius of 30° in pronation resulted in a supination deficit of only 14°. Similarly, a rotational malalignment of 30° in supination resulted in a pronation deficit of only 11° [20]. Malrotation of the ulna is well tolerated since the ulna is a relatively straight bone. Thus, this leads to less restriction in forearm rotation than malrotation of the radius [11,21]. A study by Tynan et al. created malrotations of the ulna of 30°, which led to a decrease in forearm rotation of less than 20° [21].

In our study, there were a few cases with considerable residual malalignment or malrotation (Cases 1, 2, 3, 4, and 13). Although all patients were operated on by two experienced orthopedic hand surgeons operating together, four out of five non-anatomic corrections occurred in the first four operated patients. This suggests a considerable learning curve exists for 3D corrective osteotomy for diaphyseal both-bone forearm malunion. Therefore, a larger series is needed to detect if the surgical experience is a source of bias in the accuracy of a 3D corrective osteotomy. Oka et al. stated, "The simple surgical procedure is another advantage of the use of PMIs" [3]. However, we advocate there are still many possible challenges during surgery. For example, the absence of bony landmarks on the forearm bones and additional soft-tissue hindrance may impede the optimal guide position, which may result in under- or over-correction, as suggested by Jeuken et al. [22].

We did not expect residual malalignment or malrotation. The drilling guides dictate screw placement proximal and distal of the planned osteotomy. They are designed with the correct amount of rotational and angular correction built in so once the osteotomies are completed, the placement of screws should provide the desired correction [23].

Therefore, we investigated our outliers in more detail. There were no manufacturing issues. Three out of five non-anatomic corrections were malunions in the proximal diaphysis, suggesting a relation with a more complex surgical approach and more soft tissue hindering snug fit positioning of the surgical guides. Furthermore, the pre-operative plan for 3D corrective osteotomy does not consider the soft-tissue issues seen in post-traumatic forearm malunion. If there is a long interval between trauma and osteotomy in a growing child, soft-tissue contractures of the IOM, proximal and distal radioulnar joint capsule (DRUJ) can be seen [5]. Previously, persisting deficits in pro-supination after corrective osteotomy in longstanding forearm malunions have been seen, regardless of full geometric restoration of bony anatomy [2,24]. The IPD meta-analysis results supported soft tissue contracture's role in a longstanding malunion [25]. A long interval between trauma and corrective osteotomy compromised the functional gain in pro-supination, which was confirmed in our previous publication [8].

Limitations

This study has some limitations. First, there was no control group that underwent conventional corrective osteotomy using 2D radiographic planning without patient-specific 3D printed surgical guides. However, we find using only 2D radiographic planning for the correction of a 3D deformity unethical, as inferior results can unequivocally be expected. A previous meta-analysis showed the use of 3D computer-assisted techniques is a predictor of superior functional outcome after corrective osteotomy for a malunited pediatric forearm fracture [25].

Additionally, we included a relatively small number of patients. However, severe limitation in forearm rotation due to a pediatric malunited both-bone forearm fracture fortunately occurs seldomly. Therefore, a corrective osteotomy is rarely indicated.

Another limitation is if 3D corrective osteotomy did not provide full pro-supination, additional IOM or DRUJ release was performed during surgery. Thus, post-operative outcomes were not solely determined by correcting the bony anatomy. In the previous studies, no additional soft-tissue releases were performed [2,3,5,6,18,23]. Yet, this surgical plan does reflect our clinical approach to treating a post-traumatic forearm rotation: correct the bony deformity first, then solve the soft-tissue problems.

Furthermore, the post-operative CT scan was obtained one year after surgery. Thus, in children with remaining growing potential, additional remodeling could occur. Eight out of fifteen patients were aged <15 years at the time of 3D corrective osteotomy.

Lastly, there were only a few outliers to investigate due to the overall high accuracy of the correction and excellent functional outcome after 3D corrective osteotomy. Therefore, perhaps there are other unknown predictors for an inferior outcome we have yet to identify. Larger series are needed.

5. Conclusions

Three-dimensional corrective osteotomy using patient-specific instruments results in an accurate correction of pediatric malunited forearm fractures. A close to normal pro-supination was obtained in the majority of patients. Patients with an anatomic correction of the radius had better forearm rotation than non-anatomic corrections. Residual malrotation of the radius after a 3D corrective osteotomy is associated with an inferior outcome. Although PSIs simplify the operative procedure, a considerable learning curve still exists for 3D corrective osteotomy.

Desirable future research is a randomized controlled trial (RCT) comparing the outcomes after 3D-planned corrective osteotomy with or without PSIs because cost increases are substantially due to the 3D printing of PSIs. Future studies on 3D corrective osteotomy should provide patient-reported outcomes measures, functional outcomes, as well as radiographic outcomes on the accuracy of the achieved correction.

Author Contributions: Conceptualization, K.R., E.v.E., D.E., J.C. and F.S.; methodology, K.R., E.v.E., G.K., D.E., J.C. and F.S.; software, K.R. and E.v.E.; validation, K.R. and E.v.E.; formal analysis, K.R.; investigation, K.R., E.v.E., D.E., J.C. and F.S.; resources, K.R. data curation, K.R., E.v.E., D.E., J.C. and F.S.; writing—original draft preparation, K.R., writing—review and editing, K.R., E.v.E., G.K., D.E., J.C. and F.S.; visualization, K.R., E.v.E., D.E., J.C. and F.S.; supervision, D.E., J.C. and F.S.; project administration, K.R., E.v.E., D.E., J.C. and F.S. All authors have read and agreed to the published version of the manuscript.

Funding: This research received no external funding.

Institutional Review Board Statement: The study was conducted in accordance with the Declaration of Helsinki and approved by the Institutional Ethics Committee of Erasmus University Medical Center (NL52987.078.15 and date of approval: 10 December 2015).

Informed Consent Statement: Informed consent was obtained from all subjects and parents involved in the study.

Data Availability Statement: Data are contained within the article.

Acknowledgments: The authors thank Edwin Oei and the radiology department of Erasmus MC University for their involvement in this study (scanning protocols, discussion regarding study design).

Conflicts of Interest: The authors declare no conflict of interest.

References

1. Hughstone, J.C. Fractures of the forearm in children. *J. Bone Jt. Surg.-Am. Vol.* **1962**, *44*, 1678. [CrossRef]
2. Murase, T.; Oka, K.; Moritomo, H.; Goto, A.; Yoshikawa, H.; Sugamoto, K. Three-dimensional corrective osteotomy of malunited fractures of the upper extremity with use of a computer simulation system. *J. Bone Jt. Surg. Ser. A* **2008**, *90*, 2375–2389. [CrossRef] [PubMed]
3. Oka, K.; Tanaka, H.; Okada, K.; Sahara, W.; Myoui, A.; Yamada, T.; Yamamoto, M.; Kurimoto, S.; Hirata, H.; Murase, T. Three-Dimensional Corrective Osteotomy for Malunited Fractures of the Upper Extremity Using Patient-Matched Instruments: A Prospective, Multicenter, Open-Label, Single-Arm Trial. *J. Bone Jt. Surg. Am.* **2019**, *101*, 710–721. [CrossRef] [PubMed]
4. Jayakumar, P.; Jupiter, J.B. Reconstruction of malunited diaphyseal fractures of the forearm. *Hand* **2014**, *9*, 265–273. [CrossRef]
5. Miyake, J.; Murase, T.; Oka, K.; Moritomo, H.; Sugamoto, K.; Yoshikawa, H. Computer-assisted corrective osteotomy for malunited diaphyseal forearm fractures. *J. Bone Jt. Surg. Ser. A* **2012**, *94*, e150.151–e150.111. [CrossRef]
6. Kataoka, T.; Oka, K.; Murase, T. Rotational Corrective Osteotomy for Malunited Distal Diaphyseal Radius Fractures in Children and Adolescents. *J. Hand Surg.* **2017**, *3*, 286.e1–286.e8. [CrossRef]
7. Byrne, A.M.; Impelmans, B.; Bertrand, V.; Van Haver, A.; Verstreken, F. Corrective Osteotomy for Malunited Diaphyseal Forearm Fractures Using Preoperative 3-Dimensional Planning and Patient-Specific Surgical Guides and Implants. *J. Hand Surg.* **2017**, *42*, e836.e1–e836.e12. [CrossRef]
8. Roth, K.C.; van Es, E.M.; Kraan, G.A.; Verhaar, J.A.N.; Stockmans, F.; Colaris, J.W. Outcomes of 3-D corrective osteotomies for paediatric malunited both-bone forearm fractures. *J. Hand Surg. Eur. Vol.* **2021**, *47*, 164–171. [CrossRef]
9. Nagy, L.; Jankauskas, L.; Dumont, C.E. Correction of forearm malunion guided by the preoperative complaint. *Clin. Orthop. Relat. Res.* **2008**, *466*, 1419–1428. [CrossRef]
10. Krettek, C.; Miclau, T.; Grun, O.; Schandelmaier, P.; Tscherne, H. Intraoperative control of axes, rotation and length in femoral and tibial fractures. Technical note. *Injury* **1998**, *29* (Suppl. S3), C29–C39. [CrossRef]
11. Blossey, R.D.; Krettek, C.; Liodakis, E. [Posttraumatic torsional deformities of the forearm: Methods of measurement and decision guidelines for correction]. *Unfallchirurg* **2018**, *121*, 206–215. [CrossRef] [PubMed]
12. MacDermid, J.; Solomon, G.; Valdes, K.; American Society of Hand, T. *Clinical Assessment Recommendations*; American Society of Hand Therapists: Chicago, IL, USA, 2015.
13. Wu, G.; van der Helm, F.C.; Veeger, H.E.; Makhsous, M.; Van Roy, P.; Anglin, C.; Nagels, J.; Karduna, A.R.; McQuade, K.; Wang, X.; et al. ISB recommendation on definitions of joint coordinate systems of various joints for the reporting of human joint motion–Part II: Shoulder, elbow, wrist and hand. *J. Biomech.* **2005**, *38*, 981–992. [CrossRef] [PubMed]
14. Vroemen, J.C.; Dobbe, J.G.; Strackee, S.D.; Streekstra, G.J. Positioning evaluation of corrective osteotomy for the malunited radius: 3-D CT versus 2-D radiographs. *Orthopedics* **2013**, *36*, e193–e199. [CrossRef] [PubMed]
15. Graham, T.J.; Fischer, T.J.; Hotchkiss, R.N.; Kleinman, W.B. Disorders of the forearm axis. *Hand Clin.* **1998**, *14*, 305–316. [CrossRef] [PubMed]

16. Tarr, R.R.; Garfinkel, A.I.; Sarmiento, A. The effects of angular and rotational deformities of both bones of the forearm. An in vitro study. *J. Bone Jt. Surg. Am.* **1984**, *66*, 65–70. [CrossRef]
17. Abe, S.; Murase, T.; Oka, K.; Shigi, A.; Tanaka, H.; Yoshikawa, H. In Vivo Three-Dimensional Analysis of Malunited Forearm Diaphyseal Fractures with Forearm Rotational Restriction. *J. Bone Jt. Surg. Am.* **2018**, *100*, e113. [CrossRef]
18. Kataoka, T.; Oka, K.; Miyake, J.; Omori, S.; Tanaka, H.; Murase, T. 3-Dimensional prebent plate fixation in corrective osteotomy of malunited upper extremity fractures using a real-sized plastic bone model prepared by preoperative computer simulation. *J. Hand Surg. Am.* **2013**, *38*, 909–919. [CrossRef]
19. Tevanov, I.; Liciu, E.; Chirila, M.; Dusca, A.; Ulici, A. The use of 3D printing in improving patient-doctor relationship and malpractice prevention. *Rom. J. Leg. Med.* **2017**, *25*, 279–282. [CrossRef]
20. Kasten, P.; Krefft, M.; Hesselbach, J.; Weinberg, A.M. How does torsional deformity of the radial shaft influence the rotation of the forearm? A biomechanical study. *J. Orthop. Trauma.* **2003**, *17*, 57–60. [CrossRef]
21. Tynan, M.C.; Fornalski, S.; McMahon, P.J.; Utkan, A.; Green, S.A.; Lee, T.Q. The effects of ulnar axial malalignment on supination and pronation. *J. Bone Jt. Surg. Ser. A* **2000**, *82*, 1726–1731. [CrossRef]
22. Jeuken, R.M.; Hendrickx, R.P.M.; Schotanus, M.G.M.; Jansen, E.J. Near-anatomical correction using a CT-guided technique of a forearm malunion in a 15-year-old girl: A case report including surgical technique. *Orthop. Traumatol. Surg. Res.* **2017**, *103*, 783–790. [CrossRef] [PubMed]
23. Bauer, A.S.; Storelli, D.A.R.; Sibbel, S.E.; McCarroll, H.R.; Lattanza, L.L. Preoperative computer simulation and patient-specific guides are safe and effective to correct forearm deformity in children. *J. Pediatr. Orthop.* **2017**, *37*, 504–510. [CrossRef] [PubMed]
24. Trousdale, R.T.; Linscheid, R.L. Operative treatment of malunited fractures of the forearm. *J. Bone Jt. Surg. Ser. A* **1995**, *77*, 894–902. [CrossRef] [PubMed]
25. Roth, K.C.; Walenkamp, M.M.J.; van Geenen, R.C.I.; Reijman, M.; Verhaar, J.A.N.; Colaris, J.W. Factors determining outcome of corrective osteotomy for malunited paediatric forearm fractures: A systematic review and meta-analysis. *J. Hand Surg. Eur.Vol.* **2017**, *42*, 810–816. [CrossRef] [PubMed]

Disclaimer/Publisher's Note: The statements, opinions and data contained in all publications are solely those of the individual author(s) and contributor(s) and not of MDPI and/or the editor(s). MDPI and/or the editor(s) disclaim responsibility for any injury to people or property resulting from any ideas, methods, instructions or products referred to in the content.

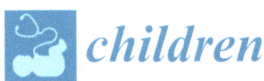

Article

Stabilisation of Pathologic Proximal Femoral Fracture near the Growth Plate with Use of a Locking Plate and Transphyseal Screws

Roman Michalik, Frank Hildebrand * and Heide Delbrück

Department of Orthopaedic, Trauma and Reconstructive Surgery, University Hospital RWTH Aachen, D-52074 Aachen, Germany
* Correspondence: fhildebrand@ukaachen.de

Abstract: Aneurysmal bone cyst (ABC) is a benign osseus lesion with a high pathologic fracture risk. The described treatment options are varied and inconsistent. For successful treatment results, it is essential to prevent recurrence and sufficiently stabilise the weakened bone. Lesions close to the growth plates, especially in the femoral neck region, are challenging to stabilise in children. In this study, 27 clinics, including 11 sarcoma centres, 15 paediatric orthopaedic clinics, and one sarcoma/paediatric orthopaedic centre, were surveyed and asked about their treatment approaches for an exemplary case of ABC in the femoral neck causing a pathological fracture in a 20-month-old infant, with a response rate of 81%. The heterogeneity of treatment options described in the literature is consistent with the survey results. The most favoured approach was curettage, defect filling of any kind, and surgical stabilisation. However, the lesion stabilisation option introduced in this paper, which involves the use of transphyseal screws, was not mentioned in the survey and has not been reported in the literature. Contrary to the existing concepts, our technique offers high stability without significant growth restriction. Transphyseal screws are also suitable for the treatment of femoral neck fractures of other aetiologies in children.

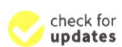

Citation: Michalik, R.; Hildebrand, F.; Delbrück, H. Stabilisation of Pathologic Proximal Femoral Fracture near the Growth Plate with Use of a Locking Plate and Transphyseal Screws. *Children* **2022**, *9*, 1932. https://doi.org/10.3390/children9121932

Academic Editors: Christiaan J. A. van Bergen and Joost W. Colaris

Received: 14 November 2022
Accepted: 7 December 2022
Published: 9 December 2022

Publisher's Note: MDPI stays neutral with regard to jurisdictional claims in published maps and institutional affiliations.

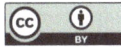

Copyright: © 2022 by the authors. Licensee MDPI, Basel, Switzerland. This article is an open access article distributed under the terms and conditions of the Creative Commons Attribution (CC BY) license (https://creativecommons.org/licenses/by/4.0/).

Keywords: bone cyst; paediatric orthopaedics; osteosyntheses in children; growth plate; transphyseal screws

1. Introduction

Aneurysmal bone cyst (ABC) is a benign tumorous lesion. Approximately 70% of lesions are found in patients between the ages of 5 and 20 years, with little predilection to the female sex [1,2]. The lesion can occur in almost any bone, although the long bones are preferentially affected [3,4]. Mankin et al. analysed 150 cases of ABC over 20 years, with the lesions occurring predominantly in the tibia, femur, fibula, pelvis, humerus, clavicle, foot, and lumbar spine, in descending order [5]. The lesion occasionally becomes symptomatic with local swelling or pain but frequently presents with a pathological fracture due to the thinned cortical bone. Various treatment methods are available, as the high risk of recurrence, which has been described in up to 60% of cases in 24–50 months [6], has constantly led to the development of new approaches.

For the therapy of the cyst itself, bloc resection of the lesion, radiation, sclerotherapy (e.g., with polidocanol), and curettage are used alone or in combination. In a prospective randomised study, Varshney et al. investigated the effectiveness of repeated polidocanol sclerotherapy in comparison with that of curettage in combination with spongiosaplasty and additional filling with synthetic hydroxyapatite. The authors concluded that, although the therapeutic strategies had equal healing rates, recurrent sclerotherapy had the advantages of outpatient feasibility, faster pain reduction, and better functional outcomes [7]. However, other studies have advocated the open procedure using curettage and, if necessary, cancellous bone or cement filling [5,8,9].

Cure rates increase with the number of procedures. In addition to therapy for the cystic lesion itself, stabilisation of the bone is often required. A challenge here is the localisation in the femoral neck and proximal femur region. In epiphyseal localisations of the heavily loaded femoral neck and proximal femur, osteosynthesis using the usual procedures of elastic stable intramedullary nailing (ESIN) and Kirschner wires during the growing age is limited. In addition, immobilisation in a hip spica cast (HSC) would result in complete immobilisation of the child for weeks.

In this work, we present a surgical one-stage treatment of an ABC with a pathologic fracture at the proximal femur and femoral neck in a 20-month-old patient. We present the case in a nationwide survey among certified German sarcoma centres and children orthopaedic departments to determine their preferred diagnostics and treatment. In our surgical approach, we performed osteosynthesis using a locking plate with so-called transphyseal screws, which could cross the growth plate at the femoral neck owing to their shape (metaphyseal thread with smooth threadless epiphyseal shape).

2. Materials and Methods

2.1. Case Report

A 20-month-old boy presented with a limping gait pattern and sparing of the left leg. Radiological examination revealed osteolysis of the femoral neck and proximal femur, adjacent to the growth plate, with a typical multiseptated aspect, marked cortical weakening, or interruption in the axial image. Magnetic resonance imaging (MRI) clearly revealed the mirror formation of the cyst contents (Figure 1).

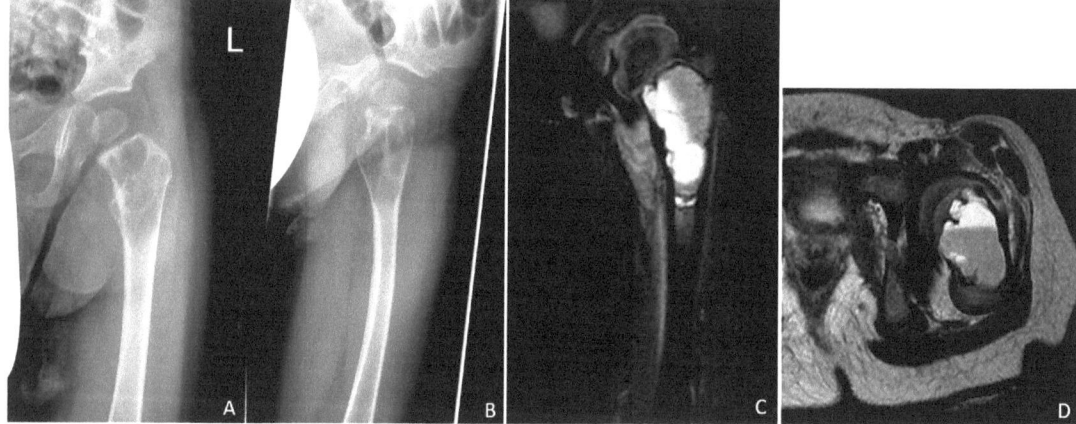

Figure 1. Conventional radiographs of the left hip joint showing the septated cystic lesion of the proximal femur extending immediately to the growth plate in two planes (**A**,**B**). Perforation of the thinned cortical bone is indicated in the lateral image (**B**). The magnetic resonance image clearly shows the multichambered fluid-filled cyst, which is confined to the proximal femur (**C**,**D**). In the axial section, the fluid levels are clearly visible (**D**).

In the otherwise healthy patient, after a biopsy and an intraoperative frozen section investigation, a one-step surgical treatment was performed by subsequent curettage of the cyst (Figure 2A–C), irrigation with polidocanol, filling with allogen cancellous bone, and subsequent osteosynthesis using a locking proximal femoral plate (OrthoPediatrics PediLoc) and transphyseal locking screws (OrthoPediatrics Corp., Warsaw, IN, USA; Figure 2D–F).

The follow-up treatment could be designed without a cast with pain-dependent mobilization.

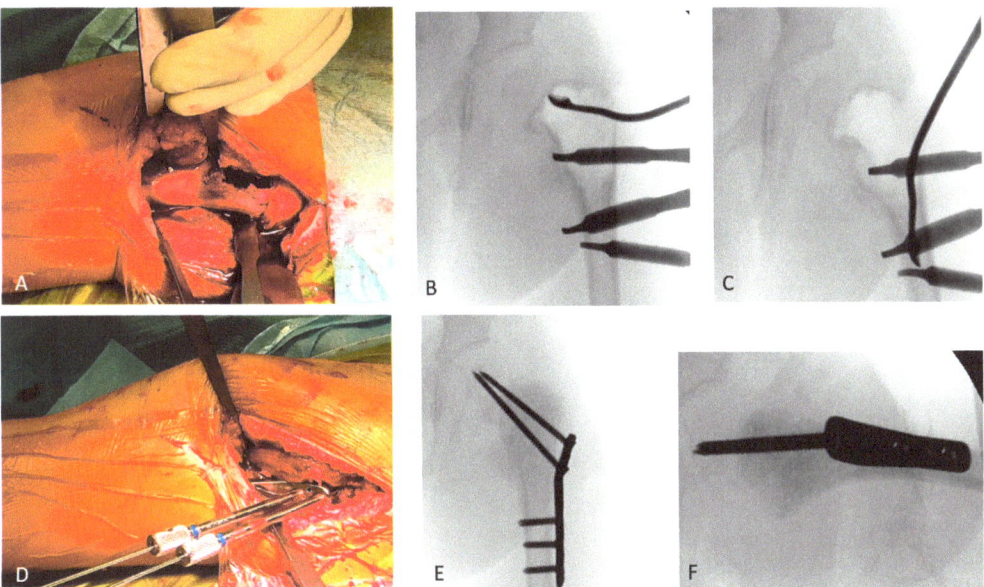

Figure 2. The femur is reached via a lateral approach. The cyst has already perforated the ventral cortex (**A**). The cyst is excochleated with a flexible sharp curette, which is documented with the image intensifier (**B**,**C**). After exclusion of malignancy in the frozen section and subsequent excochleation, rinsing with polidocanol and filling of the cyst with allogen spongiosa an osteosynthetic stabilisation is performed (**D**). After completion of the osteosynthesis, the X-ray control is carried out in two planes (**E**,**F**), showing the correct central position of the transphyseal screws in the epiphysis.

At the first outpatient visit, 6 weeks after the operation, the boy presented without pain, with an unremarkable gait pattern, and with unrestricted hip mobility. He had already returned to kindergarten. The final immuno-histopathological results confirmed the suspected diagnosis of ABC. A translocation of the *GNP6* gene was found, which is known to be linked to primary ABC [10]. The radiological examination revealed good cyst filling and screw position (Figure 3A,B). Six months after the operation, the screw tips, which were originally located in the epiphysis, had almost migrated towards the metaphysis, but a recurrence was suspected (Figure 3C,D).

However, the patient still had no pain and an unremarkable clinical examination finding. Therefore, a short-term clinical and radiological control was agreed, which showed no significant cyst progression even after 3 months; thus, further follow-up controls were scheduled (Figure 3E,F). No evidence of growth disorders or femoral head necrosis was found. There is also no need to assume any risk to stability if there is no pain and the screws are in place and thus no urgent need for action.

2.2. Conducted Survey

The anonymised preoperative images (Figure 1A–D) were sent with the abovementioned medical history to the medical directors of all 11 German sarcoma centres certified by the German Cancer Society (www.oncomap.de) at that time (accessed on 27 August 2021). They were also sent to the heads of all 16 children orthopaedic departments listed in "KlinikKompass" (www.klinikkompass.com, accessed on 27 August 2021) as the best clinics for paediatric orthopaedics in Germany. This is a platform founded in November 2018 by a journalist to help find a specialist clinic. This list was based on high case numbers for the searched field, patient safety, and, according to the surveys by the health insurance companies, high patient satisfaction. The text of inquiry was the following: "Attached are pictures of a 20-month-old boy who was already walking safely but now has a clear limp and left leg rest. We are contacting you because you are considered a certified sarcoma centre/leading clinic for paediatric orthopaedics in Germany, and in this case, there are certainly several possible approaches. How would you proceed or treat the existing bone cyst?" The entity of the lesion was not known at this time. The corresponding survey results were analysed with the consent of the participating clinics. The data protection regulations were complied with.

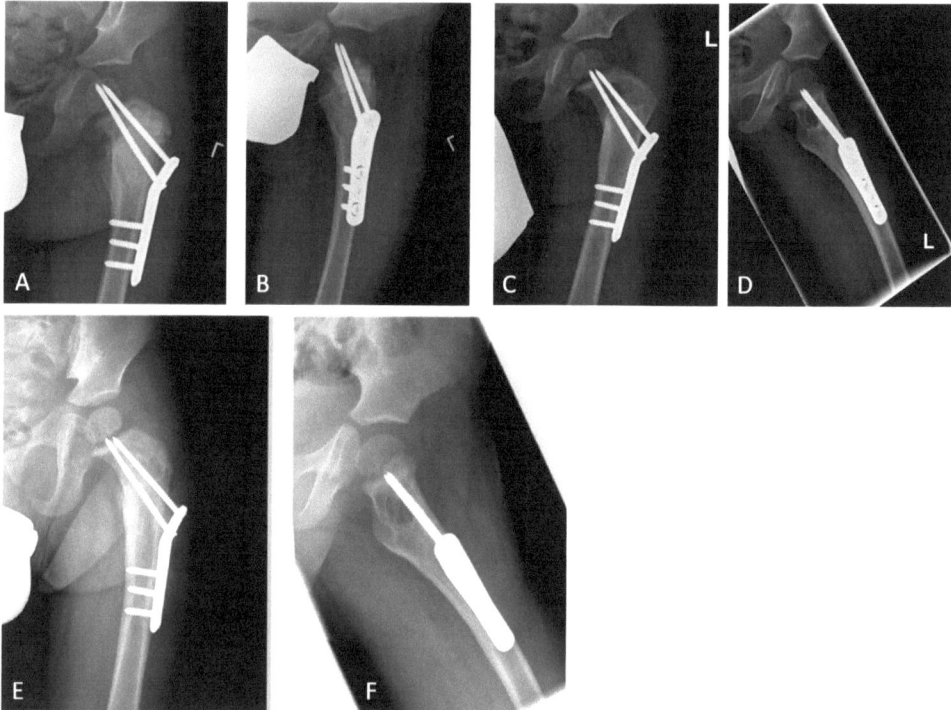

Figure 3. Radiological follow-up examination in the short and medium terms. After 6 weeks (**A**,**B**), the desired result was achieved, with a regular material position and filled cyst. The growth of the proximal femur over the physeal screws can been seen clearly in the displayed radiographs (**A**–**F**). However (**C**,**D**), radiological evidence suggests a recurrence, with the findings remaining stable for another 4 months (**E**,**F**).

3. Results

3.1. Survey Results

A nationwide survey was conducted among 11 sarcoma centres, 15 paediatric orthopaedic clinics, and one sarcoma/paediatric orthopaedic centre in Germany. A total of 22 clinics gave their assessments (response rate, 81%).

3.1.1. Entity Assessment

To the question about entity estimation, 18 clinics responded. On the basis of the provided native radiological images and MRI scan, a suspicion of ABC (36.4%) was predominantly expressed, and a differential diagnosis of juvenile bone cyst (JBC; 22.7%) or telangiectatic osteosarcoma (OS; 4.5%) was also mentioned. The sole suspected diagnosis of a juvenile bone cyst (JBC) was expressed by 18% of the hospitals (Figure 4A).

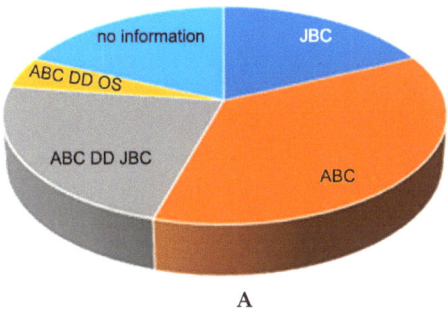 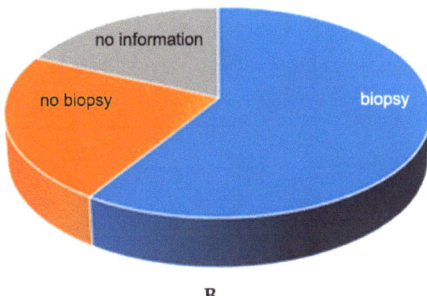

Figure 4. (**A**) Entity assessment: Most participating clinics (n = 22) classified the lesion as an aneurysmal bone cyst (ABC; 36.4%) or considered it in the differential diagnosis (ABC, DD, or juvenile bone cyst [JBC]: 22.7%; ABC, DD, or osteosarcoma (4.5%). Thus, JBC (n = 4) was the next most frequently mentioned differential diagnosis or sole diagnosis. Overall, four responding hospitals did not provide any information on this question. (**B**) Regarding the need for biopsy, of the responding hospitals, 59.1% wanted a biopsy, 22.7% did not consider it necessary, and 18.2% did not provide any information on this.

3.1.2. Assessment of the Need for Biopsy

An additional biopsy confirmation of the diagnosis before initiating therapy was requested by most clinics (59.1%), 9% recommended an MRI follow-up as an alternative, 22.7% denied a biopsy, and 18.2% did not provide any information (Figure 4B).

3.1.3. Entity-Specific Local Therapy

The answers to the question about entity-specific therapy were more heterogeneous (Figure 5A). Most hospitals recommended a primary surgical procedure (72.7%). Only 22.7% of the clinics preferred adjuvant injection in the cyst alone. Some respondents (4.5%) stated that the healing of the cyst is stimulated by the fracture that has occurred and that a wait-and-see behavior can be adopted.

Curettage was predominantly mentioned as a therapy for the cyst (68.2%). In 4.5% of cases, the therapy was extended with an adjuvant injection. In 4.5% of cases, curettage was mentioned as a therapy in the event of persistent findings after immobilisation using an HSC. Further treatment options were sole instillation (22.7%) of an adjuvant such as polidocanol (4.5%) or phenol (4.5%) for a suspected ABC or methylprednisolone acetate (9%) for JBC. In the case of biopsy-proven osteosarcoma, a Borggreve-Van Nes-Winkelmann rotationplasty was recommended as a treatment option (4.5%).

3.1.4. Defect Filling

Regarding defect filling (Figure 5B), 77% of the 22 participating clinics gave their assessment, with the remaining having either previously recommended conservative therapy (13.6%) or not provided any information (9%).

Filling with allogen spongiosa alone (13.6%) or in combination with bone replacement material (13.6%) or autologous bone (4.5%) was mentioned with a similar frequency as the recommendation to use bone replacement material alone (27.3%) or fibula interposition with/without bone replacement material (9%). Among the respondents, 9% recommended a finding-dependent procedure with allogen spongiosa or bone substitute material. A multiple-stage procedure using a bone cement (Palacos) seal and, after an observation interval, a secondary filling with spongiosa was also recommended by 9% of the participating clinics.

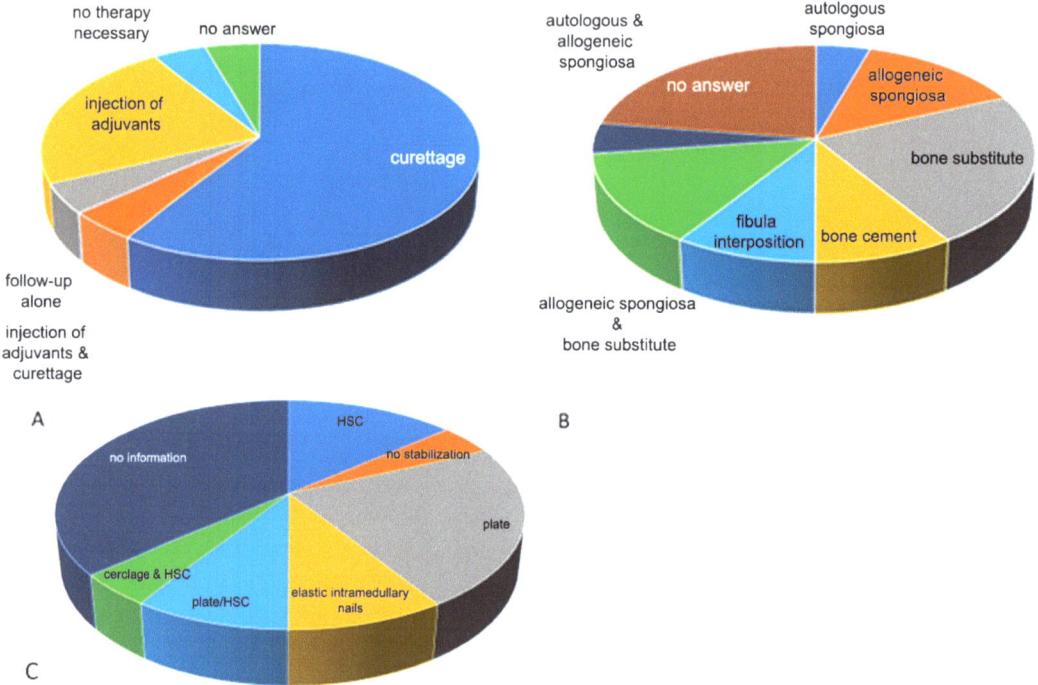

Figure 5. (**A**) As local therapy, the following were recommended by the respondents: curettage, 68.2%; adjuvant injection and curettage, 4.5%; follow-up alone, 4.5%; injection of adjuvants, 22.7%; no therapy necessary, 4.5%; and no information, 4.5%. (**B**) For defect filling, autologous spongiosa was recommended by 4.5% of the respondents; allogeneic spongiosa, by 13.6%; bone substitute, by 27.3%; bone cement, by 9%; fibula interposition, by 9%; allogeneic spongiosa and bone substitute, by 13.6%; and autologous and allogeneic spongiosa, by 4.5%. Of the respondents, 22.7% gave no answer. (**C**) For osteosynthesis/stabilisation, most of the 22 hospitals recommended surgical stabilisation (40.9%), 9% of the clinics preferred immobilisation with an HSC only; 9% did not commit themselves and recommended a procedure (plate osteosynthesis or HSC as a secondary alternative) depending on the findings and completion of the cyst removal and filling; and 4.5% saw no need for immobilisation or stabilisation. Surgical stabilisation using plate osteosynthesis (27%), elastic intramedullary nails (9%), or cerclage and additional HSC immobilisation were mentioned. Of the participating hospitals, 36.4% did not provide any information on this question.

3.1.5. Stabilisation/Osteosynthesis

Of the responding clinics, 40.9% clearly recommended stabilisation (Figure 5C); 13.6% preferred osteosynthesis-free treatment, with an HSC being the most recommended; 9% recommended the use of an HSC as an alternative to surgical treatment with a plate osteosynthesis. Osteosynthesis with a plate was mainly recommended (27%), whereby the classic locking screws should be inserted over the growth plate (GP). Retrograde ESIN (9%) was suggested as an alternative, with one clinic recommending ESIN and a plate. A GP-bridging osteosynthesis using Kirschner wires and additional application of an HSC was recommended as a treatment procedure by 4.5% of the hospitals.

4. Discussion

From our point of view, the presented case of ABC that caused a pathological fracture in the femoral neck and proximal femur region in a 20-month-old boy is unique in several aspects: First, ABCs are usually found in children at ages between 5 and 20 years [1,2];

thus, the presented case of ABC in a 20-month-old boy is rare. Other differential diagnoses must also be considered initially. Furthermore, because of the large extent of the lesion, including the hole femoral neck and proximal femur, and its localisation up to the growth plate of the femoral neck, treatment was challenging, as in addition to treating the lesion, the pathological fracture, which was in the immediate vicinity of the growth plate, must also be stabilised.

Owing to the mentioned peculiarities of this case and as treatment strategies for bone cysts, especially ABCs, are inconsistent, we asked paediatric orthopaedic specialist clinics and sarcoma centres for recommendations on how to proceed as part of an open inquiry. The high response rate of our survey of 81% shows the interest and the need for discussion of this topic and our presented case. Considering the survey results and discussing the treatment options with the patient's parents, we chose a one-stage treatment approach consisting of a biopsy and intraoperative frozen section investigation (for exclusion of malignancy and confirmation of the suspected diagnosis of ABC), extension of the approach, subtle curettage, polidocanol injection, defect filling with allogenous spongiosa, and osteosynthesis with a locking plate and the described special transphyseal screws.

The diagnosis of ABC can be made based on the combination of conventional radiography and MRI, with almost 83% sensitivity and 70% specificity [11]. The imaging diagnostic findings of our case, which showed multiple septation and mirror formation on MRI, were highly indicative of ABC. However, in our survey, only 36.4% favoured this diagnosis, whereas 27.2% considered ABC as a differential diagnosis on the basis of the presented radiography and MRI results. As mentioned earlier, only one third of the respondents suspected ABC as a diagnosis possibly because of the untypical young age of the patient. Furthermore, we suspected that highly specialised clinics want to avoid misdiagnosis in cases where suspected lesions are initially diagnosed as benign but are actually malignant. This has certainly affected a high number of respondents who aimed for a biopsy prior to further treatment (59.1%). Only 22.7% of the respondents did not consider a biopsy of the lesion. To reduce surgical burden, we chose an intraoperative frozen section analysis, which none of the interviewees mentioned as a possibility. Their reason could be the limited value of the use of frozen sections in the detailed entity classification of bone lesions. However, on the basis of contradicting study results, we believe that a first assessment of the dignity can be expected [12,13].

Regarding the treatment of the cyst itself, we decided to perform a curettage because of bone instability and the large extent of the lesion. Thus, we could immediately fill the defect with allogenous spongiosa to provide a more stable bone stock. Instillation of polidocanol as a sole therapy seemed inappropriate, although sequential percutaneous instillations of polidocanol are seemingly equally effective as intralesional curettage in the therapy of primary ABCs [7,14]. The repeated necessary procedure is considered an apparent disadvantage of polidocanol instillation. The apparently more aggressive open surgical procedure that we performed was also appropriate owing to the planned additional plate osteosynthesis. We also dabbed the lesion with polidocanol before filling. To our knowledge, the outcome of the combination of curettage and polidocanol instillation has not been evaluated. Furthermore, possible growth arrest or delay has to be kept in mind when using sclerotherapy near the growth plates because injection site necrosis was previously reported [7].

Regarding defect-filling bone substitutes, in our survey, cement or spongiosa was proposed for use in approximately equal parts to fill up the cyst. This result is representative of the reports in the literature and corresponds to the recommendations of the German S1 guideline "Bone cysts" [15]. Moreover, the combined use of allogenic bone grafting and artificial bone graft substitutes was reported by Tomaszewski et al. [16]. We decided to fill the defect in our case with allogenic spongiosa alone because the advantages with regard to consolidation and healing of the bone stock of one of the mentioned substitutes or compositions have not been completely evaluated [17].

Most of the 22 respondent hospitals recommended surgical stabilisation with a plate or intramedullary nails. Three clinics preferred immobilisation with a cast alone. Stabilisation techniques of the weakened bone in comparable situations have been rarely discussed in the literature. In their study, Vergel De Dios et al. examined 238 ABCs, with the femur (40 patients) being the most frequently affected among the long bones; the proximal femur was involved in 10 cases [18]. The authors identified "numerous forms of therapy" independent of localisation, including curettage and radiation but no stabilisation techniques. In the recently published retrospective multicentre EPOS study, in which 79 patients with ABC on the proximal femur were examined, no detailed information on the selection of the osteosynthesis technique, especially in the immediate vicinity of the growth plate, was provided [19]. The transphyseal screws we used were also not mentioned. Tomaszewski et al. reported their results from 30 children with bone cysts, tumour-like lesions of the proximal femur region, and pathological fractures [16]. They also used a locking or angular plate for stabilisation but did not mention the use of transphyseal screws.

As an open procedure was chosen by 43% of our respondents and 44% of the participants of the EPOS multicentre study [19], in our opinion, there is nothing to be said against a plate osteosynthesis, which does not significantly exceed the extent of the intervention. From our point of view, immobilisation using an HSC offers, at best, an alternative if the procedure is not open. However, above a certain lesion size, the extent at which the usual wearing time of 6 weeks is sufficient is questionable, as bone consolidation cannot be assumed within this time in the case of the present entity and lesion size. Retrograde ESIN as an alternative can hardly bridge the growth plate. Kirschner wires alone do not provide sufficient stability in an epi-meta-diaphyseal position.

Locking plate osteosynthesis, or a blade plate, is used as a more stable alternative. This is used for corrective osteotomies of the intertrochanter region in elective orthopaedics in children and can also be implanted in the event of a fracture. However, if the fully threaded locking screws used for this purpose are passed over the growth plate, growth disorders are to be expected [20,21].

The transphyseal locking screws used are characterised by a thread-free zone at the distal end of the screw, which enables length growth in this area and offers the ideal implant for the case described, such as femoral neck fractures of all origins in children with an open growth plate. None of the clinics suggested the implant in the initial survey, and the implant was not described in the above-mentioned studies. According to the current state of knowledge, growth disorders, femoral head necrosis, or biomechanical problems are not to be expected from the implant itself, as the plate design corresponds to that of the plates used for corrective osteotomies and the end of the screws corresponds to that of Kirschner wires. The benefits of immediate pain-adapted loading are significant. The disadvantage that must be mentioned is that the screws and plates are made of steel, which makes follow-up examination using MRI unsuitable. However, because cyst recurrences that require revision are sufficiently visible on conventional radiography, this aspect does not seem to be of primary importance to us.

This study has several limitations. Although in our case, we can report a good treatment result in the short term without radiologically detectable growth disturbances of the femoral epiphysis and femoral neck, longer follow-up studies and a larger number of cases in different age groups are necessary to provide definitive conclusions on the unrestricted use of transphyseal screws. Longer follow-up is needed to determine whether a progredient cyst recurrence will occur in turn requires follow-up operations that would lead to growth problems caused by the intervention but also by the disease itself.

5. Conclusions

As part of the treatment of bone cysts in the femoral neck, near the open growth plate, and femoral neck fractures of other origins, stable osteosynthesis with transphyseal screws and a locking plate should be considered. This method of osteosynthesis was obviously not widely known in the context of our survey of specialised hospitals. In addition, we advocate the feasibility of a one-stage procedure for cystic bone lesions in children, accompanied with an intraoperative frozen section investigation when in doubt of the suspected histology, which, however, requires the operation to be performed in clinics with the appropriate expertise and equipment.

Author Contributions: Conceptualization: R.M. and H.D.; data collection: H.D.; statistics: R.M.; writing of the manuscript: R.M., H.D. and F.H. All authors have read and agreed to the published version of the manuscript.

Funding: This research received no external funding.

Institutional Review Board Statement: This study was approved by the ethics commission of the medical faculty of RWTH Aachen University (reference No. EK 22-392). (approve date: 22 November 2022).

Informed Consent Statement: Informed consent was obtained from all subjects involved in the study. Written informed consent has been obtained from the patient's parents to publish this paper.

Data Availability Statement: The data that support the findings of this study are available from Roman Michalik and Heide Delbrück, but restrictions apply to the availability of these data, which were used under license for the present study and so are not publicly available.

Conflicts of Interest: The authors declare no conflict of interest.

References

1. Freiberg, A.A.; Loder, R.T.; Heidelberger, K.P.; Hensinger, R.N. Aneurysmal bone cysts in young children. *J. Pediatr. Orthop.* **1994**, *14*, 86–91. [CrossRef] [PubMed]
2. Ozaki, T.; Hillmann, A.; Lindner, N.; Winkelmann, W. Aneurysmal bone cysts in children. *J. Cancer Res. Clin. Oncol.* **1996**, *122*, 767–769. [CrossRef]
3. Dorfman, H.; Czerniak, B. Bone Tumors. Mosby: St. Louis, MI, USA, 1998; pp. 855–879.
4. Campanacci, M.; Bertoni, F.; Bacchini, P. *Bone and Soft Tissue Tumors*; Springer: Berlin, Germany, 1990; pp. 725–751.
5. Mankin, H.J.; Hornicek, F.J.; Ortiz-Cruz, E.; Villafuerte, J.; Gebhardt, M.C. Aneurysmal bone cyst: A review of 150 patients. *J. Clin. Oncol.* **2005**, *23*, 6756–6762. [CrossRef]
6. Basarr, K.; Piskin, A.; Güçlü, B.; Yldz, Y.; Sagglk, Y. Aneurysmal bone cyst recurrence in children: A review of 56 patients. *J. Pediatr. Orthop.* **2007**, *27*, 938–943. [CrossRef]
7. Puthoor, D.; Francis, L.; Ismail, R. Is sclerotherapy with polidocanol a better treatment option for aneurysmal bone cyst compared to conventional curettage and bone grafting? *J. Orthop.* **2021**, *25*, 265–270. [CrossRef]
8. Campanacci, M.; Capanna, R.; Picci, P. Unicameral and aneurysmal bone cysts. *Clin. Orthop. Relat. Res.* **1986**, *204*, 25–36. [CrossRef]
9. Dormans, J.P.; Hanna, B.G.; Johnston, D.R.; Khurana, J.S. Surgical treatment and recurrence rate of aneurysmal bone cysts in children. *Clin. Orthop. Relat. Res.* **2004**, *421*, 205–211. [CrossRef]
10. Oliveira, A.M.; Perez-Atayde, A.R.; Inwards, C.Y.; Medeiros, F.; Derr, V.; Hsi, B.L.; Gebhardt, M.C.; Rosenberg, A.E.; Fletcher, J.A. USP6 and CDH11 oncogenes identify the neoplastic cell in primary aneurysmal bone cysts and are absent in so-called secondary aneurysmal bone cysts. *Am. J. Pathol.* **2004**, *165*, 1773–1780. [CrossRef] [PubMed]
11. Mahnken, A.; Nolte-Ernsting, C.; Wildberger, J.; Heussen, N.; Adam, G.; Wirtz, D.; Piroth, W.; Bücker, A.; Biesterfeld, S.; Haage, P. Aneurysmal bone cyst: Value of MR imaging and conventional radiography. *Eur. Radiol.* **2003**, *13*, 1118–1124. [CrossRef]
12. Miwa, S.; Yamamoto, N.; Hayashi, K.; Takeuchi, A.; Igarashi, K.; Tada, K.; Higuchi, T.; Yonezawa, H.; Morinaga, S.; Araki, Y.; et al. Diagnostic accuracies of intraoperative frozen section and permanent section examinations for histological grades during open biopsy of bone tumors. *Int. J. Clin. Oncol.* **2021**, *26*, 613–619. [CrossRef]
13. Mohaidat, Z.M.; Al-gharaibeh, S.R.; Aljararhih, O.N.; Nusairat, M.T.; Al-omari, A.A. Challenges in the diagnosis and treatment of aneurysmal bone cyst in patients with unusual features. *Adv. Orthop.* **2019**, *2019*, 2905671. [CrossRef]
14. Deventer, N.; Schulze, M.; Gosheger, G.; de Vaal, M.; Deventer, N. Primary aneurysmal bone cyst and its recent treatment options: A comparative review of 74 cases. *Cancers* **2021**, *13*, 2362. [CrossRef]
15. Kaiser, M.M. (Coordinator), S1-Leitlinie AWMF: Knochenzysten 006-029. Available online: https://register.awmf.org/de/leitlinien/detail/006-029 (accessed on 1 December 2022).
16. Tomaszewski, R.; Rutz, E.; Mayr, J.; Dajka, J. Surgical treatment of benign lesions and pathologic fractures of the proximal femur in children. *Arch. Orthop. Trauma Surg.* **2022**, *142*, 615–624. [CrossRef] [PubMed]
17. Li, J.; Rai, S.; Ze, R.; Tang, X.; Liu, R.; Hong, P. Injectable calcium sulfate vs mixed bone graft of autologous iliac bone and allogeneic bone: Which is the better bone graft material for unicameral bone cyst in humerus? *Medicine* **2020**, *99*, e20563. [CrossRef] [PubMed]
18. Vergel De Dios, A.M.; Bond, J.R.; Shives, T.C.; McLeod, R.A.; Unni, K.K. Aneurysmal bone cyst. A clinicopathologic study of 238 cases. *Cancer* **1992**, *69*, 2921–2931. [CrossRef] [PubMed]

19. van Geloven, T.P.G.; van der Heijden, L.; Laitinen, M.K.; Campanacci, D.A.; Döring, K.; Dammerer, D.; Badr, I.T.; Haara, M.; Beltrami, G.; Kraus, T.; et al. Do's and don'ts in primary aneurysmal bone cysts of the proximal femur in children and adolescents: Retrospective multicenter EPOS study of 79 patients. *J. Pediatr. Orthop.* 2022, *in press*. [CrossRef] [PubMed]
20. Bagatur, A.E.; Zorer, G. Complications associated with surgically treated hip fractures in children. *J. Pediatr. Orthop. B* **2002**, *11*, 219–228. [CrossRef] [PubMed]
21. Togrul, E.; Bayram, H.; Gulsen, M.; Kalaci, A.; Ozbarlas, S. Fractures of the femoral neck in children: Long-term follow-up in 62 hip fractures. *Injury* **2005**, *36*, 123–130. [CrossRef] [PubMed]

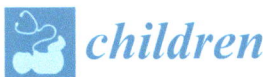

Review

Tibial Spine Avulsion Fractures in Paediatric Patients: A Systematic Review and Meta-Analysis of Surgical Management

Mehak Chandanani [1], Raian Jaibaji [2], Monketh Jaibaji [3] and Andrea Volpin [4,*]

1. School of Medicine, Medical Sciences and Nutrition, University of Aberdeen, Aberdeen AB25 2ZD, UK; m.chandanani.21@abdn.ac.uk
2. University College London, London WC1E 6BT, UK; raian.jaibaji.19@ucl.ac.uk
3. Health Education North East, Newcastle upon Tyne NE15 8NY, UK; monketh.jaibaji@nhs.net
4. NHS Grampian, Aberdeen AB15 6RE, UK
* Correspondence: andrea.volpin@nhs.scot

Abstract: Background: Tibial spine avulsion fractures (TSAFs) account for approximately 14% of anterior cruciate ligament injuries. This study aims to systematically review the current evidence for the operative management of paediatric TSAFs. Methods: A search was carried out across four databases: MEDLINE, Embase, Scopus, and Google Scholar. Studies discussing the outcomes of the surgical management of paediatric TSAFs since 2000 were included. Results: Of 38 studies included for review, 13 studies reported outcomes of TSAF patients undergoing screw fixation only, and 12 studies used suture fixation only. In total, 976 patients underwent arthroscopic reduction and internal fixation (ARIF), and 203 patients underwent open reduction and internal fixation (ORIF). The risk of arthrofibrosis with the use of ARIF ($p = 0.45$) and screws ($p = 0.74$) for TSAF repair was not significant. There was a significantly increased risk of knee instability ($p < 0.0001$), reoperation ($p = 0.01$), and post-operative pain ($p = 0.007$) with screw fixation compared to sutures. Conclusions: While the overall benefits of sutures over screws and ARIF over ORIF are unclear, there is clear preference for ARIF and suture fixation for TSAF repair in practice. We recommend large-scale comparative studies to delineate long-term outcomes for various TSAF fixation techniques.

Keywords: tibial spine avulsion; paediatric fracture; arthroscopy

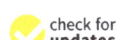

Citation: Chandanani, M.; Jaibaji, R.; Jaibaji, M.; Volpin, A. Tibial Spine Avulsion Fractures in Paediatric Patients: A Systematic Review and Meta-Analysis of Surgical Management. *Children* **2024**, *11*, 345. https://doi.org/10.3390/children11030345

Academic Editors: Christiaan J. A. van Bergen and Joost W. Colaris

Received: 18 February 2024
Revised: 6 March 2024
Accepted: 12 March 2024
Published: 14 March 2024

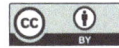

Copyright: © 2024 by the authors. Licensee MDPI, Basel, Switzerland. This article is an open access article distributed under the terms and conditions of the Creative Commons Attribution (CC BY) license (https:// creativecommons.org/licenses/by/ 4.0/).

1. Introduction

Tibial eminence fractures (TEFs), also referred to as tibial spine avulsion fractures (TSAFs) and anterior cruciate ligament (ACL) avulsion fractures, have been defined as bony avulsions of the ACL from its point of insertion on the intercondylar eminence of the tibia [1]. These injuries are most common in skeletally immature paediatric patients, accounting for approximately 14% of ACL injuries across paediatric and adult populations overall [2].

TSAFs are commonly sports-related injuries, with higher occurrence in sports such as cycling and skiing. The higher occurrence rates in children have been attributed to many causes, including the greater degree of elasticity in ligaments of young people and the weakness of incomplete ossification of the tibial eminence in relation to ACL fibres in this population [3].

TSAFs are classified in accordance with the Meyers and McKeevers (MM) classification system into type I, type II, and type III [4]. This was later modified by Zaricznyj, with the addition of type IV [5]. Details of this modified MM classification can be found in Table 1. Other classification systems include the Green Tuca classification, which uses a quantitative, magnetic resonance imaging (MRI)-based system to guide the treatment and management of TSAFs, as compared to plain radiograph evaluation in the MM system [6]. However, both systems have shown good inter-reliability [6].

Table 1. Overview of Meyers and McKeever Classification System [4,5].

Type	Description
Type 1	Non- or minimally displaced (<3 mm)
Type 2	Minimally displaced with intact posterior hinge
Type 3a	Completely displaced involving a small portion of the eminence
Type 3b	Completely displaced involving the majority of the tibial spine
Type 4	Completely displaced, rotated, and comminuted

There is broad consensus about the non-operative management of MM type I TSAFs, using casting and immobilization for 6–12 weeks, followed by a gradual transition to weight bearing and range of motion exercises [7]. The use of operative management to treat type II fractures is controversial, with a lack of consensus. Operative management is considered for types II, III, and IV TSAFs with unsuccessful closed reduction [7].

Multiple techniques exist for the operative fixation, which include arthroscopic (ARIF) and open (ORIF) approaches. There is a lack of consensus in the literature regarding the best method of fixation. Fixation materials most commonly include sutures, K-wires, and screws. With varying degrees of complications—including arthrofibrosis, non-union, mal-union, instability, and pain—with different procedures, there is currently a lack of consensus around the indications for use of different materials and approaches [8].

This study aims to systematically review the evidence base regarding the operative management of TSAFs in a paediatric population, with a focus on various approaches, subjective and objective outcomes, and complication rates. All the reporting is in accordance with the Preferred Reporting Items for Systematic Reviews and Meta-Analysis (PRISMA) guidelines.

2. Materials and Methods

2.1. Eligibility Criteria

The following inclusion criteria were applied: (i) Studies conducted after the year 2000 (ii) assessing outcomes of surgical management (including ORIF and ARIF approaches) of TSAFs (iii) in a skeletally immature population. Literature reviews, technical notes, cadaveric studies, conference abstracts, and case reports were excluded. Studies were only included if they had a minimum of five patients.

2.2. Information Sources and Search Strategy

A literature search was carried out on 9 January 2024 across four databases, namely MEDLINE (Ovid), Embase, Scopus, and Google Scholar. The search was carried out using relevant medical subject headings (MeSH) and synonyms for the following keywords: ('Tibial' AND 'Spine' AND 'Fracture') AND 'Surgical' AND 'Paediatrics'. Further details of the search strategy can be found in Appendix A. Articles with no fully published English Language text were excluded; however, a language restriction was not applied to the search itself. Fully published articles for conference abstracts were sought and included. Reference lists of systematic and literature reviews were also searched for relevant texts for inclusion. The search results were transferred to the Rayyan systematic review software for de-duplication and screening [9].

2.3. Selection Process

Following removal of duplicates, all search results were screened by two independent reviewers in two stages: (i) title and abstract stage, (ii) full manuscript review according to pre-defined inclusion and exclusion criteria. Reviewers were blinded to each other's

2.4. Data Collection Process and Data Items

To ensure standardization of the data collection process, a data extraction form was designed. Data was extracted under the following domains: (i) Study characteristics—study design, author conflicts of interest, year of publication, country of origin, and level of evidence; (ii) Participant characteristics—number of participants, mean age, MM classification of fracture, surgical technique used, materials used, mean follow-up time; and (iii) Outcomes—pre- and post-surgery outcome scores (including the International Knee Documentation Committee (IKDC) scores and Lysholm scores). Data was independently extracted from the included texts simultaneously by two reviewers. Upon completion, agreement between reviewers was checked through discussion in the presence of an adjudicator and consensus was reached following any discrepancies.

2.5. Study Risk of Bias Assessment

The quality of studies was assessed using the Methodological Index for Non-Randomized Studies (MINORS) criteria for non-randomized studies [10]. All quality assessment was conducted by two independent reviewers. The reviewers were blinded to each other's decisions until completion. Upon completion, concordance was checked between reviewers, and any discrepancies were resolved by discussion in the presence of a third adjudicator.

2.6. Data Synthesis and Measures of Effect

Data was presented in the form of four tables, namely: (i) Study Characteristics, (ii) Critical Appraisal, (iii) Population Characteristics, and (iv) Outcomes. Analysis of data was presented narratively. Statistical analysis was conducted using a random-effects model, with the use of Odds Ratios (OR), 95% Confidence Intervals (95% CI), and *p* values. A random effects model was used to control for unobserved heterogeneity. A *p* value of <0.05 was determined to be statistically significant. All statistical analysis was done using RevMan v 5.4.1.

2.7. Heterogeneity and Subgroup Analysis

Heterogeneity was measured using the I^2 statistic, where an I^2 of 0%, 25%, 50%, and 75% correspond to no, low, moderate, and high levels of heterogeneity, respectively.

3. Results

3.1. Search Results and Study Characteristics

The process of selection and inclusion of studies has been detailed in Figure 1. Of 2845 studies initially retrieved from the database search, 1906 studies were included for title and abstract screening after de-duplication. A total of 261 studies were screened by full text for inclusion within the study, of which 38 studies were found eligible for inclusion. The characteristics of the included studies have been detailed in Table 2.

Table 2. Study characteristics table.

(Author, Year of Publication)	Title of Paper	Country of Origin	Journal of Publication	Level of Evidence
(Abdelkafy and Said, 2014) [11]	Neglected ununited tibial eminence fractures in the skeletally immature: arthroscopic management	Egypt	International Orthopaedics	4
(Brunner et al., 2016) [12]	Absorbable and non-absorbable suture fixation results in similar outcomes for tibial eminence fractures in children and adolescents	Switzerland	Knee Surgery, Sports Traumatology, Arthroscopy	3

Table 2. *Cont.*

(Author, Year of Publication)	Title of Paper	Country of Origin	Journal of Publication	Level of Evidence
(Caglar et al., 2021) [13]	Mid-term outcomes of arthroscopic suture fixation technique in tibial spine fractures in the paediatric population	Turkey	Ulusal Travma va Acil Cerrahi Dergisi	4
(Callanan et al., 2019) [14]	Suture Versus Screw Fixation of Tibial Spine Fractures in Children and Adolescents: A Comparative Study	USA	The Orthopaedic Journal of Sports Medicine	3
(Casalonga et al., 2010) [15]	Tibial intercondylar eminence fractures in children: The long-term perspective	France	Orthopaedics and Traumatology: Surgery and Research	4
(Chalopin et al., 2022) [16]	Arthroscopic suture-fixation of anterior tibial intercondylar eminence fractures by retensioning of the ACL and hollowing of the tibial footprint: Objective and subjective clinical results in a paediatric population	France	Orthopaedics and Traumatology: Surgery and Research	4
(Chotel et al., 2016) [17]	Cartilaginous tibial eminence fractures in children: which recommendations for management of this new entity?	France	Knee Surgery, Sports Traumatology, Arthroscopy	4
(D'ambrosio et al., 2022) [18]	Anatomical fixation of tibial intercondylar eminence fractures in children using a threaded pin with an adjustable lock	France	Orthopaedics and Traumatology: Surgery and Research	4
(Edmonds et al., 2015) [19]	Results of Displaced Paediatric Tibial Spine Fractures: A Comparison Between Open, Arthroscopic, and Closed Management	USA	Journal of Paediatric Orthopedics	3
(Furlan et al., 2010) [20]	Paediatric Tibial Eminence Fractures: Arthroscopic Treatment using K-Wire	Croatia	Scandinavian Journal of Surgery	4
(Hirschmann et al., 2009) [21]	Physeal sparing arthroscopic fixation of displaced tibial eminence fractures: a new surgical technique	Switzerland	Knee Surgery, Sports Traumatology, Arthroscopy	4
(Jaaskela et al., 2023) [22]	Long-term Outcomes of Tibial Spine Avulsion Fractures after Open Reduction with Osteosuturing Versus Arthroscopic Screw Fixation: A Multicenter Comparative Study	Italy	The Orthopaedic Journal of Sports Medicine	3
(Kieser et al., 2011) [23]	Displaced tibial intercondylar eminence fractures	New Zealand	Journal of Orthopaedic Surgery	4
(Kim et al., 2007) [24]	Arthroscopic Internal Fixation of Displaced Tibial Eminence Fracture Using Cannulated Screw	Republic of Korea	The Journal of The Korean Orthopaedic Association	4
(Kristinsson et al., 2021) [25]	Satisfactory outcomes following arthroscopic fixation of tibial intercondylar eminence fractures in children and adolescents using bioabsorbable nails	Denmark	Archives of Orthopaedic and Trauma Surgery	4
(Liljeros et al., 2009) [26]	Arthroscopic Fixation of Anterior Tibial Spine Fractures with Bioabsorbable Nails in Skeletally Immature Patients	Sweden	The American Journal of Sports Medicine	4

Table 2. Cont.

(Author, Year of Publication)	Title of Paper	Country of Origin	Journal of Publication	Level of Evidence
(Marie-Laure et al., 2008) [27]	Surgical management of type II tibial intercondylar eminence fractures in children	France	Journal of Paediatric Orthopaedics B	4
(Memisoglu et al., 2016) [28]	Arthroscopic fixation with intra-articular button for tibial intercondylar eminence fractures in skeletally immature patients	Turkey	Journal of Paediatric Orthopaedics B	4
(Momaya et al., 2017) [29]	Outcomes after arthroscopic fixation of tibial eminence fractures with bioabsorbable nails in skeletally immature patients	USA	Journal of Paediatric Orthopaedics B	4
(Najdi et al., 2016) [30]	Arthroscopic treatment of intercondylar eminence fractures with intraepiphyseal screws in children and adolescents	France	Orthopaedics and Traumatology: Surgery and Research	4
(Perugia et al., 2009) [31]	Clinical and radiological results of arthroscopically treated tibial spine fractures in childhood	Italy	International Orthopaedics (SICOT)	4
(Russu et al., 2021) [32]	Arthroscopic Repair in Tibial Spine Avulsion Fractures Using Polyethylene Terephthalate Suture: Good to Excellent Results in Paediatric Patients	Romania	Journal of Personalized Medicine	4
(Scrimshire et al., 2018) [33]	Management and outcomes of isolated paediatric tibial spine fractures	UK	Injury: International Journal of the Care of the Injured	4
(Sharma et al., 2008) [34]	An analysis of different types of surgical fixation for avulsion fractures of the anterior tibial spine	UK	Acta Orthopaedica Belgica	4
(Shimberg et al., 2022) [35]	A Multicenter Comparison of Open Versus Arthroscopic Fixation for Paediatric Tibial Spine Fractures	USA	Journal of Paediatric Orthopedics	3
(Shin et al., 2018) [36]	Clinical and radiological outcomes of arthroscopically assisted cannulated screw fixation for tibial eminence fracture in children and adolescents	Republic of Korea	BMC Musculoskeletal Disorders	4
(Sinha et al., 2017) [37]	Arthroscopic Fixation of Tibial Spine Avulsion in Skeletally Immature: The Technique	India	Journal of Orthopaedic Case Reports	4
(Tudisco et al., 2010) [38]	Intercondylar eminence avulsion fracture in children: long-term follow-up of 14 cases at the end of skeletal growth	Italy	Journal of Paediatric Orthopaedics B	4
(Uboldi et al., 2022) [39]	Arthroscopic treatment of tibial intercondylar eminence fractures in skeletally immature patients with bioabsorbable nails	Italy	La Pediatria Medica e Chirugica	4
(Vega et al., 2008) [40]	Arthroscopic Fixation of Displaced Tibial Eminence Fractures: A New Growth Plate-Sparing Method	Chile	Arthroscopy: The Journal of Arthroscopic and Related Surgery	4
(Watts et al., 2016) [41]	Open Versus Arthroscopic Reduction for Tibial Eminence Fracture Fixation in Children	USA	Journal of Paediatric Orthopedics	3
(Wiegand et al., 2014) [42]	Arthroscopic treatment of tibial spine fracture in children with a cannulated Herbert screw	Hungary	The Knee	4

Table 2. Cont.

(Author, Year of Publication)	Title of Paper	Country of Origin	Journal of Publication	Level of Evidence
(Wiktor and Tomaszewski, 2022) [43]	Results of Anterior Cruciate Ligament Avulsion Fracture by Treatment Using Bioabsorbable Nails in Children and Adolescents	Poland	Children	4
(Wouters et al., 2010) [44]	The arthroscopic treatment of displaced tibial spine fractures in children and adolescents using Mensicus Arrows®	The Netherlands	Knee Surgery, Sports Traumatology, Arthroscopy	4
(Xu et al., 2017) [45]	Arthroscopic fixation of paediatric tibial eminence fractures using suture anchors: A mid-term follow-up	China	Archives of Orthopaedic and Trauma Surgery	4
(Zhang et al., 2020) [46]	Arthroscopic tri-pulley Technology reduction and internal fixation of paediatric Tibial Eminence: a retrospective analysis	China	BMC Musculoskeletal Disorders	4
(Zheng et al., 2021) [47]	Arthroscopically Assisted Cannulated Screw Fixation for Treating Type III Tibial Intercondylar Eminence Fractures: A Short-Term Retrospective Controlled Study	China	Frontiers in Surgery	3
(Zhou et al., 2023) [48]	Arthroscopic percutaneous pullout suture transverse tunnel technique repair for tibial spine fractures in skeletally immature patients	China	International Orthopaedics	3

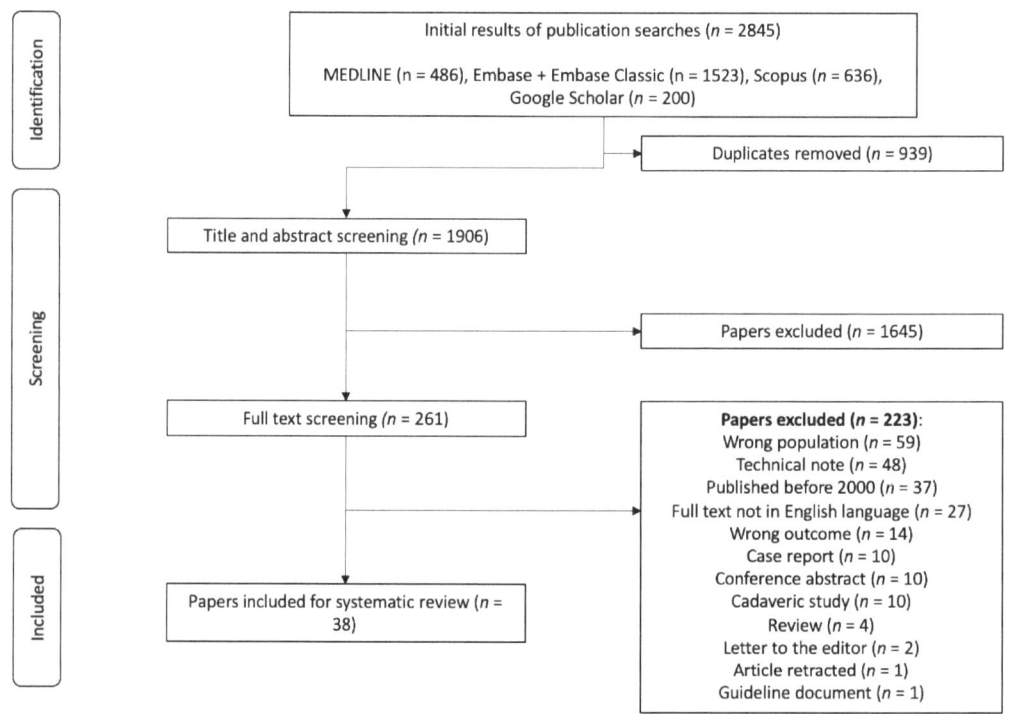

Figure 1. PRISMA Flow Diagram for Systematic Reviews. Summary of search screening progress.

3.2. Critical Appraisal

The quality of evidence was generally low. The main reasons for this include the retrospective nature of studies, the lack of control groups, and short follow-up periods. Studies also failed to calculate prospective sample sizes. The MINORS critical appraisal has been reported in Table 3.

Table 3. MINORS Critical Appraisal Results. 0 = not reported, 1 = reported but inadequate, 2 = reported and adequate.

(Author, Year of Publication)	Item 1	Item 2	Item 3	Item 4	Item 5	Item 6	Item 7	Item 8	Item 9 [1]	Item 10 [1]	Item 11 [1]	Item 12 [1]	Total [2]
(Abdelkafy and Said, 2014) [11]	2	1	2	2	0	2	2	0	NA [3]	NA	NA	NA	11
(Brunner et al., 2016) [12]	2	1	0	2	0	2	2	0	2	0	2	2	15
(Caglar et al., 2021) [13]	2	1	0	1	0	1	2	0	NA	NA	NA	NA	7
(Callanan et al., 2019) [14]	2	2	1	2	0	2	2	0	2	2	2	2	19
(Casalonga et al., 2010) [15]	1	1	0	2	1	2	2	0	NA	NA	NA	NA	9
(Chalopin et al., 2022) [16]	2	1	0	2	1	2	1	0	NA	NA	NA	NA	9
(Chotel et al., 2016) [17]	2	1	0	2	0	2	2	0	NA	NA	NA	NA	9
(D'ambrosio et al., 2022) [18]	2	1	0	2	0	2	1	0	NA	NA	NA	NA	8
(Edmonds et al., 2015) [19]	2	1	1	1	0	2	2	0	2	2	1	2	16
(Furlan et al., 2010) [20]	1	2	0	2	0	2	2	0	NA	NA	NA	NA	9
(Hirschmann et al., 2009) [21]	2	0	0	2	0	2	2	0	NA	NA	NA	NA	8
(Jaaskela et al., 2023) [22]	2	2	2	2	0	2	2	0	2	2	2	2	20
(Kieser et al., 2011) [23]	1	0	0	1	0	1	2	0	NA	NA	NA	NA	5
(Kim et al., 2007) [24]	2	0	0	2	0	1	2	0	NA	NA	NA	NA	7
(Kristinsson et al., 2021) [25]	2	2	1	2	0	2	2	0	NA	NA	NA	NA	11
(Liljeros et al., 2009) [26]	2	2	1	2	0	0	1	0	NA	NA	NA	NA	8
(Marie-Laure et al., 2008) [27]	2	1	0	2	0	2	2	0	NA	NA	NA	NA	9
(Memisoglu et al., 2016) [28]	2	0	0	2	0	2	2	0	NA	NA	NA	NA	8
(Momaya et al., 2017) [29]	2	1	1	2	0	2	2	0	NA	NA	NA	NA	10
(Najdi et al., 2016) [30]	2	1	0	2	0	2	2	0	NA	NA	NA	NA	9
(Perugia et al., 2009) [31]	2	0	0	2	0	2	2	0	NA	NA	NA	NA	8
(Russu et al., 2021) [32]	2	2	2	2	1	1	2	0	NA	NA	NA	NA	12
(Scrimshire et al., 2018) [33]	2	1	0	2	0	2	1	0	NA	NA	NA	NA	8
(Sharma et al., 2008) [34]	2	1	0	2	0	2	2	0	NA	NA	NA	NA	9
(Shimberg et al., 2022) [35]	2	2	1	2	0	1	2	0	2	2	2	2	18
(Shin et al., 2018) [36]	2	2	0	2	0	2	2	0	NA	NA	NA	NA	10
(Sinha et al., 2017) [37]	1	0	0	2	0	1	2	0	NA	NA	NA	NA	6
(Tudisco et al., 2010) [38]	2	1	0	2	0	2	2	0	1	2	0	0	12
(Uboldi et al., 2022) [39]	2	1	0	2	0	2	2	0	NA	NA	NA	NA	9
(Vega et al., 2008) [40]	2	1	0	2	0	1	2	0	NA	NA	NA	NA	8
(Watts et al., 2016) [41]	2	2	1	2	0	1	2	0	2	2	2	2	18

Table 3. Cont.

(Author, Year of Publication)	Item 1	Item 2	Item 3	Item 4	Item 5	Item 6	Item 7	Item 8	Item 9 [1]	Item 10 [1]	Item 11 [1]	Item 12 [1]	Total [2]
(Wiegand et al., 2014) [42]	2	1	1	2	0	1	2	0	NA	NA	NA	NA	9
(Wiktor and Tomaszewski, 2022) [43]	2	1	0	2	0	2	2	0	NA	NA	NA	NA	9
(Wouters et al., 2010) [44]	2	2	1	2	0	2	2	0	NA	NA	NA	NA	11
(Xu et al., 2017) [45]	2	2	1	2	1	2	2	0	NA	NA	NA	NA	12
(Zhang et al., 2020) [46]	2	2	1	2	1	2	2	0	NA	NA	NA	NA	12
(Zheng et al., 2021) [47]	1	1	0	2	0	2	2	0	NA	NA	NA	NA	8
(Zhou et al., 2023) [48]	2	2	1	2	0	2	2	0	NA	NA	NA	NA	11

[1] Items 9–12 were only considered for comparative studies. Studies with no comparison group were critically appraised using items 1–8 only. [2] The maximum MINORS score was 16 for non-comparative studies and 24 for comparative studies. [3] NA = Not Applicable.

3.3. Population Characteristics

Across 38 studies, a total of 1237 participants were included for TSAF repair. Of these, 34 patients had MM type I TSAFs (2.7%), 473 had MM type II TSAFs (38.2%), 637 had MM type III TSAFs (51.4%), and 37 had MM type IV TSAFs (2.9%). Three studies did not report the classification of their participants' TSAFs, accounting for 59 uncategorized participants (4.7%) [19,37,41]. A total of 976 TSAF patients were treated using ARIF (78.9%), 203 patients were managed using ORIF (16.4%), 54 patients were managed conservatively using closed reduction and casting (4.3%), and 4 patients were managed using a mixed approach (0.3%). A detailed description of participant characteristics of individual studies can be found in Table 4.

Table 4. Participant Characteristics. NR = Not Reported.

(Author, Year of Publication)	Number of Participants	Mean Age	Meyers and McKeever Classification	Surgical Approach	Fixation Method	Mean Follow-Up Time
(Abdelkafy and Said, 2014) [11]	13	10 ± 2.6	I: 0 II: 0 III: 13 IV: 0	Arthroscopic: 13 Open: 0	Screw: 0 Suture: 13	10.8 ± 6.8 months
(Brunner et al., 2016) [12]	25	Group A: 11.1 ± 3.3 Group B: 11.7 ± 3.3	I: 0 II: 11 III: 14 IV: 0	Arthroscopic: 25 Open: 0	Screw: 10 (non-absorbable suture with screw; Group B) Suture: 15 (absorbable with transosseus fixation; Group A)	Group A: 28.1 ± 4.6 months Group B: 47.4 ± 20.7 months
(Caglar et al., 2021) [13]	28	14.2 (8–18)	I: 0 II: 16 III: 10 IV: 2	Arthroscopic: 28 Open: 0	Screw: 0 Suture: 28	4.64 years
(Callanan et al., 2019) [14]	68	11.8 ± 2.99	I: 0 II: 14 III: 50 IV: 0	Arthroscopic: 68 Open: 0	Screw: 35 Suture: 33	26 (17–47) months
(Casalonga et al., 2010) [15]	32	12.0	I: 8 II: 17 III: 5 IV: 2	Arthroscopic: 0 Open: 7 Conservative: 25	Screw: 3 Suture: 4	14 years and 11 months (5–21 years)
(Chalopin et al., 2022) [16]	17	12 (7–15)	I: 0 II: 5 III: 9 IV: 3	Arthroscopic: 17 Open: 0	Screw: 0 Suture: 17 (Single sutures: 11, Double sutures: 6)	28 months (16–48 months)
(Chotel et al., 2016) [17]	15	6.5 ± 1.4	I: 0 II: 3 III: 6 IV: 6	Arthroscopic: 6 Open: 0 Mixed: 4 Conservative: 2	Screw: 0 Suture: 8	4.6 years (1–18.5)

Table 4. Cont.

(Author, Year of Publication)	Number of Participants	Mean Age	Meyers and McKeever Classification	Surgical Approach	Fixation Method	Mean Follow-Up Time
(D'ambrosio et al., 2022) [18]	34	11.5 ± 2.7	I: 0 II: 19 III: 12 IV: 3	Arthroscopic: 34 Open: 0	Screw: 34 Suture: 0	8.8 ± 6 years
(Edmonds et al., 2015) [19]	18	Arthroscopic: 18.3 ± 2.0 Open: 18.2 ± 3.0 Conservative: 17.4 ± 5.0	NR	Arthroscopic: 5 Open: 7 Conservative: 6	Screw: 0 Suture: 12	Arthroscopic: 5.6 ± 2.0 years Open: 6.8 ± 2.0 years Conservative: 5.8 ± 2.0 years
(Furlan et al., 2010) [20]	10	15 (12–17)	I: 0 II: 5 III: 4 IV: 1	Arthroscopic: 10 Open: 0	NR (K-wire fixation)	42 (9–78) months
(Hirschmann et al., 2009) [21]	6	14 ± 2	I: 0 II: 2 III: 3 IV: 1	Arthroscopic: 6 Open: 0	Screw: 6 Suture: 0	5 ± 2 years
(Jaaskela et al., 2023) [22]	61	11.2 ± 2.6	I: 1 II: 26 III: 34 IV: 0	Arthroscopic: 29 Open: 32	Screw: 29 Suture: 32	87.0 ± 47.1 months
(Kieser et al., 2011) [23]	9	12 (6–15)	I: 0 II: 2 III: 7 IV: 0	Arthroscopic: 2 Open: 7	Screw: 2 Suture: 6	45 (6–260) weeks
(Kim et al., 2007) [24]	10	10.5 (7–13)	I: 0 II: 4 III: 6 IV: 0	Arthroscopic: 10 Open: 0	Screw: 10 Suture: 0	22.4 (12–81) months

Table 4. *Cont.*

(Author, Year of Publication)	Number of Participants	Mean Age	Meyers and McKeever Classification	Surgical Approach	Fixation Method	Mean Follow-Up Time
(Kristinsson et al., 2021) [25]	13	11 (4–15)	I: 0 II: 9 III: 2 IV: 2	Arthroscopic: 13 Open: 0	Screw: 13 Suture: 0	6.5 (1–10) years
(Liljeros et al., 2009) [26]	13	11 (7–15)	I: 0 II: 1 III: 12 IV: 0	Arthroscopic: 13 Open: 0	Screw: 13 Suture: 0	NR
(Marie-Laure et al., 2008) [27]	17	2.1 (6–16)	I: 0 II: 17 III: 0 IV: 0	Arthroscopic: 0 Open: 17	NR	3 (0.5–7) years
(Memisoglu et al., 2016) [28]	11	12.2 (10–16)	I: 0 II: 1 III: 9 (A), 1 (B) IV: 1	Arthroscopic: 11 Open: 0	Screw: 0 Suture: 0 Both: 11 (+ Endobutton)	69 (60–84) months
(Momaya et al., 2017) [29]	7	11.6 (8–15)	I: 0 II: 1 III: 6 IV: 0	Arthroscopic: 7 Open: 0	Screw: 7 Suture: 0	31 (24–36) months
(Najdi et al., 2016) [30]	24	1 (6–15)	I: 0 II: 15 III: 9 IV: 0	Arthroscopic: 24 Open: 0	Screw: 24 Suture: 0	2 (1.5–3) years
(Perugia et al., 2009) [31]	10	13.5 (2–15)	I: 0 II: 3 III: 7 IV: 0	Arthroscopic: 10 Open: 0	Screw: 0 Suture: 10	85.8 (20–188) months

Table 4. *Cont.*

(Author, Year of Publication)	Number of Participants	Mean Age	Meyers and McKeever Classification	Surgical Approach	Fixation Method	Mean Follow-Up Time
(Russu et al., 2021) [32]	12	14.3 ± 2.1	I: 0 II: 0 III: 12 IV: 0	Arthroscopic: 12 Open: 0	Screw: 0 Suture: 12	6 months
(Scrimshire et al., 2018) [33]	40	11.8	I: 3 II: 13 III: 24 IV: 0	Arthroscopic: 0 Open: 30 Conservative: 10	Screw: 30 Suture: 0	36 months
(Sharma et al., 2008) [34]	14 (children), 11 (adults)	13 (8–16)	I: 0 II: 0 III: 19 IV: 6	Arthroscopic: 0 Open: 24	Screw: 7 (children), 6 (adults) Suture: 6 (children), 3 (adults) Stainless steel loop: 2 (children), 2 (adults)	44 months
(Shimberg et al., 2022) [35]	477	Arthroscopic: 12.1 Open: 12.5	I: 14 II: 211 III: 252 IV: 0	Arthroscopic: 420 Open: 57	NR	1.12 years
(Shin et al., 2018) [36]	27	10.1 ± 2.2	I: 0 II: 12 III: 13 IV: 2	Arthroscopic: 27 Open: 0	Screw: 27 Suture: 0	3.9 ± 2.2 years
(Sinha et al., 2017) [37]	10	12.1 ± 1.9	NR	Arthroscopic: 10 Open: 0	Screw: 0 Suture: 10	12 months
(Tudisco et al., 2010) [38]	14	12.25 (7–16)	I: 4 II: 3 III: 7 IV: 0	Arthroscopic: 6 Open: 1 Conservative: 7	Screw: 0 Suture: 14	29 (12–42) years

Table 4. *Cont.*

(Author, Year of Publication)	Number of Participants	Mean Age	Meyers and McKeever Classification	Surgical Approach	Fixation Method	Mean Follow-Up Time
(Uboldi et al., 2022) [39]	19	10 (6–13)	I: 0 II: 5 III: 14 IV: 0	Arthroscopic: 19 Open: 0	Screw: 19 Suture: 0	27 (6–60) months
(Vega et al., 2008) [40]	7	11.8	I: 0 II: 0 III: 5 IV: 2	Arthroscopic: 7 Open: 0	Screw: 0 Suture: 0 Both: 7	6 (6–24) months
(Watts et al., 2016) [41]	31	Arthroscopic group: 12.9 (7–18) Open group: 11.5 (7–16)	NR	Arthroscopic: 18 Open: 13	Screw: 17 Suture: 11 Both: 3	Arthroscopic: 13.9 (3–33) months Open: 12.7 (3–50) months
(Wiegand et al., 2014) [42]	8 (+4 treated conservatively)	12.5	I: 4 II: 3 III: 5 IV: 0	Arthroscopic: 8 Open: 0 Conservative: 4	Screw: 8 Suture: 0	1 year
(Wiktor and Tomaszewski, 2022) [43]	17	13.1 (5–15.2)	I: 0 II: 5 III: 10 IV: 2	Arthroscopic: 10 Open: 7	Screw: 17 Suture: 0	28 ± 21.9 months
(Wouters et al., 2010) [44]	12	12.0 (6–15)	NR	Arthroscopic: 12 Open: 0	NR	3–10 years
(Xu et al., 2017) [45]	20	15.3 (13–17)	I: 0 II: 10 III: 6 IV: 4	Arthroscopic: 20 Open: 0	Screw: 0 Suture: 20	43.4 (40–47) months
(Zhang et al., 2020) [46]	21	12.5 (8–16)	I: 0 II: 14 III: 3 (A), 4 (B) IV: 0	Arthroscopic: 21 Open: 0	Screw: 0 Suture: 21	28.4 ± 5.6 months

Table 4. *Cont.*

(Author, Year of Publication)	Number of Participants	Mean Age	Meyers and McKeever Classification	Surgical Approach	Fixation Method	Mean Follow-Up Time
(Zheng et al., 2021) [47]	Group 1 (arthroscopically assisted cannulated screw fixation) = 12 Group 2 (open reduction and cannulated screw internal fixation) = 10	Group 1: 10.94 ± 2.00 Group 2: 10.85 ± 1.53	I: 0 II: 12 III: 22 IV: 0	Arthroscopic: 12 Open: 10	Screw: 22 Suture: 0	27.5 (12–58) months
(Zhou et al., 2023) [48]	Group 1 (transtibial pullout suture technique) = 21 Group 2 (percutaneous pullout suture transverse tunnel) = 20	Group 1: 12.5 ± 2.6 Group 2: 11.3 ± 2.9	I: 0 II: 19 III: 22 IV: 0	Arthroscopic: 41 Open: 0	Screw: 0 Suture: 41	Group 1: 33.27 ± 4.18 months Group 2: 34.15 ± 3.65 months

3.4. Screw vs. Suture Fixation

Treatment with screws was reported for 333 cases, while 313 cases used sutures. A total of 21 cases used both screws and sutures. Thirteen studies reported outcomes with the use of screws only, of which ten studies used ARIF [18,21,24–26,29,30,36,39,42], one study used ORIF [33], and two studies used both ARIF and ORIF [43,47]. Twelve studies reported outcomes with the use of sutures only, of which nine studies used ARIF [11,13,16,31,32,37,45,46,48], and three studies used both ARIF and ORIF [17,19,38]. Four studies directly compared the use of sutures with the use of screws [12,14,22,34].

Of patients undergoing ARIF, 5 patients had complications with suture fixation (5/172, 2.9%), and 21 patients had complications with screw fixation (21/161, 13.0%); the difference was statistically significant (OR 5.01 [95% CI 2.0–12.4], p.0006). The study outcomes have been detailed in Table 5, and the related complications have been detailed in Table 6.

3.5. Screw vs. Suture Risk of Arthrofibrosis

After pooling the outcomes of the studies comparing screw and suture interventions [12,14], the results revealed an increased risk of screw fixation over suture fixation for development of arthrofibrosis however, this did not reach the threshold for statistical significance (OR [95% CI] = 1.18 [0.45, 3.15], $p = 0.74$). A representation of this can be seen in Figure 2.

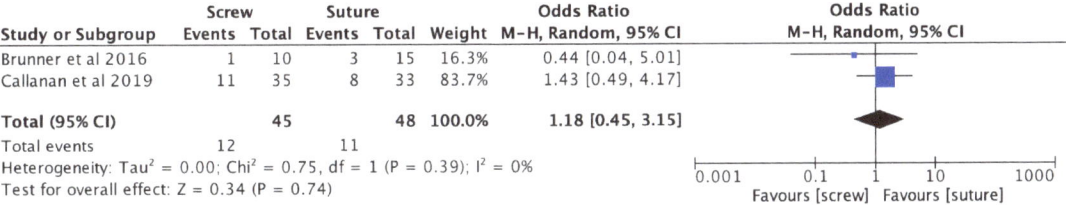

Figure 2. Forest Plot Comparison of Screw vs. Suture for Arthrofibrosis [12,14].

3.6. Screw vs. Suture Risk of Reoperation

After pooling the outcomes of the studies comparing screw and suture interventions [14,22], the results revealed a significantly increased risk of screw fixation over suture fixation for reoperation (OR [95% CI] = 2.81 [1.23, 6.40], $p = 0.01$). A representation of this can be seen in Figure 3.

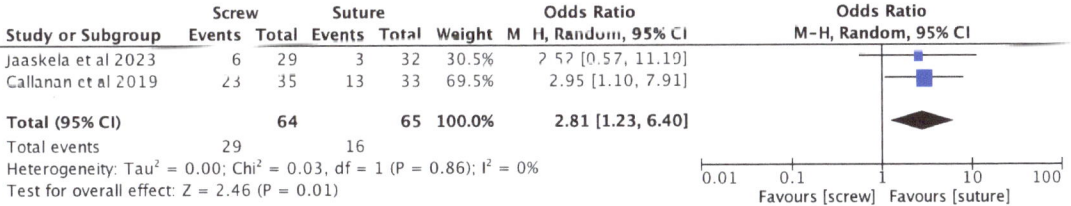

Figure 3. Forest Plot Comparison of Screw vs. Suture for Reoperation [14,22].

Table 5. Study Outcomes. International Knee Documentation Committee (IKDC), Visual Analog Scale (VAS), Association pour la Recherche et la Promotion de l'Étude du Genou (ARPEGE), Knee Injury and Osteoarthritis Outcome Score (KOOS), Activities of Daily Living (ADL), Quality of Life (QOL). NR = Not Reported.

(Author, Year of Publication)	Pre-Surgery IKDC Score	Post-Surgery IKDC Score	Pre-Surgery Lysholm Score	Post-Surgery Lysholm Score	Other Outcomes Pre-Surgery	Other Outcomes Post-Surgery
(Abdelkafy and Said, 2014) [11]	Objective: Grade B (1), Grade C (10), Grade D (2) Subjective: 15.4 ± 4.2	Objective: Grade A (12), Grade B (1) Subjective: 80.5 ± 16.7	3.8 ± 2.5	91.2 ± 8.9	VAS: 8.5 ± 1.2 (pain)	VAS: 9.6 ± 0.5 (operation satisfaction), 0.4 ± 0.5 (pain)
(Brunner et al., 2016) [12]	NR	Objective Group A: Grade A (10), Grade B (5) Objective Group B: Grade A (7), Grade B (3) Subjective: NA	NR	Group A: 94.1 ± 8.1 Group B: 90.1 ± 10.2	NR	Rollimeter difference to ipsilateral knee (mm): Group A: 0.5 ± 0.8 Group B: 0.5 ± 0.7
(Caglar et al., 2021) [13]	NR	Objective: NR Subjective: 6 months: 82.3 (68–91); 12 months: 91.4 (81–100); 24 months: 95.7 (89–100)	NR	NR	NR	NR
(Callanan et al., 2019) [14]	NR	NR	NR	NR	NR	Time to radiographic union: 2.1 years (suture); 4.3 years (screw)
(Casalonga et al., 2010) [15]	NR	Objective: Grade A (4), Grade B (4), Grade C (4), Grade D (1) Subjective: 91 (mailed, n = 10), 81 (at follow-up, n = 13)	NR	NR	NR	ARPEGE Score: 8.3
(Chalopin et al., 2022) [16]	NR	Objective: Grade A (14), Grade B (3) Subjective: 97 ± 2.46	NR	99.1 ± 1.62	NR	NR
(Chotel et al., 2016) [17]	NR	Objective: Grade A (9), Grade B (3), Grade C (1) Subjective: 97 (91–100)	NR	97.36 (94–100)	NR	NR

Table 5. *Cont.*

(Author, Year of Publication)	Pre-Surgery IKDC Score	Post-Surgery IKDC Score	Pre-Surgery Lysholm Score	Post-Surgery Lysholm Score	Other Outcomes Pre-Surgery	Other Outcomes Post-Surgery
(D'ambrosio et al., 2022) [18]	NR	Objective: NR Subjective: 93.8 ± 6.4	NR	93.1 ± 9.8	NR	Average return to sport time: 9.1 ± 9.5 months Average Tegner Score: 5.6 ± 1.5
(Edmonds et al., 2015) [19]	NR	NR	NR	Arthroscopic: 95 Open: 97.4 Conservative: 86	NR	Pain (0–10): Arthroscopic: 0.2 Open: 0.7 Conservative: 2.7
(Furlan et al., 2010) [20]	NR	Objective: Grade A (8), Grade B (2) Subjective: 96 (85–100)	NR	NR	NR	NR
(Hirschmann et al., 2009) [21]	NR	Objective: Grade A (5), Grade B (1) Subjective: 197 ± 4	NR	97 ± 3	Tegner Score: 8 (6–9)	VAS: 0.5 ± 0.8 (pain), 9.5 ± 1.5 (satisfaction) Tegner Score: 8 (6–9)
(Jaaskela et al., 2023) [22]	NR	Objective: NR Subjective: 93.1 ± 13.5 (open osteosuture), 90.4 ± 14.5 (arthroscopic screw)	NR	NR	NR	Time to return to sport (weeks): 8.0 (8–12) (open osteosuture), 21.0 (12–36.3) (arthroscopic screw)
(Kieser et al., 2011) [23]	NR	NR	NR	NR	NR	NR
(Kim et al., 2007) [24]	NR	NR	NR	96.3 (92.6–99.0)	NR	NR
(Kristinsson et al., 2021) [25]	NR	NR	NR	NR	NR	KOOS Scores: (1) Pain: 100 (19–100) (2) Symptoms: 91.0 (54–100) (3) ADL: 100 (22–100) (4) Sport: 90.0 (0–100) (5) QOL: 88.0 (13–100) EQ5D-5L index value: 1.0 (0.225–1) EQ5D-5L VAS–92.0 (50–100)

Table 5. Cont.

(Author, Year of Publication)	Pre-Surgery IKDC Score	Post-Surgery IKDC Score	Pre-Surgery Lysholm Score	Post-Surgery Lysholm Score	Other Outcomes Pre-Surgery	Other Outcomes Post-Surgery
(Liljeros et al., 2009) [26]	NR	NR	NR	93.69	Activity Level (1–3): 2 (1–3)	Activity Level (1–3): 2 (1–3)
(Marie-Laure et al., 2008) [27]	NR	NR	NR	99.7 (95–100)	NR	NR
(Memisoglu et al., 2016) [28]	NR	Objective: Grade A (7), Grade B (4) Subjective: 94.3 (85–100)	NR	95.7 ± 6.6	NR	NR
(Momaya et al., 2017) [29]	NR	Objective: NR Subjective: 97.3 ± 3.5	NR	95.6 ± 5.2	NR	NR
(Najdi et al., 2016) [30]	NR	NR	NR	99.1 ± 1.9	NR	NR
(Perugia et al., 2009) [31]	NR	Objective: Grade A (3), Grade B (4), Grade C (3) Subjective: 92.4 ± 3.3	NR	95.9 ± 2.9	NR	NR
(Russu et al., 2021) [32]	Objective: NR Subjective: 33.4 ± 23.3	Objective: NR Subjective: 84.2 ± 14.3	53.7 ± 17.3	87.7 ± 9.9	Tegner Score: 3.8 ± 1.1	Tegner Score: 6.7 ± 2.2
(Scrimshire et al., 2018) [33]	NR	NR	NR	Operative: 94 (washer used = 92, no washer used = 96) Non-operative: 95	NR	Cincinnati Score: Operative: 96 Non-operative: 96
(Sharma et al., 2008) [34]	NR	NR	NR	Screw and wire (non-absorbable): 89 (69–100) Suture (absorbable): 100 (85–100)	NR	NR
(Shimberg et al., 2022) [35]	NR	NR	NR	NR	NR	NR
(Shin et al., 2018) [36]	NR	NR	NR	94.8 ± 6.8	NR	NR
(Sinha et al., 2017) [37]	NR	NR	50.8 ± 1.4	96.3 ± 2.9	NR	NR

Table 5. Cont.

(Author, Year of Publication)	Pre-Surgery IKDC Score	Post-Surgery IKDC Score	Pre-Surgery Lysholm Score	Post-Surgery Lysholm Score	Other Outcomes Pre-Surgery	Other Outcomes Post-Surgery
(Tudisco et al., 2010) [38]	NR	Objective: Grade A (2), Grade B (11), Grade C (1) Subjective: NR	NR	NR	NR	NR
(Uboldi et al., 2022) [39]	NR	Objective: Grade A (18), Grade B (19) Subjective: 88.45 (80–95)	NR	NR	Tegner Activity Scale: 5.51 (3–7)	Tegner Activity Scale: 5.61 (4–7)
(Vega et al., 2008) [40]	NR	Objective: Grade A (4), Grade B (3) Subjective: 92 (86–98)	29	94	NR	NR
(Watts et al., 2016) [41]	NR	NR	NR	NR	NR	NR
(Wiegand et al., 2014) [42]	NR	NR	NR	Conservative (Type I): 97.00 Arthroscopic (Type II): 94.97 Arthroscopic (Type III): 94.20	NR	NR
(Wiktor and Tomaszewski, 2022) [43]	NR	Objective: NR Subjective: 84.64 ± 3.10	NR	96.64 ± 4.54	NR	NR
(Wouters et al., 2010) [44]	NR	NR	NR	NR	NR	NR
(Xu et al., 2017) [45]	Objective: Grade C (15), Grade D (5) Subjective: NR	Objective: Grade A (13), Grade B (7) Subjective: NR	57.5 ± 11.2	91.0 ± 7.2	Tegner Score: 4.6 ± 1.4	Tegner Score: 8.0 ± 1.7
(Zhang et al., 2020) [46]	Objective: NR Subjective: 43.1 ± 13.2	Objective: NR Subjective: 83.8 ± 6.3	48.3 ± 6.21	87.1 ± 9.8	NR	NR

Table 5. Cont.

(Author, Year of Publication)	Pre-Surgery IKDC Score	Post-Surgery IKDC Score	Pre-Surgery Lysholm Score	Post-Surgery Lysholm Score	Other Outcomes Pre-Surgery	Other Outcomes Post-Surgery
(Zheng et al., 2021) [47]	NR	Objective: NR Subjective: Group 1: 92.06 ± 3.55 Group 2: 86.07 ± 5.81	NR	Group 1: 93.33 ± 3.55 Group 2: 86.20 ± 4.52	NR	Tegner Score: Group 1: 7.75 ± 0.87 Group 2: 6.40 ± 0.52
(Zhou et al., 2023) [48]	Objective: NR Subjective: Group 1: 46.16 ± 12.57 Group 2: 47.27 ± 11.87	Objective: NR Subjective: Group 1: 90.15 ± 8.12 Group 2: 92.14 ± 7.89	Group 1: 43.23 ± 9.54 Group 2: 41.62 ± 10.15	Group 1: 91.08 ± 7.65 Group 2: 92.54 ± 9.17	Tegner Score: Group 1: 3.26 ± 1.54 Group 2: 3.02 ± 1.34 VAS Score: Group 1: 4.86 ± 0.53 Group 2: 5.13 ± 0.71	Tegner Score: Group 1: 5.76 ± 1.12 Group 2: 5.52 ± 1.01 VAS Score: Group 1: 1.23 ± 0.41 Group 2: 1.31 ± 0.51

Table 6. Complications NR = Not Reported.

(Author, Year of Publication)	Wound Infection	Post-Surgical Pain	Stiffness	Instability	Arthrofibrosis	Reoperation	Leg Length Discrepancy	Deep Venous Thrombosis
(Abdelkafy and Said, 2014) [11]	1 (superficial)	0	0	0	0	0	0	0
(Brunner et al., 2016) [12]	0	Group B: 8 (pain around screw)	0	0	Group A: 3 Group B: 1	0	0	0
(Caglar et al., 2021) [13]	0	0	1	1	1	1	0	0
(Callanan et al., 2019) [14]	0	0	Suture: 8 Screw: 11	Suture: 3 Screw: 22	Suture: 8 Screw: 11	Suture: 13 Screw: 23	0	1
(Casalonga et al., 2010) [15]	0	0	3 (Type II)	0	0	1	0	0
(Chalopin et al., 2022) [16]	0	0	0	0	0	0	0	0
(Chotel et al., 2016) [17]	0	0	1	0	0	4	6	0
(D'ambrosio et al., 2022) [18]	0	0	0	5	0	0	0	0
(Edmonds et al., 2015) [19]	0	Conservative: 3	0	0	0	0	0	0
(Furlan et al., 2010) [20]	0	0	0	0	0	0	0	0
(Hirschmann et al., 2009) [21]	0	0	0	0	0	0	0	0
(Jaaskela et al., 2023) [22]	0	Arthroscopic screw: 3	0	Arthroscopic screw: 2	0	Arthroscopic screw: 6 Open osteosuture: 3	0	0
(Kieser et al., 2011) [23]	0	0	0	0	1	2	0	0
(Kim et al., 2007) [24]	0	0	0	0	0	0	0	0
(Kristinsson et al., 2021) [25]	0	0	0	0	0	0	0	0
(Liljeros et al., 2009) [26]	0	1	0	1	0	0	0	0
(Marie-Laure et al., 2008) [27]	0	0	0	0	0	0	0	0
(Memisoglu et al., 2016) [28]	0	0	0	0	0	2	0	0
(Momaya et al., 2017) [29]	0	0	0	0	1	0	0	0
(Najdi et al., 2016) [30]	0	0	1	0	0	0	0	0
(Perugia et al., 2009) [31]	0	0	0	0	0	0	0	0

Table 6. Cont.

(Author, Year of Publication)	Wound Infection	Post-Surgical Pain	Stiffness	Instability	Arthrofibrosis	Reoperation	Leg Length Discrepancy	Deep Venous Thrombosis
(Russu et al., 2021) [32]	NR	NR	NR	NR	NR	NR	NR	NR
(Scrimshire et al., 2018) [33]	0	1	5	0	0	9	0	0
(Sharma et al., 2008) [34]	1	0	0	6	0	1	0	0
(Shimberg et al., 2022) [35]	Arthroscopic: 2 (0.5%)	0	0	0	Arthroscopic: 29 (6.9%) Open: 4 (7.0%)	Arthroscopic: 90 (21%) Open: 18 (32%)	Arthroscopic: 6 (1.4%)	0
(Shin et al., 2018) [36]	0	0	1	0	0	0	10	0
(Tudisco et al., 2010) [38]	0	0	0	Conservative: 1	2	Conservative: 1	0	0
(Uboldi et al., 2022) [39]	0	0	0	0	0	0	0	0
(Vega et al., 2008) [40]	NR	NR	NR	NR	NR	NR	NR	NR
(Watts et al., 2016) [41]	0	0	0	0	Arthroscopic: 7 Open: 1	10	0	0
(Wiegand et al., 2014) [42]	0	0	0	0	1	0	0	0
(Wiktor and Tomaszewski, 2022) [43]	0	0	4	0	0	0	0	0
(Wouters et al., 2010) [44]	0	0	0	0	0	1	0	0
(Xu et al., 2017) [45]	0	0	0	0	0	0	0	0
(Zhang et al., 2020) [46]	0	0	0	0	0	0	0	0
(Zheng et al., 2021) [47]	0	0	0	0	0	0	0	0
(Zhou et al., 2023) [48]	0	0	0	0	0	0	0	0

3.7. Screw vs. Suture Risk of Post-Operative Pain

After pooling the outcomes of the studies comparing screw and suture interventions [12,22], the results revealed a significantly increased risk of screw fixation over suture fixation for post-operative pain (OR [95% CI] = 28.75 [2.45, 337.10], $p = 0.007$). A representation of this can be seen in Figure 4.

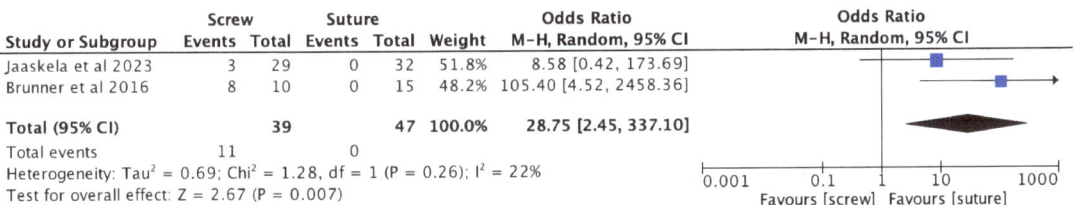

Figure 4. Forest Plot Comparison of Screw vs. Suture for Post-operative Pain [12,22].

3.8. Screw vs. Suture Risk of Instability

The pooled data from the studies comparing screw and suture fixation [14,22] revealed a significantly increased risk of post-operative knee instability with screw fixation over suture fixation (OR [95% CI] = 14.31 [4.09, 50.05], $p < 0.0001$). See Figure 5.

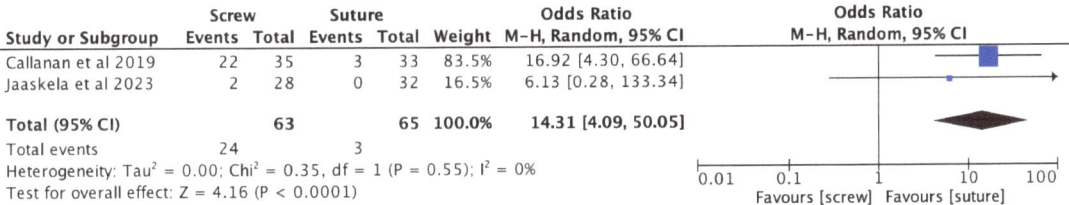

Figure 5. Forest Plot Comparison of Screw vs. Suture for Knee Instability [14,22].

3.9. ORIF vs. ARIF Risk of Arthrofibrosis

The pooled outcomes of the studies comparing ORIF and ARIF fixation techniques [35,41] demonstrated no difference in the risk of arthrofibrosis between ARIF and ORIF (OR [95% CI] = 0.46 [0.06, 3.35], $p = 0.45$). See Figure 6.

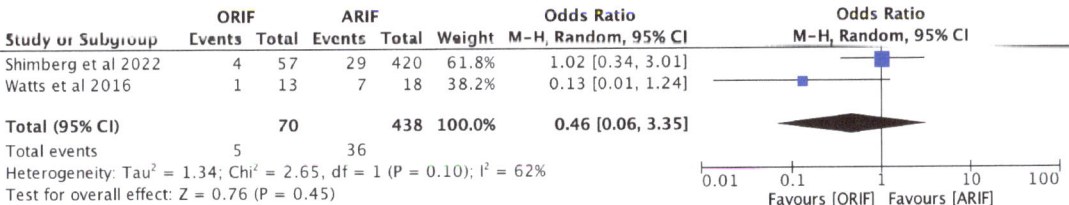

Figure 6. Forest Plot Comparison of ORIF vs. ARIF for Risk of Arthrofibrosis [35,41].

4. Discussion

We present a systematic review of the literature discussing outcomes of ORIF and ARIF techniques for the fixation of paediatric TSAFs using suture and screw materials. TSAFs are increasingly common injuries in adolescents. If left untreated, they can result in significant pain and deformity, with further complications of non-union and malunion [49]. As can be seen across all these studies, the complication rate is low, and good outcomes have been reported with all methods of fixation. There has been a general trend towards arthroscopic management, as evidenced by the current literature. This has several key advantages.

First, there is reduced soft tissue dissection, which may facilitate an earlier range of motion and reduced post-operative pain. The second and perhaps most important advantage is the ability to perform a thorough inspection of the knee joint. In Shimberg et al.'s study, 7% of patients who underwent preoperative MRI had further injuries identified during fixation [50]. There are other studies that have called into question the under-sensitivity of MRI in paediatric cases. Kocher et al. found MRI had a sensitivity of 71% in partial ACL ruptures in adolescents [51]. In a larger cohort study in 2022, Dawkins et al. reported MRI scanning had moderate diagnostic ability to predict meniscal injuries with associated ACL ruptures in adolescents [52]. The performance was particularly poor with lateral meniscal tears (51% sensitivity). This is contrary to the original dogma, which states that MRI is a highly sensitive study for soft tissue near injuries. It appears true that, when ACL or meniscal injuries are present in isolation, MRI is highly sensitive and specific, but the diagnostic accuracy declines in cases where concomitant injuries are present [53]. The sensitivity declines to around 50–75% [52,54–56]. This could have significant implications for management. ARIF would therefore facilitate adequate inspection of the joint prior to proceeding with fixation. While concomitant injuries can be identified with an open approach, diagnostic arthroscopy would likely facilitate more thorough inspection of the joint, particularly the posteromedial and posterolateral corners. What remains unclear from the literature is whether these missed injuries would have significantly impacted the outcomes. However, diagnostic accuracy does remain a priority, and we would certainly recommend preoperative MRI in all cases, especially where the treating surgeon is planning an open approach. While it can be argued that MRI is not necessary in ARIF, we would still advise it for two reasons. First, MRI can facilitate operative planning. Second, MRI has the potential to demonstrate extension of the fracture line into the tibial plateau, which can often be missed on plain radiographs [57].

There was no clear difference in the overall complications between arthroscopic and open approaches. The traditional concern of increased risk of arthrofibrosis with ARIF appears to be unfounded. In Watts et al.'s study, prolonged time to surgery was the more significant factor in the development of arthrofibrosis [41]. This is perhaps more likely to occur in cases of ARIF, as there may be a delay until a surgeon with the appropriate skill set becomes available. Early range of motion is also important in preventing ongoing stiffness and should be encouraged post-operatively, where appropriate [58]. While ARIF provides a minimally invasive approach to fixation, along with shorter hospital stays and lower risks of infection, the surgical outcomes between ORIF and ARIF techniques remain similar. Hence, the choice of fixation technique would be heavily reliant on the experience of the surgeon.

Suture vs. screw fixation is the other key controversy in management. This review demonstrated a higher overall complication risk with screw fixation—reoperation rates were higher due to the need for metalware in screw fixation. Screw fixation can increase the risk of anterior impingement and can damage the femoral notch, but this can be mitigated with the use of a bioabsorbable screw [59]. From the studies in the review, it appears that arthroscopic suture fixation is the most common practice. Suture fixation has been shown to be biomechanically superior to screw fixation when considering the cyclical loads the knee is subjected to [60]. However, there was no difference in load required for overall failure [60]. While there is no clinical evidence to suggest one method is superior to the other with respect to fracture healing and overall outcomes, suture fixation has several additional advantages. First, sutures can be used for more comminuted MM type IV injuries; the degree of comminution may have been underestimated in preoperative imaging [60]. Second, there is a theoretical increased risk of physeal damage with screw placement, which could lead to growth arrest [50]. An all-epiphyseal approach to fixation is essential to avoid growth arrest. A review by Osti et al. also highlighted the controversy between choice of screw versus suture fixation, with screws allowing for more early mobilization and weight bearing compared to sutures [61]. However, the potential to treat small and comminuted fractures with sutures, while avoiding risks of reoperation and impaired bone growth, underlines the need to consider a risk–benefit ratio while choosing fixation materials.

This review was limited by the retrospective nature of the studies, the lack of adequate control groups in many of the studies, and the short overall follow-up. In addition, many studies had low patient numbers. This limited the depth of the meta-analysis possible. However, it is clear that TSAFs have a good prognosis if treated well, regardless of the operative approach or fixation method. We would advocate preoperative MRI in all cases, and arthroscopic suture fixation where possible, as it will allow for the most thorough inspection of the joint, and suture fixation offers superior biomechanical support and greater versatility along with a lower risk of impingement. However, we would caveat this by emphasising that all recognised approaches appear to give good outcomes with low risk of complications when performed well, and the treating surgeon should perform the procedure that best matches their skillset.

5. Conclusions

Overall, good outcomes are reported in TSAFs regardless of the approach or surgical fixation. There is no clear evidence to advocate one method of fixation over another. However, we would recommend arthroscopic suture fixation due to the diagnostic utility of arthroscopy and the biomechanical superiority of suture fixation. Preoperative MRI scans are essential in all cases of operative management, but surgeons should be cognisant of the limitations of MRI. Further evidence is needed to investigate the long-term outcomes and evaluate the significance of concomitant injuries that may be present.

Author Contributions: Conceptualization, A.V. and M.J.; methodology, M.C.; software, M.C.; validation, M.C., R.J. and A.V.; formal analysis, M.C.; investigation, M.C.; resources, M.C.; data curation, M.C.; writing—original draft preparation, M.C. and R.J.; writing—review and editing, M.C., M.J. and A.V.; visualization, M.C.; supervision, A.V.; project administration, M.C. All authors have read and agreed to the published version of the manuscript.

Funding: This research received no external funding.

Institutional Review Board Statement: Not applicable.

Informed Consent Statement: Not applicable.

Conflicts of Interest: The authors declare no conflicts of interest.

Appendix A

Table A1. Detailed Search Strategy with search terms. ? = wild card used to account for missing characters, * = truncation tool used to account for alternative forms of the root word.

Tibial Spine Avulsion Fracture AND	Surgical Management AND	Paediatric Patients
(Tibial OR Tibia) AND (spine OR eminence OR inter?condylar OR inter?condyle) AND fracture OR avulsion Tibial eminence avulsion Tibial eminence fracture Intercondylar fracture Intercondylar avulsion Anterior cruciate ligament avulsion ACL avulsion	Surgery Surgical treatment Surgical management Operative treatment Operative management Surgical technique Management Treatment Fracture fixation Surgical fixation	Paediatric * Child * Youth High school Adolescent * Paediatric surgery Juvenile

References

1. Poncet, A. Arrachement de l'epine du tibia a l'insertion du ligament croise anterieur. *Bull Mem. Soc. Chir. Paris.* **1875**, 883–884.
2. Kendall, N.; Hsu, S.; Chan, K. Fracture of the tibial spine in adults and children. A review of 31 cases. *J. Bone Joint Surg. Br.* **1992**, *74-B*, 848–852. [CrossRef] [PubMed]
3. Sapre, V.; Bagari, V. Tibial Spine Avulsion Fractures: Current Concepts and Technical Note on Arthroscopic Techniques Used in Management of These Injuries. In *Regional Arthroscopy*; InTech: London, UK, 2013. [CrossRef]
4. Meyers, M.H.; McKeever, F.M. Fracture of the Intercondylar Eminence of the Tibia. *J. Bone Jt. Surg.* **1959**, *41*, 209–222. [CrossRef]
5. Zaricznyj, B. Avulsion fracture of the tibial eminence: Treatment by open reduction and pinning. *J Bone Joint Surg. Am.* **1977**, *59*, 1111–1114. [CrossRef] [PubMed]
6. Green, D.; Tuca, M.; Luderowski, E.; Gausden, E.; Goodbody, C.; Konin, G. A new, MRI-based classification system for tibial spine fractures changes clinical treatment recommendations when compared to Myers and Mckeever. *Knee Surg. Sports Traumatol. Arthrosc.* **2019**, *27*, 86–92. [CrossRef] [PubMed]
7. Meyers, A.L.; Tiwari, V.; Nelson, R. *Tibial Eminence Fractures*; StatPearls: St. Petersburg, FL, USA, 2024.
8. Coyle, C.; Jagernauth, S.; Ramachandran, M. Tibial eminence fractures in the paediatric population: A systematic review. *J. Child Orthop.* **2014**, *8*, 149–159. [CrossRef] [PubMed]
9. Ouzzani, M.; Hammady, H.; Fedorowicz, Z.; Elmagarmid, A. Rayyan—A web and mobile app for systematic reviews. *Syst. Rev.* **2016**, *5*, 210. [CrossRef] [PubMed]
10. Slim, K.; Nini, E.; Forestier, D.; Kwiatkowski, F.; Panis, Y.; Chipponi, J. Methodological Index for Non-Randomized Studies (MINORS): Development and Validation of A New Instrument. *ANZ J. Surg.* **2003**, *73*, 712–716. [CrossRef]
11. Abdelkafy, A.; Said, H.G. Neglected ununited tibial eminence fractures in the skeletally immature: Arthroscopic management. *Int. Orthop.* **2014**, *38*, 2525–2532. [CrossRef]
12. Brunner, S.; Vavken, P.; Kilger, R.; Vavken, J.; Rutz, E.; Brunner, R.; Camathias, C. Absorbable and non-absorbable suture fixation results in similar outcomes for tibial eminence fractures in children and adolescents. *Knee Surg. Sports Traumatol. Arthrosc.* **2016**, *24*, 723–729. [CrossRef]
13. Çağlar, C.; Yagar, H.; Emre, F.; Ugurlu, M. Mid-term Outcomes of Arthroscopic Suture Fixation Technique in Tibial Spine Fractures in the Pediatric Population. *Turk. J. Trauma Emerg. Surg.* **2020**, *27*, 571–576. [CrossRef]
14. Callanan, M.; Allen, J.; Flutie, B.; Tepolt, F.; Miller, P.E.; Kramer, D.; Kocher, M.S. Suture Versus Screw Fixation of Tibial Spine Fractures in Children and Adolescents: A Comparative Study. *Orthop. J. Sports Med.* **2019**, *7*, 232596711988196. [CrossRef] [PubMed]
15. Casalonga, A.; Bourelle, S.; Chalencon, F.; De Oliviera, L.; Gautheron, V.; Cottalorda, J. Tibial intercondylar eminence fractures in children: The long-term perspective. *Orthop. Traumatol. Surg. Res.* **2010**, *96*, 525–530. [CrossRef]
16. Chalopin, A.; Geffroy, L.; Decante, C.; Noailles, T.; Hamel, A. Arthroscopic suture fixation of anterior tibial intercondylar eminence fractures by retensioning of the ACL and hollowing of the tibial footprint: Objective and subjective clinical results in a paediatric population. *Orthop. Traumatol. Surg. Res.* **2022**, *108*, 103270. [CrossRef]
17. Chotel, F.; Raux, S.; Accadbled, F.; Gouron, R.; Pfirrmann, C.; Bérard, J.; Seil, R. Cartilaginous tibial eminence fractures in children: Which recommendations for management of this new entity? *Knee Surg. Sports Traumatol. Arthrosc.* **2016**, *24*, 688–696. [CrossRef] [PubMed]
18. D'Ambrosio, A.; Schneider, L.; Bund, L.; Gicquel, P. Anatomical fixation of tibial intercondylar eminence fractures in children using a threaded pin with an adjustable lock. *Orthop. Traumatol. Surg. Res.* **2022**, *108*, 103021. [CrossRef] [PubMed]
19. Edmonds, E.W.; Fornari, E.D.; Dashe, J.; Roocroft, J.H.; King, M.M.; Pennock, A.T. Results of Displaced Pediatric Tibial Spine Fractures: A Comparison Between Open, Arthroscopic, and Closed Management. *J. Pediatr. Orthop.* **2015**, *35*, 651–656. [CrossRef] [PubMed]
20. Furlan, D.; Pogorelic, Z.; Biocic, M.; Juric, I.; Mestrovic, J. Pediatric tibial eminence fractures: Arthroscopic treatment using K-wire. *Scand. J. Surg.* **2010**, *99*, 38–44. [CrossRef]
21. Hirschmann, M.T.; Mayer, R.R.; Kentsch, A.; Friederich, N.F. Physeal sparing arthroscopic fixation of displaced tibial eminence fractures: A new surgical technique. *Knee Surg. Sports Traumatol. Arthrosc.* **2009**, *17*, 741–747. [CrossRef]
22. Jääskelä, M.; Turati, M.; Lempainen, L.; Bremond, N.; Courvoisier, A.; Henri, A.; Accadbled, F.; Sinikumpu, J. Long-term Outcomes of Tibial Spine Avulsion Fractures After Open Reduction with Osteosuturing Versus Arthroscopic Screw Fixation: A Multicenter Comparative Study. *Orthop. J. Sports Med.* **2023**, *11*, 23259671231176991. [CrossRef]
23. Kieser, D.C.; Gwynne-Jones, D.; Dreyer, S. Displaced tibial intercondylar eminence fractures. *J. Orthop. Surg.* **2011**, *19*, 292–298. [CrossRef]
24. Kim, K.T.; Shon, S.K.; Kim, S.S.; Song, C.G.; Ha, I.S. Arthroscopic Internal Fixation of Displaced Tibial Eminence Fracture Using Cannulated Screw. *J. Korean Orthop. Assoc.* **2007**, *42*, 659–664. [CrossRef]
25. Kristinsson, J.; Elsoe, R.; Jensen, H.P.; Larsen, P. Satisfactory outcome following arthroscopic fixation of tibial intercondylar eminence fractures in children and adolescents using bioabsorbable nails. *Arch. Orthop. Trauma Surg.* **2021**, *141*, 1945–1951. [CrossRef]
26. Liljeros, K.; Werner, S.; Janarv, P.-M. Arthroscopic Fixation of Anterior Tibial Spine Fractures with Bioabsorbable Nails in Skeletally Immature Patients. *Am. J. Sports Med.* **2009**, *37*, 923–928. [CrossRef]

27. Marie-Laure, L.; Jean-Marc, G.; Franck, L.; Christophe, T.; Jean-Luc, J.; Gérard, B. Surgical management of type II tibial intercondylar eminence fractures in children. *J. Pediatr. Orthop. B* **2008**, *17*, 231–235.
28. Memisoglu, K.; Muezzinoglu, U.S.; Atmaca, H.; Sarman, H.; Kesemenli, C.C. Arthroscopic fixation with intra-articular button for tibial intercondylar eminence fractures in skeletally immature patients. *J. Pediatr. Orthop. B* **2016**, *25*, 31–36. [CrossRef]
29. Momaya, A.M.; Read, C.; Steirer, M.; Estes, R. Outcomes after arthroscopic fixation of tibial eminence fractures with bioabsorbable nails in skeletally immature patients. *J. Pediatr. Orthop. B* **2018**, *27*, 8–12. [CrossRef]
30. Najdi, H.; Thévenin-lemoine, C.; Sales de gauzy, J.; Accadbled, F. Arthroscopic treatment of intercondylar eminence fractures with intraepiphyseal screws in children and adolescents. *Orthop. Traumatol. Surg. Res.* **2016**, *102*, 447–451. [CrossRef]
31. Perugia, D.; Basiglini, L.; Vadalà, A.; Ferretti, A. Clinical and radiological results of arthroscopically treated tibial spine fractures in childhood. *Int. Orthop.* **2009**, *33*, 243–248. [CrossRef]
32. Russu, O.M.; Pop, T.S.; Ciorcila, E.; Gergely, I.; Zuh, S.-G.; Trâmbițas, C.; Borodi, P.G.; Incze-Bartha, Z.; Feier, A.M.; Georgeanu, V.A. Arthroscopic Repair in Tibial Spine Avulsion Fractures Using Polyethylene Terephthalate Suture: Good to Excellent Results in Pediatric Patients. *J. Pers. Med.* **2021**, *11*, 434. [CrossRef]
33. Scrimshire, A.B.; Gawad, M.; Davies, R.; George, H. Management and outcomes of isolated paediatric tibial spine fractures. *Injury* **2018**, *49*, 437–442. [CrossRef]
34. Sharma, A.; Lakshmannan, P.; Peehal, J.; David, H. An analysis of different types of surgical fixation for avulsion fractures of the anterior tibial spine. *Acta Orthop. Belg.* **2008**, *74*, 90–97.
35. Shimberg, J.L.; Leska, T.M.; Cruz, A.I.; Patel, N.M.; Ellis, H.B.; Ganley, T.J.; Johnson, B.; Milbrandt, T.A.; Yen, Y.-M.; Mistovich, R.J. A Multicenter Comparison of Open Versus Arthroscopic Fixation for Pediatric Tibial Spine Fractures. *J. Pediatr. Orthop.* **2022**, *42*, 195–200. [CrossRef]
36. Shin, C.H.; Lee, D.J.; Choi, I.H.; Cho, T.-J.; Yoo, W.J. Clinical and radiological outcomes of arthroscopically assisted cannulated screw fixation for tibial eminence fracture in children and adolescents. *BMC Musculoskelet. Disord.* **2018**, *19*, 41. [CrossRef]
37. Sinha, S.; Meena, D.; Naik, A.K.; Selvamari, M.; Arya, R.K. Arthroscopic Fixation of Tibial Spine Avulsion in Skeletally Immature: The Technique. *J. Orthop. Case Rep.* **2017**, *7*, 80–84.
38. Tudisco, C.; Giovarruscio, R.; Febo, A.; Savarese, E.; Bisicchia, S. Intercondylar eminence avulsion fracture in children: Long-term follow-up of 14 cases at the end of skeletal growth. *J. Pediatr. Orthop. B* **2010**, *19*, 403–408. [CrossRef]
39. Uboldi, F.M.; Trezza, P.; Panuccio, E.; Memeo, A. Arthroscopic treatment of tibial intercondylar eminence fractures in skeletally immature patients with bioabsorbable nails. *La Pediatr. Medica E Chir.* **2022**, *44*. [CrossRef]
40. Vega, J.R.; Irribarra, L.A.; Baar, A.K.; Iñiguez, M.; Salgado, M.; Gana, N. Arthroscopic Fixation of Displaced Tibial Eminence Fractures: A New Growth Plate–Sparing Method. *Arthrosc. J. Arthrosc. Relat. Surg.* **2008**, *24*, 1239–1243. [CrossRef]
41. Watts, C.D.; Larson, A.N.; Milbrandt, T.A. Open Versus Arthroscopic Reduction for Tibial Eminence Fracture Fixation in Children. *J. Pediatr. Orthop.* **2016**, *36*, 437–439. [CrossRef]
42. Wiegand, N.; Naumov, I.; Vámhidy, L.; Nöt, L.G. Arthroscopic treatment of tibial spine fracture in children with a cannulated Herbert screw. *Knee* **2014**, *21*, 481–485.
43. Wiktor, Ł.; Tomaszewski, R. Results of Anterior Cruciate Ligament Avulsion Fracture by Treatment Using Bioabsorbable Nails in Children and Adolescents. *Children* **2022**, *9*, 1897. [CrossRef] [PubMed]
44. Wouters, D.B.; de Graaf, J.S.; Hemmer, P.H.; Burgerhof, J.G.M.; Kramer, W.L.M. The arthroscopic treatment of displaced tibial spine fractures in children and adolescents using Meniscus Arrows®. *Knee Surg. Sports Traumatol. Arthrosc.* **2011**, *19*, 736–739. [CrossRef] [PubMed]
45. Xu, X.; Liu, Z.; Wen, H.; Pan, X. Arthroscopic fixation of pediatric tibial eminence fractures using suture anchors: A mid term follow-up. *Arch. Orthop. Trauma Surg.* **2017**, *137*, 1409–1416. [CrossRef]
46. Zhang, L.; Zhang, L.; Zheng, J.; Ren, B.; Kang, X.; Zhang, X.; Dang, X. Arthroscopic tri-pulley Technology reduction and internal fixation of pediatric Tibial Eminence fracture: A retrospective analysis. *BMC Musculoskelet. Disord.* **2020**, *21*, 408. [CrossRef]
47. Zheng, C.; Han, H.; Cao, Y. Arthroscopically Assisted Cannulated Screw Fixation for Treating Type III Tibial Intercondylar Eminence Fractures: A Short-Term Retrospective Controlled Study. *Front. Surg.* **2021**, *8*, 639270. [CrossRef]
48. Zhou, Y.; Deng, G.; She, H.; Zhou, Y.; Xiang, B.; Bai, F. Arthroscopic percutaneous pullout suture transverse tunnel technique repair for tibial spine fractures in skeletally immature patients. *Int. Orthop.* **2023**, *47*, 1353–1360. [CrossRef]
49. Vannabouathong, C.; Ayeni, O.R.; Bhandari, M. A Narrative Review on Avulsion Fractures of the Upper and Lower Limbs. *Clin. Med. Insights Arthritis Musculoskelet. Disord.* **2018**, *11*, 1179544118809050. [CrossRef]
50. Shimberg, J.L.; Aoyama, J.T.; Leska, T.M.; Ganley, T.J.; Fabricant, P.D.; Patel, N.M.; Cruz, A.I.; Ellis, H.B.; Schmale, G.A.; Green, D.W.; et al. Tibial Spine Fractures: How Much Are We Missing Without Pretreatment Advanced Imaging? A Multicenter Study. *Am. J. Sports Med.* **2020**, *48*, 3208–3213. [CrossRef] [PubMed]
51. Kocher, M.S.; Micheli, L.J.; Zurakowski, D.; Luke, A. Partial Tears of the Anterior Cruciate Ligament in Children and Adolescents. *Am. J. Sports Med.* **2002**, *30*, 697–703. [CrossRef]
52. Dawkins, B.J.; Kolin, D.A.; Park, J.; Fabricant, P.D.; Gilmore, A.; Seeley, M.; Mistovich, R.J. Sensitivity and Specificity of MRI in Diagnosing Concomitant Meniscal Injuries with Pediatric and Adolescent Acute ACL Tears. *Orthop. J. Sports Med.* **2022**, *10*, 232596712210793. [CrossRef]
53. Bouju, Y.; Carpentier, E.; Bergerault, F.; De Courtivron, B.; Bonnard, C.; Garaud, P. The concordance of MRI and arthroscopy in traumatic meniscal lesions in children. *Orthop. Traumatol. Surg. Res.* **2011**, *97*, 712–718. [CrossRef]

54. Samora, W.P.; Palmer, R.; Klingele, K.E. Meniscal Pathology Associated with Acute Anterior Cruciate Ligament Tears in Patients with Open Physes. *J. Pediatr. Orthop.* **2011**, *31*, 272–276. [CrossRef]
55. Gans, I.; Baldwin, K.D.; Ganley, T.J. Treatment and Management Outcomes of Tibial Eminence Fractures in Pediatric Patients. *Am. J. Sports Med.* **2014**, *42*, 1743–1750. [CrossRef]
56. Munger, A.M.; Gonsalves, N.R.; Sarkisova, N.; Clarke, E.; VandenBerg, C.D.; Pace, J.L. Confirming the Presence of Unrecognized Meniscal Injuries on Magnetic Resonance Imaging in Pediatric and Adolescent Patients with Anterior Cruciate Ligament Tears. *J. Pediatr. Orthop.* **2019**, *39*, e661–e667. [CrossRef]
57. Cirrincione, P.M.; Salvato, D.; Chipman, D.E.; Mintz, D.N.; Fabricant, P.D.; Green, D.W. Extension of Tibial Spine Fractures Beyond the Tibial Spine: An MRI Analysis of 54 Patients. *Am. J. Sports Med.* **2023**, *51*, 2085–2090. [CrossRef] [PubMed]
58. Kushare, I.; Lee, R.J.; Ellis, H.B.; Fabricant, P.D.; Ganley, T.J.; Green, D.W.; McKay, S.; Patel, N.M.; Schmale, G.A.; Weber, M.; et al. Tibial Spine Fracture Management—Technical Tips and Tricks from the Tibial Spine Fracture Research Interest Group. *J. Pediatr. Orthop. Soc. N. Am.* **2020**, *2*, 68. [CrossRef]
59. Salvato, D.; Green, D.W.; Accadbled, F.; Tuca, M. Tibial spine fractures: State of the art. *J. ISAKOS* **2023**, *8*, 404–411. [CrossRef] [PubMed]
60. Eggers, A.K.; Becker, C.; Weimann, A.; Herbort, M.; Zantop, T.; Raschke, M.J.; Petersen, W. Biomechanical Evaluation of Different Fixation Methods for Tibial Eminence Fractures. *Am. J. Sports Med.* **2007**, *35*, 404–410.
61. Osti, L.; Buda, M.; Soldati, F.; Del Buono, A.; Osti, R.; Maffulli, N. Arthroscopic treatment of tibial eminence fracture: A systematic review of different fixation methods. *Br. Med. Bull.* **2016**, *118*, 77–94. [CrossRef] [PubMed]

Disclaimer/Publisher's Note: The statements, opinions and data contained in all publications are solely those of the individual author(s) and contributor(s) and not of MDPI and/or the editor(s). MDPI and/or the editor(s) disclaim responsibility for any injury to people or property resulting from any ideas, methods, instructions or products referred to in the content.

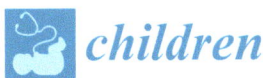

Article

Treatment of Refractory Congenital Pseudoarthrosis of Tibia with Contralateral Vascularized Fibular Bone Graft and Anatomic Distal Tibial Locking Plate: A Case Series and Literature Review

Te-Feng Arthur Chou [1,2,3], Ting-Yu Liu [1,2,4], Matthew N. Wang [1,4] and Chen-Yuan Yang [1,4,*]

1. Department of Orthopaedics, Kuang Tien General Hospital, Taichung 433401, Taiwan
2. Department of Orthopaedics and Traumatology, Taipei Veterans General Hospital, Taipei 112201, Taiwan
3. Department of Orthopaedic Surgery, Montefiore Medical Center, Albert Einstein College of Medicine, The Bronx, NY 10461, USA
4. Department of Nursing, Hungkuang University, Taichung 433304, Taiwan
* Correspondence: chenyuanyangmd@gmail.com; Tel.: +886-4-2662-5111

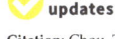

Citation: Chou, T.-F.A.; Liu, T.-Y.; Wang, M.N.; Yang, C.-Y. Treatment of Refractory Congenital Pseudoarthrosis of Tibia with Contralateral Vascularized Fibular Bone Graft and Anatomic Distal Tibial Locking Plate: A Case Series and Literature Review. *Children* 2023, *10*, 503. https://doi.org/10.3390/children10030503

Academic Editor: Johannes Mayr

Received: 6 February 2023
Revised: 27 February 2023
Accepted: 28 February 2023
Published: 3 March 2023

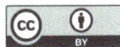

Copyright: © 2023 by the authors. Licensee MDPI, Basel, Switzerland. This article is an open access article distributed under the terms and conditions of the Creative Commons Attribution (CC BY) license (https://creativecommons.org/licenses/by/4.0/).

Abstract: Background: Congenital pseudoarthrosis of the tibia (CPT) remains a challenge for physicians. Several treatment options have been proposed, but the standard of care remains inconclusive. In this study, we present three patients for whom the failure of prior treatments was managed with a contralateral vascularized fibular bone graft (VFG) and an anatomic distal tibial locking plate. Methods: Between 2017 and 2021, three patients were referred for failed treatment of CPT. All patients had undergone multiple prior surgeries, including tumor excision and fixation with ring external fixators, plates, and screws. We performed radical tumor resection and reconstruction of bone defects with a VFG. The construct was fixed with an anatomic locking plate, and the patients were followed up for a mean of 45.7 months. Results: All three patients were able to obtain graft union at 19.3 weeks. At the final follow-up, all grafts achieved bony hypertrophy without evidence of bone resorption or local tumor recurrence. There was a mean leg length difference of 8.5 cm preoperatively, compared with 6.3 cm postoperatively. The average lower leg angulation was 7.4 degrees and the average ankle range of motion was 58.3 degrees. The mean VAS score was 0 and the mean AOFAS score was 88.3. No significant complications were noted. Conclusions: Implantation of a VFG and an anatomic distal tibia locking plate can be considered an option for treatment-refractory CPT. Patients can expect to achieve bone consolidation, ambulate as tolerated, and have a low complication rate.

Keywords: congenital pseudoarthrosis of tibia; autologous vascularized bone graft; free-fibular bone graft; tibial nonunion; neurofibromatosis; anatomic distal tibia locking plate

1. Introduction

Congenital pseudoarthrosis of the tibia (CPT) remains one of the most challenging conditions to manage [1]. The incidence is reported to be between 1:140,000 and 1:250,000 live births, and is frequently associated with neurofibromatosis (NF) [2]. Other conditions, such as fibrous dysplasia and osteofibrous dysplasia, may also be associated with CPT [3]. Although the cause of CPT remains inconclusive, several hypotheses, such as vascular compromise, soft tissue interposition, and a lack of osteoblastic activity have been considered as the initial pathologic process [3]. CPT is characterized by spontaneous fracture of the tibia in the pediatric population, and the probability of achieving unequivocal union, without refracture, with the index procedure is only about 50% [4]. Therefore, the ideal treatment remains inconclusive [3]. The standard procedure generally involves resection of the pseudoarthrosis site, the pathologic osseous tissue, and the surrounding fibrous hamartoma [3]. The remaining bone defect can be reconstructed with a bone graft, a bone transport, and/or a free vascularized fibular bone graft (VFG), and stabilized with either an internal device or external fixation [5–8]. A VFG has the advantage of restoring the extensive defect with strut bone and healthy periosteum simultaneously, while fixation methods such as screws, smooth intramedullary (IM) rods, or an external fixator are also used to stabilize the CPT lesion [7–10]. However, concerns with IM rods include difficulty with nail entry and passage due to osseous deformities, the inadequate purchase of the distal tibial fragment, and the risk of nail exchange due to skeletal development [3]. With the advancements in anatomic plate designs and surgical techniques, most studies have confirmed that tibial plating and intramedullary devices yield comparable outcomes for traumatic fractures of the distal tibia [11]. Moreover, biomechanical analysis revealed that plating can be more advantageous than intramedullary nails for a distal tibial fracture, for which it provides a sufficient amount of axial interfragmentary movement [12]. In this study, we present three CPT patients for whom multiple prior surgical treatments that were performed at other institutions failed. All three patients were managed with radical excision of the diseased bone, while reconstruction with a contralateral VFG and fixation with an anatomic distal tibia locking plate were achieved. In addition, a literature review was completed to review the current management options for CPT.

2. Materials and Methods

This is a retrospective review of 3 patients who underwent revision open reduction and internal fixation (re-ORIF) with a VFG and a distal tibia locking plate for non-united CPT. The study was designed in accordance with the Declaration of Helsinki, and approved by the ethics committee of our institution. The surgeries were performed by a single fellowship-trained (microsurgery and trauma) orthopaedic surgeon (CYY) at a regional medical center in Taichung, Taiwan. Each patient had a confirmed diagnosis of neurofibromatosis type 1 (NF-1), a nonunion of CPT that was previously managed with multiple surgical interventions, and had a minimum follow-up of more than 30 months. We excluded patients with other causes of tibia pseudoarthrosis, CPT patients who did not have prior surgical treatments, patients with ongoing infections, and patients that had vascular disorders and coagulopathies. The age, gender, affected side, and number and type of prior surgeries were recorded for each patient.

Preoperative evaluation:

All patients underwent standard anteroposterior and lateral radiographs of the lower leg. A full lower-extremity scanogram was also performed to assess for leg length discrepancy (LLD) (Figure 1). The Crawford Classification was used to determine the type of CPT [13]. In addition, a computed tomography angiography (CTA) was performed to evaluate the vascular anatomy (specifically for patent peroneal, anterior tibial, and posterior tibial vessels) of bilateral lower extremities. Ambulating distance was assessed by having the patient ambulate and recording the distance when the patient elected to stop due to discomfort.

Surgical method:

Under general anesthesia, the patient was placed in a supine position and both lower extremities were draped with a sterile technique. A sterile tourniquet was applied over the affected limb and was inflated prior to incision. The pseudoarthrosis site was confirmed and marked under fluoroscopy. A longitudinal anterolateral incision was made just lateral to the tibial crest. The incision extended 7 cm above the fracture site and ended at the level of the ankle joint. The fascia was then excised and blunt dissection was carried down to the CPT. The dense fibrotic hamartoma and diseased periosteum around the CPT lesion (Figure 2A) were radically removed until both ends of the tibia had visible bleeding with healthy bone stock and normal periosteum. The medullary canal was debrided and recanalized to improve graft incorporation. Correction of the antero-lateral deformity was then applied under direct visualization and with the assistance of fluoroscopic images. The size of the defect was measured. The tibial artery and two accompanying veins were identified and marked with vessel loops (Figure 2B). The wound was packed with moist gauze and the tourniquet was deflated.

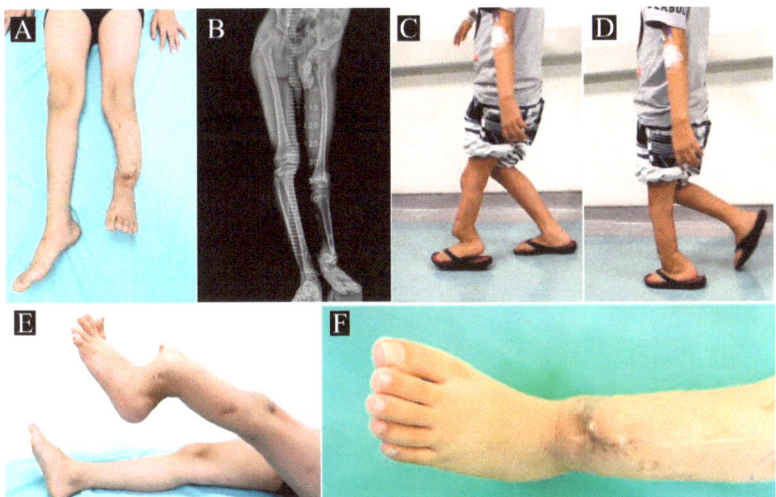

Figure 1. Preoperative evaluation of patient 2. (**A**) Leg length discrepancy (LLD) of 10.2 cm is noted; (**B**) full scanogram confirming the LLD; (**C**) left lower leg deformity prior to weight bearing; (**D**) severe deformity in left lower leg with weight bearing; (**E**) significant angulation upon leg raising; (**F**) near-penetration of the skin due to deformity.

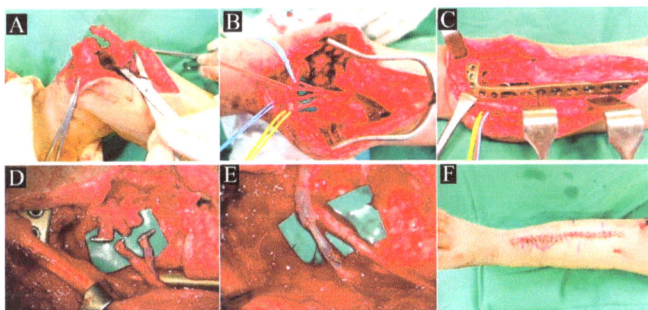

Figure 2. Intraoperative findings: (**A**) the pseudoarthrosis site; (**B**) Radical excision and identification of the anterior tibial artery (red) and veins (blue); (**C**) fibular graft implantation and placement of the anterolateral locking plate; (**D**) preparation for anastomosis of donor and recipient vessels; (**E**) completion of end-to-end anastomosis; (**F**) postoperative wound closure.

Attention was then turned to the contralateral fibula. A longitudinal incision over the midportion of the lateral calf in line with the fibula was made, and then dissection was performed between the interval of the peroneus muscle and the soleus muscle to expose the fibula. The middle third of the fibula, together with the surrounding healthy periosteum and nutrient vessels (branches of the peroneal artery and two accompanying veins), was harvested. The size of the graft was determined based on the measured defect size (Figure 3A,C). Careful attention was taken to ensure that the graft did not extend beyond the mid 1/3 of the fibula (Figure 3B) in order to preserve ankle joint stability.

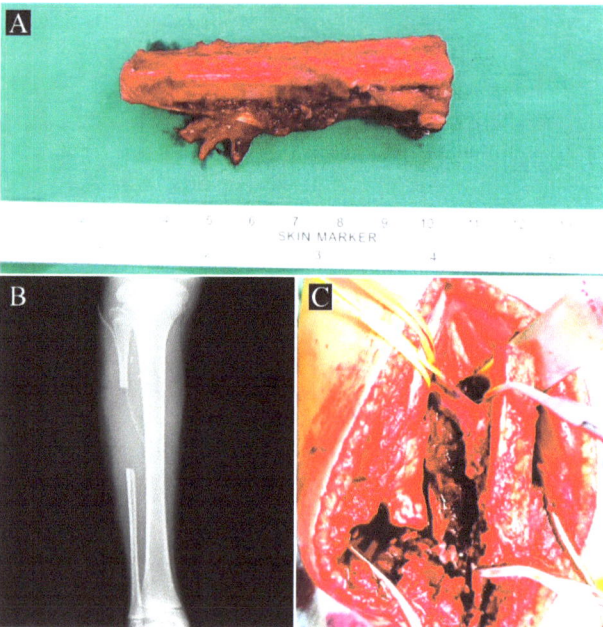

Figure 3. Harvesting the contralateral vascularized fibular graft: (**A**) harvested vascularized graft; (**B**) postoperative X-ray indicating well-preserved fibula beyond the mid-diaphysis region; (**C**) intraoperative image showing the donor peroneal artery and vein and fibular bone graft.

The tourniquet was inflated once again. Prior to inserting the VFG into the defect, the proximal end of the VFG was slightly tapered to fit the narrow intramedullary canal of the tibia shaft. The distal end of the tibia was mainly composed of the wider tibial metaphysis in which the graft could slide with ease. A 3.5 mm medial or anterolateral anatomic distal tibia locking plate® (DePuy Synthes, Raynham, MA, USA) was used to stabilize the distal tibia and VFG (Figure 2C). Tension-free end-to-end anastomoses were completed between the donor peroneal artery and the recipient anterior tibial artery, and between the donor peroneal vein and the recipient anterior tibial vein (Figure 2E). The tourniquet was deflated and a patent circulation between the donor and recipient sites was confirmed. A hemovac® (Zimmer Biomet, Warsaw, IN, USA) was inserted. The affected fibula was also treated with radical excision of the hamartoma and the diseased periosteum, then fixed with an appropriately sized Kirschner wire. The incisions were closed and the patient was placed in a below-knee short leg splint.

Postoperative care:

The patient remained immobilized and non-weight-bearing in the short leg splint for 4 weeks. Clinic follow-ups were arranged at 2 weeks, 4 weeks, 6 weeks, and every 4–6 weeks after the 6th week. Plain radiographs and neurovascular exams were completed at each follow-up visit. At 2 weeks, wound inspection and removal of the sutures were completed. At 4 weeks, the splint was removed and the passive range of motion was initiated. Partial assisted weight bearing was also permitted. The patient was allowed to weight-bear as tolerated when the following 3 criteria were met: (1) radiographic evidence of osseus formation filling in the fracture site or bridging callus surrounding the defect, (2) non-tender fracture site, and (3) pain-free upon full weight bearing. At 2.5 years after the operation, the final LLD, lower leg angulation, visual analogue pain scale (VAS), ambulation distance, range of motion in the affected knee and ankle, and AOFAS score were assessed.

3. Results

Between 2017 and 2021, a total of three patients with NF-1 complicated with nonunion of CPT were included in this study. All of the patients had a type IV CPT. The mean age was 11 years, the mean follow-up time was 45.7 months, and the mean LLD was 8.5 cm. The baseline characteristics of each patient are shown in Table 1 and the serial preoperative X-rays of patient 2 are shown in Figure 4.

Table 1. Patient demographic.

Patient	Age (Years)	Gender	Laterality	Pseudoarthrosis *	LLD (cm)	Ambulation (Meters)	Prior Surgeries	F/u Time (Months)
1	9	F	R	Type IV	11.1	50	ORIF:2 ROI:2 BG:1	65
2	11	M	L	Type IV	10.2	10	ORIF:1 IEF:3 ROI:2	42
3	13	M	L	Type IV	4.1	30	ORIF:4 ROI:1 BG:2	30
Mean	11				8.5	30	6	45.7

* Classified based on Crawford classification; LLD—limb length discrepancy; F/u—follow-up; ORIF—open reduction and internal fixation; IEF—Ilizarov external fixation; ROI—removal of implant; BG—bone graft.

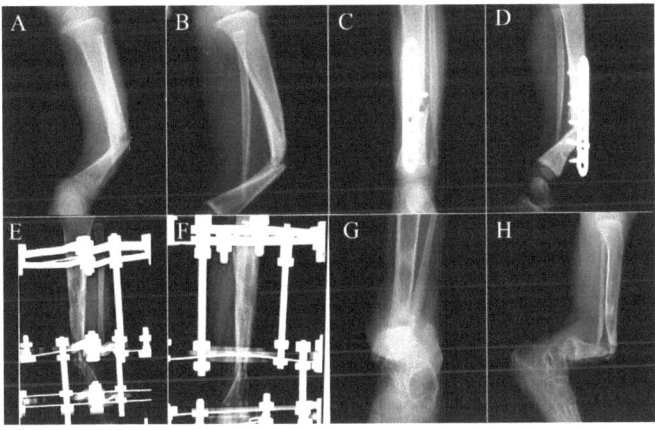

Figure 4. Serial X-rays of patient 2 prior to this correction surgery: (A) anteroposterior (AP) and (B) lateral views of left lower leg at 2 years old; recurrence of deformity (C) AP and (D) lateral views after first correction surgery at age 3; the patient was then placed in an Ilizarov frame, as seen in (E) AP and (F) lateral views, but recurrence occurred at age 4; (G) and (H) show the patient's deformity at age 11 upon presenting to our institution.

3.1. Intraoperative Findings

The procedure type and intraoperative findings are shown in Table 2. The mean operative time was 20 h. Patient 1 had a CVG graft size of 10 cm, and the tibia was fixed with an anatomic medial distal tibia locking plate ® (DePuy Synthes, Raynham, MA, USA). Patient 2 underwent a similar procedure, aside from using an anterolateral distal tibia locking plate ® (DePuy Synthes, Raynham, MA, USA). In addition, because of significant soft tissue contracture due to multiple prior surgeries and chronic LLD, we performed V-Y Achilles tendon lengthening to accommodate the soft tissue contracture. We were able to gain approximately 5 cm of soft tissue lengthening after the V-Y advancement. Patient 3 required a two-stage procedure due to secondary skin contracture after prior surgeries.

The first stage was a CPT excision and a tibia-lengthening procedure with a Taylor spatial frame. Over a 5-week period, the TSP was adjusted daily and we were able to lengthen the tibia by 4 cm. This was deemed within an acceptable range. The patient subsequently underwent a definitive second-stage procedure with VFG implantation and fixation with a similar anterolateral distal tibia locking plate. All of the patients were able to achieve primary skin closure (Figure 2F).

Table 2. Intraoperative findings.

Patient	Procedure	Graft Fixation	Graft Length (cm)	Operative Time
1	CPT excision and reconstruction with contralateral VFG	Anatomic medial distal tibia locking plate	10	16.5 h
2	CPT excision, Achilles tendon lengthening and reconstruction with contralateral VFG	Anatomic anterolateral distal tibia locking plate	7	20.5 h
3	1st stage: CPT excision and tibia lengthening with TSP 2nd stage: reconstruction with contralateral VFG	Anatomic anterolateral distal tibia locking plate	10	23 h

CPT—congenital pseudoarthrosis of the tibia; VFG—vascularized fibular graft; TSP—Taylor spatial frame.

3.2. Postoperative Follow-Up

The postoperative information for each patient is shown in Table 3. All three patients were able to achieve bone consolidation at a mean of 19.3 weeks. This was maintained to the final follow-up for all three patients. All of the fibular grafts incorporated well with bony hypertrophy without evidence of bone resorption or local CPT recurrence (Figure 5). There was a mean postoperative leg length discrepancy of 6.3 cm. The average lower leg angulation was 7.4° and the average ankle range of motion was 58.3 degrees. The mean VAS score was 0 and the mean AOFAS score was 88.3. Figure 6 shows clinical images of patient 2 at postoperative 30 months.

Patient 1 had a final LLD of 8.5 cm with a 15° right lower leg valgus deformity. Although the tibia remained consolidated, the fibula was complicated with pseudoarthrosis which was starting at the 20-month follow-up. At the final follow-up (65 months), the patient had a VAS score of 0, and was able to ambulate without restrictions. Her knee ROM was full, and ankle ROM was 75°. For patient 2, bone consolidation was noted at 20 weeks, and his residual LLD was 7.5 cm with 4.7° lower leg angulation. At the final follow-up (42 months), he was able to walk without pain (VAS 0), and was able to walk for 1000 m. However, he continued to have a progressing LLD and currently requires a 5 cm shoe lift. Since his physeal was preserved and he continues to grow taller, he will potentially require corrective surgery in the future. The postoperative clinical images are shown in Figure 6. Patient 3 achieved bone consolidation at 21 weeks. At his final follow-up (30 months), his residual bone defect was 3.0 cm with 2.3° lower leg angulation, and he was able to ambulate without pain or restrictions. The ESF incisions healed without complications. No significant disability-causing complications such as neurovascular deficits, wound dehiscence, limb edema, or donor site morbidity (e.g., peroneal nerve injury, knee or ankle joint instability, or lower extremity weakness) were noted. The preoperative and postoperative radiographs of patients 1 and 3 are displayed in Figures 7 and 8.

Table 3. Postoperative radiologic and functional outcomes (at 30 months).

Patient	Graft Consolidation	Final LLD	Angulation	VAS	Ambulation Distance	ROM	AOFAS Score
1	17 weeks	8.5 cm	valgus 15°	0	Without limitations	Knee: full/Ankle: 75°	88
2	20 weeks	7.5 cm	valgus 4.8°	0	1000 m	Knee: full/Ankle: 50°	82
3	21 weeks	3.0 cm	valgus 2.3°	0	Without limitations	Knee: full/Ankle: 50°	95

LLD—leg length discrepancy; VAS—visual analogue scale; AOFAS—American Orthopedic Foot & Ankle Society.

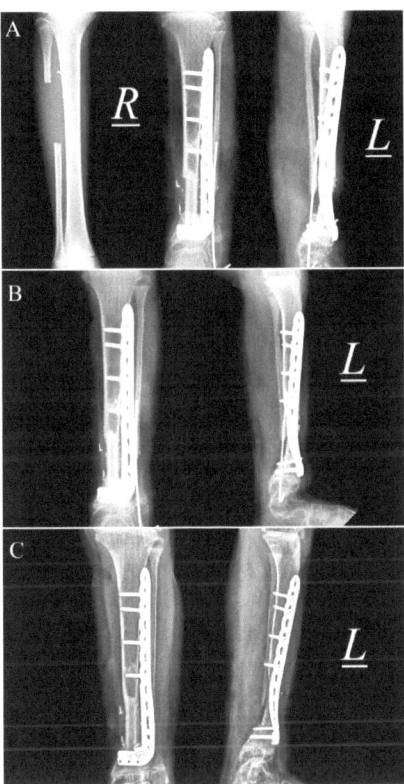

Figure 5. Postoperative follow-up X-ray images of patient 2: (**A**) postoperative 4 weeks with R indicating the right lower leg and L indicating the left. Both anteroposterior (AP) and lateral views are shown for the left. (**B**) AP and lateral X-ray of left lower leg at 3 months. (**C**) AP and lateral X-ray of left lower leg at 12 months.

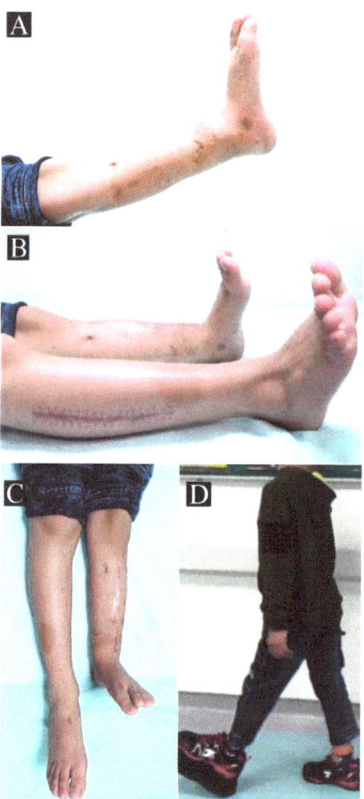

Figure 6. Postoperative clinical images for patient 2 at postoperative 30 months. (**A**) The patient is able to fully extend his knee with no gross angular deformities in the left lower leg. (**B**) Range of motion in bilateral ankles is preserved. (**C**) Leg length discrepancy around 7.5 cm is noted. (**D**) With a 5 cm shoe lift, the patient is able to ambulate with minimal discomfort.

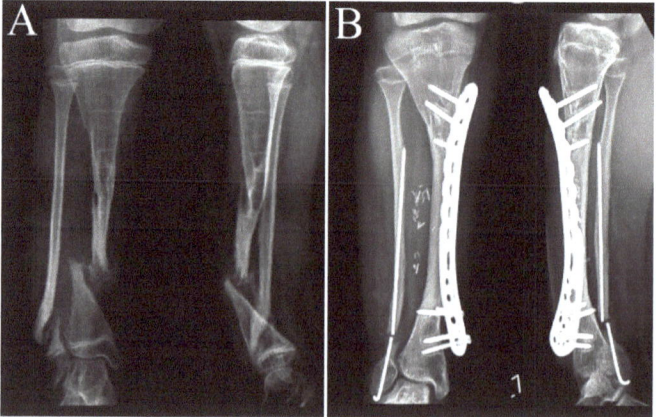

Figure 7. Radiographs of patient 1: (**A**) preoperative AP and lateral radiographs and (**B**) postoperative AP and lateral radiographs at 53 months after the surgery.

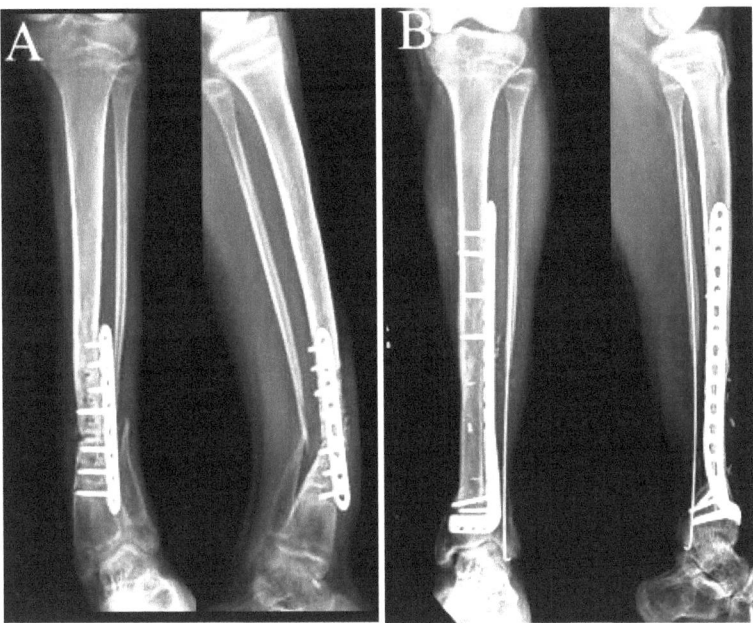

Figure 8. Radiographs of patient 3: (**A**) preoperative AP and lateral radiographs and (**B**) postoperative AP and lateral radiographs at 18 months after the surgery.

4. Discussion

In this study, we presented three patients who had NF-1 complicated with repeated failed surgical treatment of CPT, and each subsequently underwent a successful revision surgery with VFG implantation and anatomic distal tibia locking plate fixation. The most significant finding was that all three patients were able to achieve bone consolidation at a mean of 19.3 weeks, and were able to ambulate without pain and restore good ankle function by the final follow-up (mean 45.7 months). In addition, there was no evidence of recurrence during our follow-up period.

There are two main pathologic processes in CPT. The first is pathobiological, in which there is diseased soft tissue (e.g., hamartoma formation and pathologic periosteum) leading to osteolysis and vascular compromise in the local region [4]. In addition, a pathomechanical process occurs, leading to angular deformities and atrophic bone ends [4]. Therefore, treatment options that can address both pathologies is required. In the current literature, the treatment options for reconstruction following the radical excision of CPT lesions are (1) a bone graft and internal fixation with an IM rod or ring external fixator, (2) bone transport, and (3) free VFG transfer with (4) amputation reserved for refractory cases [4]. Although the optimal treatment remains inconclusive, VFG implantation theoretically provides structural support with a healthy periosteum, sufficient length, low donor site morbidities, and reliable circulation that can hasten the healing of the CPT site [3]. In two case series reports, the bone consolidation rate was reported to be near 94–100% with a very low recurrence rate [8,14]. Our results are in agreement, as we were able to achieve consolidation at an average of 19.3 weeks with no evidence of recurrence up to at least 30 months after the surgery. In our series, the short- to mid-term results are promising, but the long-term results remain to be determined.

When treating CPT, one of the most important factors is to apply rigid fixation, in order to maintain axial, rotational, and angular stability at the CPT site [4]. Most studies have favored the use of IM rods, ring external fixators, and screws as the fixation method [6–8]. The screws were the weakest mechanically, and ring external fixators have disadvantages such as Schanz screws/wires loosening or pin tract infection after long-term usage. The IM rods seemed to be an option with better fixation stability; however, in the refractory CPT cases, the lesion sites were mostly located in the very distal tibia and fibula [4,14]. This makes it very difficult to establish reliable mechanical stability with only IM devices or ring external fixators in the small distal tibia fragment after extensively resecting the fibrous hamartoma. Therefore, our experience was that fixation with a plate system was more favorable.

In this study, we elected to use distal tibia anatomic locking plates to provide a rigid construct (avoiding rotational and angular deforming forces) in order to reduce refracture and malalignment [15,16]. In the past, controversies with plating caused concern about higher failure rates. However, most of these studies utilized conventional non-locking plates, which have different mechanical properties, and the plates were generally bulkier, which would further increase soft tissue tension and obscure the anastomosing sites [7,17]. Interestingly, the three patients presented in our series were previously treated with straight-type non-anatomic locking plates® (DePuy Synthes, Raynham, MA, USA), which all failed due to distal metaphyseal fragment loosening and screw pullout. With the development of low-profile 3.5 mm anatomic distal tibia locking plates with more metaphyseal screws, these concerns seem less problematic [4]. In our study, anastomosis was achieved between the peroneal vessels on the VFG and the recipient anterior tibial vessels, which are located in the anterior leg compartment. Since the plates were relatively low-profile, they did not obscure the surgical field and we were able to complete the anastomosis with relative ease. Moreover, a lower-profile plate placed less tension on the surrounding soft tissue. This is crucial in patients with CPT to allow for wound closure.

In our first patient, a medial distal tibia LCP® (DePuy Synthes, Raynham, MA, USA) was used. Although consolidation of the CPT was achieved, insufficient mechanical support on the lateral side, together with pseudoarthrosis of the ipsilateral fibula, progressively caused a valgus deformity of up to 15 degrees to develop. In addition to the minimal soft tissue coverage on the medial aspect of the lower leg, especially in these patients with a history of multiple surgeries, this made medial plates less desirable [18]. Therefore, an anterolateral distal tibia LCP® (DePuy Synthes, Raynham, MA, USA) was used in the subsequent patients. In comparison to the medial plate, with a transverse metaphyseal screw axis, the anterolateral plate had metaphyseal screws in the anteroposterior axis, which could potentially resist screw pullout from the valgus deformity. In the diaphyseal region, the laterally placed design of the anterolateral plate provided a stronger buttress force than the medial plate, which is crucial to prevent further valgus deformity and malunion [19]. In the clinical study of distal tibia fracture with comminuted fibular fracture, the anterolateral plates also showed mechanical superiority to the medial plate [19].

In our experience, the limitations of anterolateral plating with a 3.5 mm fixed-angle distal tibia LCP are the plate width, locking screw axis, and its proximity to growth plates in the metaphyseal area. Therefore, some patients may require a slight adjustment of the plate placement, or the potential removal of one or two screw holes to adequately fit each individual patient. Moreover, the locking mechanism increased the fixation stability, but the fixed-angle screw axis and proximity to growth plates may pose a challenge during the placement of the locking plate. To prevent intraoperative physeal injuries, the locking sleeves can be preloaded onto the screw hole to help predict the metaphyseal screw axis while meticulously adjusting the plate positions. These advantages could be improved by adopting a newer version of the distal tibia LCP with more metaphyseal screw holes, a smaller diameter (2.7 mm) locking screw, variable-angle screw axis, and a lower profile design than the currently used 3.5 mm LCP systems [20].

Residual deformities after CPT correction are a frequent problem [4,21]. For instance, tibia diaphyseal malalignment, LLD, ankle arthritis, ankle valgus deformity, and calcaneal deformities can all occur [4,21]. In particular, LLD can be problematic for these patients, with the incidence said to be as high as 56% [21]. The reason for this is growth arrest secondary to the pathologic process of CPT, as well as multiple operations that could lead to physeal injuries [3,21]. In our series, the average LLD at the final follow-up was 6.3 cm. These patients were managed with a shoe lift that could partially compensate for this difference. Current options for management include shoe lifts for defects < 5 cm; epiphysiodesis of the contralateral femur, tibia, or both in defects < 5 cm; and lengthening procedures with ESF or the Ilizarov technique in defects > 5 cm [3,21]. Given the high incidence of LLD, subsequent procedures to address the LLD should be informed to the patients. Moreover, a high rate of pseudoarthrosis can be seen at these lengthening sites [21], although the significance of this remains unknown. Despite having a residual LLD up to 8.5 cm in our series, all three of our patients tolerated their LLD well with good functional outcomes (average AOFAS score 88.3) and did not require further lengthening or corrective procedures.

A potential alternative procedure to consider is the induced membrane technique (IMT) previously applied by Masquelet et al. for the treatment of septic nonunion of the tibia [22]. In a retrospective study performed by Vigouroux et al., the authors followed 18 patients for a mean of 9.5 years and revealed comparable results with patients who underwent VFG implantation [9]. The IMT, theoretically, can reduce donor site morbidity while providing a biological chamber that contains growth factors and angiogenetic factors that can promote osteointegration of the graft [9]. However, this procedure requires two stages, and further long-term results are required to further confirm the efficacy of this method.

This study is not without limitations. Given the small number of cases we presented, inherent concerns related to a small sample size are inevitable. In addition, we did not have a control or comparison group to validate our results against. Nonetheless, our results seem in line with the current literature. Moreover, given the limited resources available at smaller institutions, all of the surgeries were performed by a single surgeon. This led to a longer operative time and can be a burden for both the surgeon and the patient. Lastly, harvesting the VFG and the microvascular anastomosis of the graft can be technically demanding and requires a learning curve. Nonetheless, VFG implantation appears to have a favorable outcome in this subset group of challenging patients.

5. Conclusions

Treatment of refractory congenital pseudoarthrosis of the tibia with a contralateral vascularized fibular bone graft and anatomic distal tibial locking plate fixation appears to have satisfactory results at mid-term follow-up.

Author Contributions: Conceptualization, T.-F.A.C., M.N.W. and C.-Y.Y.; methodology, T.-F.A.C. and C.-Y.Y.; investigation, T.-Y.L. and C.-Y.Y.; surgical procedures: T.-Y.L. and C.-Y.Y.; data curation, T.-F.A.C. and T.-Y.L.; writing—original draft preparation, T.-F.A.C. and C.-Y.Y.; supervision, M.N.W. and C.-Y.Y. All authors have read and agreed to the published version of the manuscript.

Funding: This research received no external funding.

Institutional Review Board Statement: The study was conducted in accordance with the Declaration of Helsinki and approved by the Ethics Committee of Kuang-Tien General Hospital, Taiwan.

Informed Consent Statement: Informed consent was obtained from all subjects involved in the study and written informed consent has been obtained from the patient(s) to publish this paper.

Data Availability Statement: Data are unavailable due to privacy or ethical restrictions.

Conflicts of Interest: The authors declare no conflict of interest.

References

1. O'Donnell, C.; Foster, J.; Mooney, R.; Beebe, C.; Donaldson, N.; Heare, T. Congenital Pseudarthrosis of the Tibia. *JBJS Rev.* **2017**, *5*, e3. [CrossRef]
2. Hefti, F.; Bollini, G.; Dungl, P.; Fixsen, J.; Grill, F.; Ippolito, E.; Romanus, B.; Tudisco, C.; Wientroub, S. Congenital pseudarthrosis of the tibia: History, etiology, classification, and epidemiologic data. *J. Pediatr. Orthop. B* **2000**, *9*, 11–15. [CrossRef] [PubMed]
3. Khan, T.; Joseph, B. Controversies in the management of congenital pseudarthrosis of the tibia and fibula. *Bone Jt. J.* **2013**, *95-B*, 1027–1034. [CrossRef] [PubMed]

4. Paley, D. Congenital pseudarthrosis of the tibia: Biological and biomechanical considerations to achieve union and prevent refracture. *J. Child Orthop.* **2019**, *13*, 120–133. [CrossRef]
5. Weiland, A.J.; Daniel, R.K. Congenital pseudarthrosis of the tibia: Treatment with vascularized autogenous fibular grafts. A preliminary report. *Johns Hopkins Med. J.* **1980**, *147*, 89–95.
6. Weiland, A.J.; Weiss, A.P.; Moore, J.R.; Tolo, V.T. Vascularized fibular grafts in the treatment of congenital pseudarthrosis of the tibia. *J. Bone Jt. Surg. Am.* **1990**, *72*, 654–662. [CrossRef]
7. Romanus, B.; Bollini, G.; Dungl, P.; Fixsen, J.; Grill, F.; Hefti, F.; Ippolito, E.; Tudisco, C.; Wientroub, S. Free vascular fibular transfer in congenital pseudoarthrosis of the tibia: Results of the EPOS multicenter study. European Paediatric Orthopaedic Society (EPOS). *J. Pediatr. Orthop. B* **2000**, *9*, 90–93. [CrossRef] [PubMed]
8. Sakamoto, A.; Yoshida, T.; Uchida, Y.; Kojima, T.; Kubota, H.; Iwamoto, Y. Long-term follow-up on the use of vascularized fibular graft for the treatment of congenital pseudarthrosis of the tibia. *J. Orthop. Surg. Res.* **2008**, *3*, 13. [CrossRef]
9. Vigouroux, F.; Mezzadri, G.; Parot, R.; Gazarian, A.; Pannier, S.; Chotel, F. Vascularised fibula or induced membrane to treat congenital pseudarthrosis of the Tibia: A multicentre study of 18 patients with a mean 9.5-year follow-up. *Orthop. Traumatol. Surg. Res.* **2017**, *103*, 747–753. [CrossRef] [PubMed]
10. Kalra, G.D.; Agarwal, A. Experience with free fibula transfer with screw fixation as a primary modality of treatment for congenital pseudarthrosis of tibia in children—Series of 26 cases. *Indian J. Plast. Surg.* **2012**, *45*, 468–477. [CrossRef]
11. Hu, L.; Xiong, Y.; Mi, B.; Panayi, A.C.; Zhou, W.; Liu, Y.; Liu, J.; Xue, H.; Yan, C.; Abududilibaier, A.; et al. Comparison of intramedullary nailing and plate fixation in distal tibial fractures with metaphyseal damage: A meta-analysis of randomized controlled trials. *J. Orthop. Surg. Res.* **2019**, *14*, 30. [CrossRef]
12. Nourisa, J.; Rouhi, G. Biomechanical evaluation of intramedullary nail and bone plate for the fixation of distal metaphyseal fractures. *J. Mech. Behav. Biomed. Mater.* **2016**, *56*, 34–44. [CrossRef] [PubMed]
13. Crawford, A.H. Neurofibromatosis in children. *Acta Orthop. Scand. Suppl.* **1986**, *218*, 1–60. [CrossRef] [PubMed]
14. Gilbert, A.; Brockman, R. Congenital pseudarthrosis of the tibia. Long-term followup of 29 cases treated by microvascular bone transfer. *Clin. Orthop. Relat. Res.* **1995**, *314*, 37–44.
15. Vallier, H.A.; Cureton, B.A.; Patterson, B.M. Randomized, prospective comparison of plate versus intramedullary nail fixation for distal tibia shaft fractures. *J. Orthop. Trauma* **2011**, *25*, 736–741. [CrossRef] [PubMed]
16. Markolf, K.L.; Cheung, E.; Joshi, N.B.; Boguszewski, D.V.; Petrigliano, F.A.; McAllister, D.R. Plate Versus Intramedullary Nail Fixation of Anterior Tibial Stress Fractures: A Biomechanical Study. *Am. J. Sports Med.* **2016**, *44*, 1590–1596. [CrossRef]
17. Hardinge, K. Congenital anterior bowing of the tibia. The significance of the different types in relation to pseudarthrosis. *Ann. R. Coll. Surg. Engl.* **1972**, *51*, 17–30.
18. Garg, S.; Khanna, V.; Goyal, M.P.; Joshi, N.; Borade, A.; Ghuse, I. Comparative prospective study between medial and lateral distal tibial locking compression plates for distal third tibial fractures. *Chin. J. Traumatol.* **2017**, *20*, 151–154. [CrossRef]
19. Busel, G.A.; Watson, J.T.; Israel, H. Evaluation of Fibular Fracture Type vs Location of Tibial Fixation of Pilon Fractures. *Foot Ankle Int.* **2017**, *38*, 650–655. [CrossRef]
20. Aneja, A.; Luo, T.D.; Liu, B.; Domingo, M.; Danelson, K.; Halvorson, J.J.; Carroll, E.A. Anterolateral distal tibia locking plate osteosynthesis and their ability to capture OTAC3 pilon fragments. *Injury* **2018**, *49*, 409–413. [CrossRef]
21. Inan, M.; El Rassi, G.; Riddle, E.C.; Kumar, S.J. Residual deformities following successful initial bone union in congenital pseudoarthrosis of the tibia. *J. Pediatr. Orthop.* **2006**, *26*, 393–399. [CrossRef] [PubMed]
22. Masquelet, A.C.; Fitoussi, F.; Begue, T.; Muller, G.P. [Reconstruction of the long bones by the induced membrane and spongy autograft]. *Ann. Chir. Plast. Esthet.* **2000**, *45*, 346–353. [PubMed]

Disclaimer/Publisher's Note: The statements, opinions and data contained in all publications are solely those of the individual author(s) and contributor(s) and not of MDPI and/or the editor(s). MDPI and/or the editor(s) disclaim responsibility for any injury to people or property resulting from any ideas, methods, instructions or products referred to in the content.

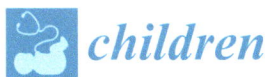

Review

Fracture through Pre-Existing Tarsal Coalition: A Narrative Review

Albert T. Anastasio [1], Emily M. Peairs [2], Caitlin Grant [2], Billy I. Kim [2], Anthony Duruewuru [3] and Samuel B. Adams [1,*]

1. Department of Orthopaedic Surgery, Duke University Medical Center, Durham, NC 27705, USA
2. Duke University School of Medicine, Durham, NC 27705, USA
3. Baylor College of Medicine, Houston, TX 77030, USA
* Correspondence: samuel.adams@duke.edu

Abstract: Tarsal coalitions are abnormal fibrous or bony connections between the tarsal bones of the foot. While not always symptomatic, coalitions can cause pain, alterations in forefoot and hindfoot morphology, and alterations in foot and ankle biomechanics. Previous research has described the association of tarsal coalitions with fractures of the lower extremity. Multiple reports of acute fracture in the presence of tarsal coalition have been presented, as have reports of stress fractures of the foot and ankle with concomitant coalition, insidious in onset and thought to be related to aberrancies in foot and ankle biomechanics. The purpose of this review is to discuss the biomechanics seen in tarsal coalitions and to describe reports of fracture occurring concomitantly with tarsal coalitions. We will discuss diagnostic options and treatment approaches in the setting of fracture with preexisting tarsal coalition.

Keywords: tarsal coalition; calcaneonavicular coalitions; talocalcaneal coalition; ankle; foot; biomechanics; stress fracture

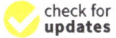

Citation: Anastasio, A.T.; Peairs, E.M.; Grant, C.; Kim, B.I.; Duruewuru, A.; Adams, S.B. Fracture through Pre-Existing Tarsal Coalition: A Narrative Review. *Children* **2023**, *10*, 72. https://doi.org/10.3390/children10010072

Academic Editor: Pasquale Farsetti

Received: 14 November 2022
Revised: 21 December 2022
Accepted: 27 December 2022
Published: 29 December 2022

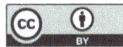

Copyright: © 2022 by the authors. Licensee MDPI, Basel, Switzerland. This article is an open access article distributed under the terms and conditions of the Creative Commons Attribution (CC BY) license (https://creativecommons.org/licenses/by/4.0/).

1. Introduction

A tarsal coalition is an abnormal connection of the tarsal bones of the foot [1,2]. This bridging can be fibrous, cartilaginous, or bony in origin, and most often involves the talocalcaneal (Figure 1) or calcaneonavicular joints (Figure 2) [1,3]. Other more rare tarsal coalitions include talonavicular, cubonavicular, naviculocunieform, and calcaneocuboid [3,4]. Congenital coalitions occur in an autosomal dominant fashion from a failure of early mesenchymal differentiation [2,4]. Recent research has identified a proline to arginine mutation in the fibroblast growth factor receptor 3 (*FGFR3*) gene in association with these malformations [5]. While tarsal coalitions can be associated with other congenital disorders such as Apert syndrome or Nievergelt-Pearlman syndrome, it is more common for these abnormalities to be isolated occurrences [6–9]. Acquired tarsal coalitions can be caused by degenerative joint disease, inflammatory arthritis, infectious sequelae, or clubfoot deformities [1,4,6].

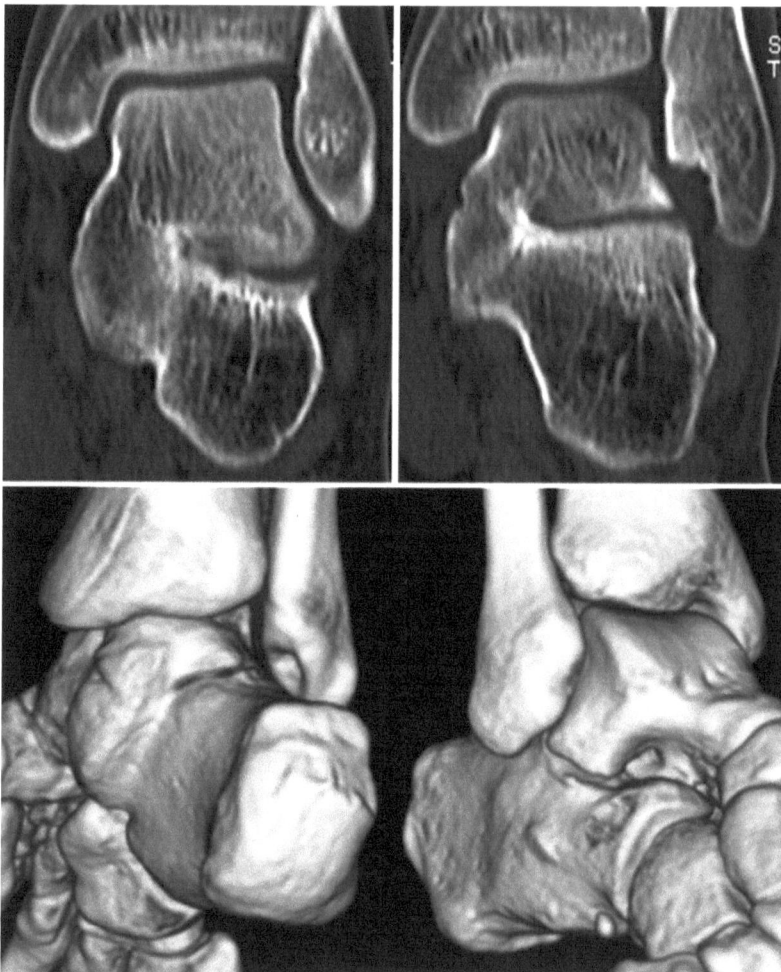

Figure 1. Talocalcaneal coalition, as viewed from two coronal CT sections (upper images) and three-dimensional (3D) reconstruction (lower image). Abnormal bony coalition is noted at the medial aspect of the posterior facet of the subtalar joint [10] (Borrowed using Creative Commons licensing).

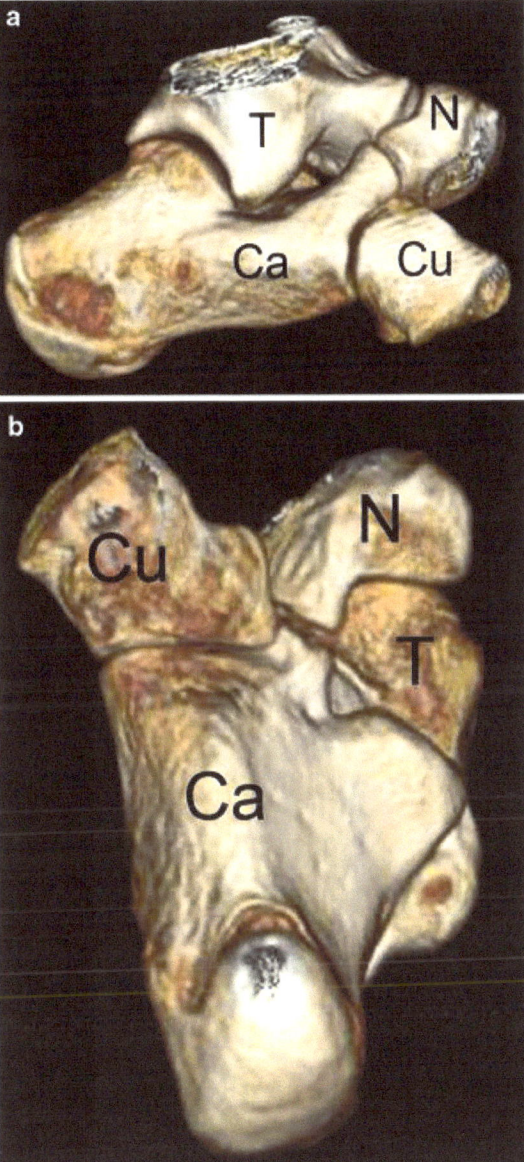

Figure 2. Cropped 3D reconstruction demonstrating sagittal (**a**) and axial (**b**) views of a calcaneonavicular coalition. (calcaneus (Ca), navicular (N), talus (T) and cuboid (Cu)) [11] (borrowed using Creative Commons licensing).

Commonly, these coalitions present in childhood and adolescence with vague hindfoot pain or recurrent sprains and other minor injuries [1,6]. Calcaneonavicular coalitions typically present earlier, from 8 to 12 years of age, while talocalcaneal present in patients 12–16 years of age [12]. The prevalence of coalitions in the United States (US) has been reported from 1–13%; the wide range is due in part to the undetermined proportion of patients who remain asymptomatic [4]. It has been reported in the literature that as many as 75% of patients are asymptomatic [13]. Patients who are symptomatic typically endorse pain that is worsened with activity and improved with rest [4]. Increased stiffness and decreased range of motion may be concurrent with pain due to progressive ossification of the foot [4,14,15]. Furthermore, patients may also report flattening of the longitudinal arch with a valgus deformity of the hindfoot that accompanies or predates symptoms [6]. The location of pain in the foot usually depends on the specific tarsal coalition, with talocalcaneal coalitions presenting with migrating medial malleolus pain and calcaneonavicular coalitions causing pain over the anterior process of the calcaneus, in the talus, or more distally [12,16]. Patients may also present with a spastic peroneal flatfoot, but there is debate within the literature on the positive predictive value of this presentation in identifying a tarsal coalition and the frequency with which patients present with this abnormality [1,17].

In addition to pain and stiffness, tarsal coalitions can cause aberrancies in normal foot and ankle biomechanics or may be seen in conjunction with foot and ankle fracture patterns. While multiple case reports and incomplete literature reviews have been published discussing fracture in the presence of tarsal coalition, a comprehensive review with thorough discussion of related biomechanical factors and their contribution to fracture patterns is indicated. Thus, the purpose of this review is to discuss the biomechanics seen with tarsal coalitions and to describe reports of fracture occurring concomitantly with tarsal coalitions. We will discuss diagnostic options and treatment approaches in the setting of a fracture with a preexisting tarsal coalition.

2. Methodology

Articles in each individual section were found via a PubMed term search between 1970–2022 or via the references in articles from the PubMed search. Search terms and inclusion criteria for each section were utilized as described in Figure 3. Articles were excluded if they were written in a non-English language, and if they were a book chapter, conference paper, extended abstract, or pre-print. All abstracts were reviewed by authors followed by a full text review prior to inclusion.

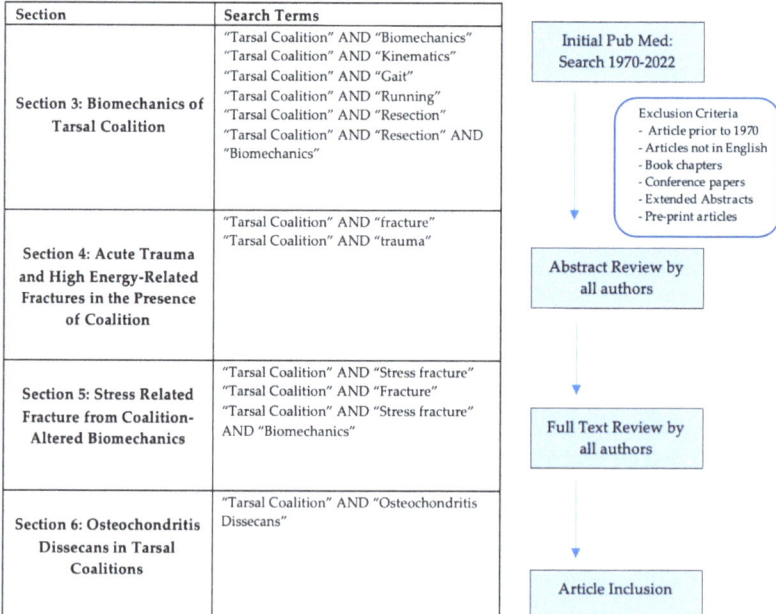

Figure 3. Study Selection and Search Criteria.

3. Biomechanics of Tarsal Coalition

Tarsal coalitions have significant and clinically relevant effects on foot and ankle biomechanics and gait. With talocalcaneal and calcaneonavicular coalitions, the two most common types of tarsal coalitions, the rotary and gliding motion of the talus against the calcaneus is restricted [18]. When examined in the coronal plane, the gait of patients with a tarsal coalition demonstrates a significantly restricted subtalar range of motion and increased subtalar angular velocity [18]. Due to these changes in subtalar kinematics, patients have restrictions in eversion and inversion of the foot and a shortened time interval from heel strike to maximum eversion, both of which increase the magnitude of impact during locomotion [18]. The difference in plantar pressure specifically in patients with tarsal coalitions has also been examined. Prior to surgical resection, patients with tarsal coalitions were found to have significantly higher medial midfoot pressures during walking and running compared to normal controls [19]. The altered biomechanics found in tarsal coalitions have been hypothesized to contribute to stress on neighboring bony anatomy and an increased risk of fracture [20,21].

Although tarsal coalition resection can improve pain and increase return to activity rates, whether patient gait biomechanics improve following surgery is less clear. Significant improvements in passive range of motion have been found in patients after tarsal coalition resection, but range of motion typically remains lower than normal in patients without previous coalitions [17,22,23]. Prior work examining foot kinematics demonstrated that following tarsal coalition resection, patients continue to have significantly reduced subtalar range of motion when compared to normal feet with no significant difference between pre-operative and post-operative motion [18]. The continuation of these altered biomechanics indicates that patients with tarsal coalitions have similar eversion-inversion motion restrictions even after surgical intervention [18]. These differences in inversion and eversion mobility can have functional consequences. Chambers et al. found a positive correlation between side-to-side mobility of the foot and functional scores based on functional tests such as single-limb standing and gait analysis [23].

When examining the effect of surgical intervention on plantar pressure, the results are mixed. A study by Hetsroni et al. found that tarsal coalition resection reduces elevated medial midfoot pressures to those of normal feet during walking [19]. However, patients continued to have persistently elevated medial midfoot mean pressures and impulses during running following surgery, indicating that running accentuates pathological loading [19]. In contrast, a study by Lyon et al. found that following tarsal coalition resection, patients continued to have significantly greater peak pressures in the midfoot and first metatarsal head compared to normal feet during walking [24]. Furthermore, patterns of muscle activity in the lower extremities remain persistently aberrant after tarsal coalition resection. Electromyography studies have found that despite close to normal gastrocnemius, peroneal, and soleus muscle strength, patients after tarsal coalition resection demonstrate continued abnormal premature and prolonged firing in the peroneus longus during walking; this aberrant activity often extended to the gastrocnemius and soleus [24].

4. Acute Trauma and High Energy-Related Fractures in the Presence of Coalition

Altered biomechanics resulting from tarsal coalitions, particularly due to subtalar joint rigidity, are thought to increase stress across structures adjacent to tarsal coalitions [25,26]. Over the last few decades, several case reports have documented acute traumatic and high energy-related fractures in the presence of preexisting talocalcaneal and calcaneonavicular coalitions [27–31]. Typically, tarsal coalitions are incidentally found after identification of the fracture with conventional radiographs for calcaneonavicular coalitions [10]. Additional cross-sectional imaging may be required for identifying subtle talocalcaneal forms or differentiating osseous, fibrous, or cartilaginous coalitions with magnetic resonance imaging (MRI) [10].

Although there are no established clinical guidelines on the treatment of tarsal coalitions in the setting of acute traumatic fractures, the decision to concomitantly address a coalition in the reported cases to date has been influenced by the presence of pre-existing symptoms and patient characteristics (e.g., age, activity), characteristics of the coalition (e.g., calcaneonavicular versus talocalcaneal), detection of degenerative changes in which arthrodesis could be performed, and the need for coalition resection to obtain adequate fracture reduction [27]. Three cases of calcaneus fractures (two closed intraarticular and one open, comminuted) in the setting of middle facet coalition (two bony, one fibrous) have been reported in the literature [27,29,30]. All three patients were treated with ORIF, of which two did not undergo excision or arthrodesis of talocalcaneal coalition due to lack of pre-traumatic symptoms while one 50-year-old male patient with preexisting mild hindfoot pain and degenerative changes in the subtalar joint received concomitant subtalar arthrodesis.

Three case reports of fractures through the calcaneonavicular bar with non-operative management of the fracture and variable treatment of the concomitant calcaneonavicular coalition have been documented [27,29,30]. Pai et al. present the case of a 43-year-old female patient treated nonoperatively in a splint for six weeks with subsequent union and return to work at the four-month follow-up visit [28]. In contrast, despite the union of the calcaneonavicular bar fracture with conservative cast treatment, one 17-year-old male had persistent pain requiring triple arthrodesis [32]. Finally, Tanaka et al. demonstrated a successful return to truck driving for a 23-year-old male after en bloc resection from the beak of the calcaneus to the fracture line. Although the authors acknowledged that conservative treatment may have been adequate, they opted for resection due to the possibility of delayed union due to subtalar joint rigidity and refracture through the calcaneonavicular coalition [31].

Two case reports of three patients with fracture of the sustentaculum tali adjacent to talocalcaneal coalitions have been published, with excellent postoperative functional outcome scores after coalition resection in all three patients [25,33]. Kehoe and Scher present two pediatric patients (11 and 12 years old) with different treatment methods for sustentaculum tali fractures: one with concomitant coalition resection and excision of a fracture fragment after chronic nonunion, and one acute fracture with resection performed after six weeks of immobilization and non-weight-bearing to provide time for healing of the acute fracture [25]. These authors surmised that in the acute setting, a simultaneous excision of both the fracture fragment and tarsal coalition would have rendered the hindfoot unstable and likely to collapse into varus. In addition, simultaneous fracture fixation and tarsal coalition excision would have been technically challenging, given inadequate sustentaculum tali fracture components to repair [25].

Further case examples include the case of a 23-year-old patient with persistent inability to weight-bear after an ankle sprain [31]. The patient was found to have a fracture through a talocalcaneal coalition and was treated with an immobilizing orthosis and weight-bearing as tolerated [31]. Hughes and Brown present a 32-year-old male with a vertical fracture through the posterior third of the talar body with posteromedial displacement of roughly 7 mm in the setting of a talocalcaneal coalition. In this case, the patient's osseous coalition had to be excised to achieve an adequate reduction of the fracture. At 1-year postoperatively, this patient returned to sports without osteonecrosis of the talus and only moderate hindfoot motion restriction [34].

Two cases of ankle fractures, one involving the tibial pilon and one involving both the medial and lateral malleoli, have been documented with incidental findings of talocalcaneal coalitions. Both patients underwent operative fixation of the fracture (one open and one percutaneous with arthroscopic guidance) and without excision of the coalition as neither patient had pre-traumatic symptoms [35,36]. One patient (53-year-old female) had subsequent hardware removal without increased pain or arthritic changes at 15 months postoperatively while another (16-year-old male) had no pain but was unable to invert his hindfoot.

5. Stress Related Fracture from Coalition-Altered Biomechanics

Stress fractures occur in the presence of repetitive mechanical stress on an affected bone, such as in the case of overuse [37]. They are a common pathology, accounting for up to 10% of all orthopedic injuries and up to 20% of injuries seen in sports medicine clinics [38]. The two imaging modalities commonly used to evaluate stress fractures in the foot and ankle are radiography and MRI, with the latter having a significantly higher sensitivity and specificity, especially in the early stages of injury [37,39]. Typical treatment for stress fractures consists of activity modification, analgesics, and potential bracing until pain symptoms resolve [40].

Although rare, stress fractures can also be seen in association with tarsal coalition [20,41–44]. It is thought that this associated stress response may be due to altered biomechanics of the foot leading to increased, abnormal load transfer and hindfoot stress-loading, leading to subsequent fracture [20]. In the case series reported by Jain et al., all six of the adolescent patients presented with diffuse pain of insidious onset and hindfoot stiffness [20]. All had a tarsal coalition of the fibrous sub-type. The locations of stress fractures or stress responses in the patients were the posterosuperior calcaneus, the posterior calcaneus, the cuboid and head of talus, the base of the third metatarsal, the posterosuperior calcaneus, and the head of talus. After using MRI to delineate stress fracture with coalition from coalition alone, the patients were started on nonoperative treatment including analgesics, activity modification and either orthotics or shoe modification [20]. Because tarsal coalitions are often found incidentally, a better understanding of the relationship between coalitions and stress response would aid in swift diagnosis and treatment.

Other case reports of talar stress fracture with preexisting talocalcaneal coalition exist in the literature. Manzotti et al. present a 24-year-old non-professional female runner presenting with left hindfoot pain without a specific area of point tenderness [41]. Initially, radiographs and CT scans were obtained and were non-illustrative. Cancellous edema of the talus due to stress fracture was revealed upon review of MRI, highlighting the utility of this imaging modality in diagnosis of stress injuries [41]. Similar to the six patient case series described above, this patient was started on nonoperative treatment, which included NSAIDs, non-weight bearing, compressive dressing, ankle training, and the use of a wooden-soled shoe [20]. With this conservative approach, the patient experienced a complete resolution of symptoms and a high degree of satisfaction with no further complications.

A case report of a concomitant calcaneal stress fracture with a rare subtalar facet coalition was documented by Moe et al. in 2006 [42]. In this article, a 48-year-old woman presented with worsening left heel pain without any prior accident or injury, a common manifestation of tarsal coalitions. Similar to the case study by Manzotti et al., initial radiographs were unreliable [41,42]. The early clinical diagnosis was presumed to be plantar fasciitis; when the patient did not respond to conservative treatment, further imaging including MRI revealed a "posterior subtalar facet coalition with associated medial and lateral calcaneal stress fractures." MRI allowed for detection of the osseous prominence that gave a "humpback appearance" of the superior posterior calcaneus on the lateral radiograph that was previously missed. These authors hypothesized that the calcaneal stress fracture was due to abnormal forces placed on the hindfoot due to coalition [20]. The treatment plan indicated for the patient to be partially weight-bearing with crutches, but there were no mentions of other treatments, follow-ups, or further complications.

Two cases of stress fractures associated with calcaneonavicular coalitions have been reported. Nilsson & Coetzee investigated a 47-year-old man with a 5-week history of pain in lateral aspect of his left foot that was exacerbated by completing a marathon [43]. Initial radiographs of the foot did not show any fracture or dislocation, but an MRI three weeks after the initial radiograph showed a fracture of the anterior process of the calcaneus and a fibrous calcaneonavicular coalition. A comparison MRI five weeks later showed the continued presence of bone marrow edema confirming the stress fracture. Similar to the previous cases, this stress fracture was treated non-operatively, incorporating non-impact and low-impact training with pool and elliptical trainer workouts for 2 months. The patient was able to run without discomfort, even later completing a marathon without symptoms. Pearce et al. documented a case of a 30-year-old rugby player with a 5-week history of foot pain [44]. An MRI scan was conducted first, which demonstrated some degenerative changes between the navicular and calcaneus. However, a CT scan clearly revealed a stress fracture across the anterior process and a fibrous calcaneonavicular coalition [44]. In contrast to the other cases, these authors decided that the risk of non-union of the stress fracture or recurrence was too high to treat conservatively and opted for surgical excision of the coalition and fixation of the fracture. The patient did well and returned to rugby 6 months later.

6. Osteochondritis Dissecans in Tarsal Coalitions

In addition to abnormal talocrural stress, hindfoot malalignment, ankle sprains and fractures, another possible co-occurring pathology with tarsal coalition is osteochondritis dissecans (OCD) of the talar dome. Cheng et al. aimed to determine the prevalence of OCDs among patients with tarsal coalition [45]. After studying ankle MRIs in 57 patients with tarsal coalitions, the study found 89% of these tarsal coalitions to be non-osseous and talar OCDs present in 29 of them. The authors concluded that talar OCD prevalence is higher in patients with tarsal coalition than the general population, attributing this occurrence to the altered biomechanics and repetitive talocrural stress due to the altered subtalar motion [45]. There is a paucity of research evaluating for presence of OCD in conjunction with tarsal coalition, and future research is indicated to further expand upon this phenomenon.

7. Discussion and Treatment Considerations

Foot and ankle injury in the form of fracture or sprain in the presence of an existing tarsal coalition is a relatively uncommon clinical entity. However, a large number of case reports outline this condition, with heterogeneous treatment options described throughout the literature. Our goal in this review was to provide a comprehensive summary of what has been published to date with regard to the co-occurrence of fracture and tarsal coalition. Given the wide array of management strategies employed to treat this condition, defining specific clinical algorithms for workup and intervention remains elusive. Moreover, given that the existing literature is limited to single patient case reports or small series, there is a high likelihood for an element of publication bias, with only positive outcomes being reported. Despite this, through careful review of the literature, some overarching principles can be gleaned for the treatment of this condition.

For patients being evaluated for foot and ankle fracture in the presence of an incidentally noted or previously symptomatic tarsal coalition, the first branch point for management should be to determine whether the fracture is acute, resulting from a recent injury, or chronic and stress-related in nature. If the fracture is stress-related and appears to be related either to altered biomechanics resulting from the tarsal coalition or from a period of intense activity increase leading to subsequent overuse, nonoperative management should trialed. Nonoperative treatment modalities which have been reported with success in the literature include NSAIDs, non-weight-bearing, compressive dressing, ankle training, and the use of a wooden-soled shoe [20]. Casting and activity modification as well as partial weight-bearing with crutches have also been utilized with positive results [42]. Except in cases of prolonged duration of pain after a trial of nonoperative management and persistent CT-confirmed nonunion, we recommend avoidance of surgical intervention for stress related fracture in the setting of tarsal coalition.

In patients who present after an acute trauma, with a fracture either to the foot or ankle, who are also found to have a tarsal coalition to the ipsilateral extremity, we recommend careful consideration of patient and fracture specific factors to guide treatment. While nonoperative management is not commonly appropriate for acute fracture in the setting of tarsal coalition, fractures which are minimally displaced, where an incidentally noted, asymptomatic tarsal coalition is present, may be managed without surgery. In this case, we recommend a period of casting and non-weight-bearing to prevent fracture displacement. Fractures involving the calcaneus, talus, tibial plafond, medial and lateral malleoli, and bones of the midfoot which are significantly displaced should be treated operatively, following standard operative protocols for these respective injuries. Any existing coalition should be evaluated through the use of advanced imaging modalities. In cases where a coalition is diagnosed and a preoperative examination is possible, a careful history should be obtained as to whether the tarsal coalition is currently symptomatic or has caused a period of symptoms at an earlier time point. Physical exam, including point tenderness at the site of the coalition or range of motion limitation from the fibrous or bony union, may be significantly limited given swelling and pain in the acute traumatic setting.

If the tarsal coalition is confirmed to be currently symptomatic or to have caused a period of prior symptomology, the coalition should be resected at the time of fracture fixation with either subcutaneous fat, extensor digitorum brevis, or bone wax interposition to prevent coalition return. However, as Kehoe et al. caution [25], tarsal coalition excision should only be performed if there is no concern for further destabilization of the midfoot or hindfoot, as achieving an appropriate reduction with adequate stability is paramount to success of fracture management, and takes precedence over coalition resection. A final consideration should be given for the presence of pre-existing osteoarthritis at the subtalar, calcaneocuboid, or talonavicular joint, especially in older patients with pre-existing pain with inversion and eversion of the ankle. In patients with symptomatic arthritis, joint arthrodesis procedures can be combined with ORIF to achieve a stable, plantigrade foot and to reduce postoperative pain and need for reoperations at the expense of joint range of motion.

8. Conclusions

Tarsal coalitions are an uncommon foot pathology that may be asymptomatic or present with vague pain and progressive stiffness. Abnormal loading forces of the mid- and hindfoot prior to surgery may contribute to recurrent ankle sprains or fractures. These altered biomechanics may still be present following surgical intervention with activities that increase the load placed on the foot and ankle, such as in running or jumping. Multiple case series have described the association of these coalitions with stress fractures, with key findings including the utility of nonoperative treatment and the superiority of MRI in visualizing these stress responses. Osteochondritis dissecans is another pathology that may commonly be seen in conjunction with tarsal coalitions, given abnormal joint biomechanics and high incidence of ankle sprains. Why some coalitions remain asymptomatic while other lead to progressive pain, stiffness, and fractures is unclear, but is a potential avenue for further research. This study summarizes the available literature regarding fracture in the presence of concomitant tarsal coalition and discusses possible nonoperative and surgical treatment to improve pain, function, and quality of life for patients with this rare, but important association.

Author Contributions: Conceptualization, A.T.A. and S.B.A.; investigation, A.T.A., E.M.P., C.G., B.I.K. and A.D.; resources, A.T.A., E.M.P., C.G., B.I.K. and A.D.; writing—original draft preparation, E.M.P., C.G., B.I.K. and A.D.; writing—review and editing, A.T.A., E.M.P. and S.B.A.; visualization, A.T.A.; supervision, S.B.A. All authors have read and agreed to the published version of the manuscript.

Funding: This research received no external funding.

Institutional Review Board Statement: Not applicable.

Informed Consent Statement: Not applicable.

Data Availability Statement: Not applicable.

Conflicts of Interest: The authors declare no conflict of interest.

References

1. Bohne, W.H. Tarsal coalition. *Curr. Opin. Pediatr.* **2001**, *13*, 29–35. [CrossRef] [PubMed]
2. Kulik, S.A.; Clanton, T.O. Tarsal Coalition. *Foot Ankle Int.* **1996**, *17*, 286–296. [CrossRef] [PubMed]
3. Stormont, D.M.; Peterson, H.A. The relative incidence of tarsal coalition. *Clin. Orthop. Relat. Res.* **1983**, *181*, 28–36. [CrossRef]
4. Soni, J.F.; Valenza, W.; Matsunaga, C. Tarsal coalition. *Curr Opin Pediatr* **2020**, *32*, 93–99. [CrossRef] [PubMed]
5. Graham, J.M., Jr.; Braddock, S.R.; Mortier, G.R.; Lachman, R.; Van Dop, C.; Jabs, E.W. Syndrome of coronal craniosynostosis with brachydactyly and carpal/tarsal coalition due to Pro250Arg mutation in FGFR3 gene. *Am. J. Med. Genet.* **1998**, *77*, 322–329. [CrossRef]
6. Mosca, V.S. Subtalar coalition in pediatrics. *Foot Ankle Clin.* **2015**, *20*, 265–281. [CrossRef]
7. Grogan, D.P.; Holt, G.R.; Ogden, J.A. Talocalcaneal coalition in patients who have fibular hemimelia or proximal femoral focal deficiency. A comparison of the radiographic and pathological findings. *JBJS* **1994**, *76*, 1363–1370. [CrossRef]
8. Spero, C.R.; Simon, G.S.; Tornetta, P.I. Clubfeet and Tarsal Coalition. *J. Pediatr. Orthop.* **1994**, *14*, 372–376. [CrossRef]
9. Mah, J.; Kasser, J.; Upton, J. The Foot in Apert Syndrome. *Clin. Plast. Surg.* **1991**, *18*, 391–397. [CrossRef]
10. Wähnert, D.; Grüneweller, N.; Evers, J.; Sellmeier, A.C.; Raschke, M.J.; Ochman, S. An unusual cause of ankle pain: Fracture of a talocalcaneal coalition as a differential diagnosis in an acute ankle sprain: A case report and literature review. *BMC Musculoskelet. Disord.* **2013**, *14*, 111. [CrossRef]
11. Upasani, V.V.; Chambers, R.C.; Mubarak, S.J. Analysis of calcaneonavicular coalitions using multi-planar three-dimensional computed tomography. *J. Child. Orthop.* **2008**, *2*, 301–307. [CrossRef]
12. Cass, A.D.; Camasta, C.A. A review of tarsal coalition and pes planovalgus: Clinical examination, diagnostic imaging, and surgical planning. *J. Foot Ankle Surg.* **2010**, *49*, 274–293. [CrossRef]
13. Khoshbin, A.; Bouchard, M.; Wasserstein, D.; Leroux, T.; Law, P.W.; Kreder, H.J.; Daniels, T.R.; Wright, J.G. Reoperations after tarsal coalition resection: A population-based study. *J. Foot Ankle Surg.* **2015**, *54*, 306–310. [CrossRef]
14. Katayama, T.; Tanaka, Y.; Kadono, K.; Taniguchi, A.; Takakura, Y. Talocalcaneal coalition: A case showing the ossification process. *Foot Ankle Int.* **2005**, *26*, 490–493. [CrossRef]
15. Lemley, F.; Berlet, G.; Hill, K.; Philbin, T.; Isaac, B.; Lee, T. Current concepts review: Tarsal coalition. *Foot Ankle Int.* **2006**, *27*, 1163–1169. [CrossRef]
16. Stuecker, R.D.; Bennett, J.T. Tarsal coalition presenting as a pes cavo-varus deformity: Report of three cases and review of the literature. *Foot Ankle* **1993**, *14*, 540–544. [CrossRef]
17. Guduri, V.; Dreyer, M.A. Talocalcaneal Coalition. In *StatPearls*; StatPearls Publishing LLC.: Treasure Island, FL, USA, 2022.
18. Hetsroni, I.; Nyska, M.; Mann, G.; Rozenfeld, G.; Ayalon, M. Subtalar kinematics following resection of tarsal coalition. *Foot Ankle Int.* **2008**, *29*, 1088–1094. [CrossRef]
19. Hetsroni, I.; Ayalon, M.; Mann, G.; Meyer, G.; Nyska, M. Walking and running plantar pressure analysis before and after resection of tarsal coalition. *Foot Ankle Int.* **2007**, *28*, 575–580. [CrossRef]
20. Jain, V.K.; Iyengar, K.P.; Botchu, R. Bone stress injuries in the presence of tarsal coalition as a cause of hindfoot pain in adolescents: Case series of 6 patients with literature review. *Skelet. Radiol.* **2022**, *51*, 991–996. [CrossRef]
21. Welck, M.J.; Hayes, T.; Pastides, P.; Khan, W.; Rudge, B. Stress fractures of the foot and ankle. *Injury* **2017**, *48*, 1722–1726. [CrossRef]
22. Mahan, S.T.; Miller, P.E.; Kasser, J.R.; Spencer, S.A. Prospective Evaluation of Tarsal Coalition Excision Show Significant Improvements in Pain and Function. *J. Pediatr. Orthop.* **2021**, *41*, e828–e832. [CrossRef] [PubMed]
23. Chambers, R.B.; Cook, T.M.; Cowell, H.R. Surgical reconstruction for calcaneonavicular coalition. Evaluation of function and gait. *J. Bone Jt. Surg. Am.* **1982**, *64*, 829–836. [CrossRef]
24. Lyon, R.; Liu, X.C.; Cho, S.J. Effects of tarsal coalition resection on dynamic plantar pressures and electromyography of lower extremity muscles. *J. Foot Ankle Surg.* **2005**, *44*, 252–258. [CrossRef] [PubMed]
25. Kehoe, C.M.; Scher, D.M. Sustentaculum Tali Fracture Adjacent to Talocalcaneal Tarsal Coalitions: A Report of 2 Cases. *JBJS Case Connect* **2021**, *11*, e20.00360. [CrossRef] [PubMed]
26. Jayakumar, S.; Cowell, H.R. Rigid flatfoot. *Clin. Orthop. Relat. Res.* **1977**, *122*, 77–84. [CrossRef]
27. Chodos, M.D.; Campbell, J.T. Intra-articular calcaneal fracture with tarsal coalition treated with open reduction, internal fixation, and isolated subtalar arthrodesis: A case report. *Foot Ankle Int.* **2007**, *28*, 1017–1020. [CrossRef]
28. Pai, S.K.; Swamy, K.; Browne, A. Tarsal coalition complicated by fracture: A case report. *J. Trauma* **2009**, *66*, 276–278. [CrossRef]
29. Berzins, U.; Hohenberger, G.M.; Vielgut, I.; Krassnig, R.; Bakota, B.; Seibert, F.J. Talocalcaneal Coalition Including Open Comminuted Calcaneal Fracture; A Case Report and Literature Review. *Bull. Emerg. Trauma* **2019**, *7*, 80–83. [CrossRef]
30. Kim, D.H.; Berkowitz, M.J. Fracture of the calcaneus associated with talocalcaneal coalition. *Foot Ankle Int.* **2004**, *25*, 426–428. [CrossRef]
31. Tanaka, Y.; Takakura, Y.; Akiyama, K.; Kamei, S.; Nukata, M.; Tamai, S. Fracture of the tarsal navicular associated with calcaneonavicular coalition: A case report. *Foot Ankle Int.* **1995**, *16*, 800–802. [CrossRef]
32. Richards, R.R.; Evans, J.G.; McGoey, P.F. Fracture of a calcaneonavicular bar: A complication of tarsal coalition. A case report. *Clin. Orthop. Relat. Res.* **1984**, *185*, 220–221. [CrossRef]
33. Moonot, P.; Sharma, G.; Kadakia, A.R. Mal-union of sustentaculum tali fracture with talo-calcaneal coalition leading to tarsal tunnel syndrome: A case report. *Foot* **2021**, *47*, 101797. [CrossRef]

34. Hughes, A.; Brown, R. Talar body fracture associated with unrecognised talocalcaneal coalition. *Foot Ankle Surg.* **2010**, *16*, e4–e7. [CrossRef]
35. Godoy, H.M.; Micciche, M.J. An Incidental Finding of a Talonavicular and Talocalcaneal Joint Coalition After a Tibial Pilon Fracture: A Case Report. *J. Foot Ankle Surg.* **2017**, *56*, 1332–1334. [CrossRef]
36. Imade, S.; Takao, M.; Nishi, H.; Uchio, Y. Unusual malleolar fracture of the ankle with talocalcaneal coalition treated by arthroscopy-assisted reduction and percutaneous fixation. *Arch. Orthop. Trauma Surg.* **2007**, *127*, 277–280. [CrossRef]
37. May, T.; Marappa-Ganeshan, R. Stress Fractures. In *StatPearls*; StatPearls Publishing LLC.: Treasure Island, FL, USA, 2022.
38. Abbott, A.; Bird, M.L.; Wild, E.; Brown, S.M.; Stewart, G.; Mulcahey, M.K. Part I: Epidemiology and risk factors for stress fractures in female athletes. *Phys. Sportsmed.* **2020**, *48*, 17–24. [CrossRef]
39. Marshall, R.A.; Mandell, J.C.; Weaver, M.J.; Ferrone, M.; Sodickson, A.; Khurana, B. Imaging Features and Management of Stress, Atypical, and Pathologic Fractures. *Radiographics* **2018**, *38*, 2173–2192. [CrossRef]
40. Patel, D.S.; Roth, M.; Kapil, N. Stress fractures: Diagnosis, treatment, and prevention. *Am. Fam. Physician* **2011**, *83*, 39–46.
41. Manzotti, A.; Deromedis, B.; Locatelli, A. Intracancellous bone stress fracture of the talus in talo-calcaneal coalition: A case report. *Foot Ankle Surg.* **1999**, *5*, 101–104. [CrossRef]
42. Moe, D.C.; Choi, J.J.; Davis, K.W. Posterior subtalar facet coalition with calcaneal stress fracture. *AJR Am. J. Roentgenol.* **2006**, *186*, 259–264. [CrossRef]
43. Nilsson, L.J.; Coetzee, J.C. Stress fracture in the presence of a calcaneonavicular coalition: A case report. *Foot Ankle Int.* **2006**, *27*, 373–374. [CrossRef] [PubMed]
44. Pearce, C.J.; Zaw, H.; Calder, J.D. Stress fracture of the anterior process of the calcaneus associated with a calcaneonavicular coalition: A case report. *Foot Ankle Int.* **2011**, *32*, 85–88. [CrossRef] [PubMed]
45. Cheng, K.Y.; Fuangfa, P.; Shirazian, H.; Resnick, D.; Smitaman, E. Osteochondritis dissecans of the talar dome in patients with tarsal coalition. *Skelet. Radiol.* **2022**, *51*, 191–200. [CrossRef] [PubMed]

Disclaimer/Publisher's Note: The statements, opinions and data contained in all publications are solely those of the individual author(s) and contributor(s) and not of MDPI and/or the editor(s). MDPI and/or the editor(s) disclaim responsibility for any injury to people or property resulting from any ideas, methods, instructions or products referred to in the content.

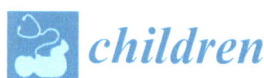
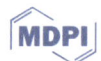

Systematic Review

A Systematic Review and Meta-Analysis on the Management and Outcome of Isolated Skull Fractures in Pediatric Patients

Lucca B. Palavani [1], Raphael Bertani [2,*], Leonardo de Barros Oliveira [3], Sávio Batista [4], Gabriel Verly [4], Filipi Fim Andreão [4], Marcio Yuri Ferreira [5] and Wellingson Silva Paiva [2]

1. Faculty of Medicine, Max Planck University Center, Indaiatuba 13343-060, Brazil; lucca.palavani730@al.unieduk.com.br
2. Faculty of Medicine, São Paulo University, São Paulo 05508-220, Brazil
3. Faculty of Medicine, State University of Ponta Grossa, Ponta Grossa 84010-330, Brazil
4. Faculty of Medicine, Federal University of Rio de Janeiro, Rio de Janeiro 21941-617, Brazil; saviobatista@ufrj.br (S.B.); gabrielverly@ufrj.br (G.V.)
5. Faculty of Medicine, Ninth July University, São Paulo 02117-010, Brazil
* Correspondence: raphael.bertani@hc.fm.usp.br

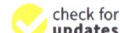

Citation: Palavani, L.B.; Bertani, R.; de Barros Oliveira, L.; Batista, S.; Verly, G.; Andreão, F.F.; Ferreira, M.Y.; Paiva, W.S. A Systematic Review and Meta-Analysis on the Management and Outcome of Isolated Skull Fractures in Pediatric Patients. *Children* **2023**, *10*, 1913. https://doi.org/10.3390/children10121913

Academic Editors: Christiaan J. A. van Bergen and Joost W. Colaris

Received: 10 October 2023
Revised: 2 November 2023
Accepted: 20 November 2023
Published: 12 December 2023

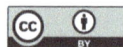

Copyright: © 2023 by the authors. Licensee MDPI, Basel, Switzerland. This article is an open access article distributed under the terms and conditions of the Creative Commons Attribution (CC BY) license (https://creativecommons.org/licenses/by/4.0/).

Abstract: Background: The impact of traumatic brain injury (TBI) on the pediatric population is profound. The aim of this study is to unveil the state of the evidence concerning acute neurosurgical intervention, hospitalizations after injury, and neuroimaging in isolated skull fractures (ISF). Materials and Methods: This systematic review was conducted in accordance with PRISMA guidelines. PubMed, Cochrane, Web of Science, and Embase were searched for papers until April 2023. Only ISF cases diagnosed via computed tomography were considered. Results: A total of 10,350 skull fractures from 25 studies were included, of which 7228 were ISF. For the need of acute neurosurgical intervention, the meta-analysis showed a risk of 0% (95% CI: 0–0%). For hospitalization after injury the calculated risk was 78% (95% CI: 66–89%). Finally, for the requirement of repeated neuroimaging the analysis revealed a rate of 7% (95% CI: 0–15%). No deaths were reported in any of the 25 studies. Conclusions: Out of 7228 children with ISF, an almost negligible number required immediate neurosurgical interventions, yet a significant 74% were hospitalized for up to 72 h. Notably, the mortality was zero, and repeat neuroimaging was uncommon. This research is crucial in shedding light on the outcomes and implications of pediatric TBIs concerning ISFs.

Keywords: isolated skull fracture in children; pediatric traumatic brain injury; pediatric

1. Introduction

The impact of traumatic brain injury (TBI) on the pediatric population is profound, as it stands as a leading cause of both fatalities and disabilities [1,2]. While TBI's severity in adults is widely acknowledged, the unique pathophysiological aspects involved in pediatric cases magnify the associated burden, making it even more substantial [1].

Pediatric brain injuries present distinctive biomechanical characteristics due to the heightened plasticity and deformability of the developing brain. The infant skull, less rigid and featuring flexible sutures that act like joints, allows for some movement in response to mechanical stress, potentially resulting in birth-related injuries such as intracranial hemorrhages caused by compression and traction during delivery [3,4]. Additionally, shaking can cause a slight deformity of the skull and redistribute forces within, potentially leading to stretching and shearing injuries. Furthermore, children's relatively larger heads make them more vulnerable to head trauma compared to adults [1,5].

An isolated skull fracture (ISF) stands as a distinct focal point within the complex spectrum of TBI. TBI, in its broad context, is associated with severe and multifaceted consequences. However, the ISF introduces its own set of distinctive characteristics that warrant specific attention. Extensive analysis, through prior comprehensive meta-analyses, has diligently explored the short-term implications of this condition. The collective findings from these studies ultimately revealed a rather low likelihood of emergent neurosurgical intervention or fatality in cases of ISF. Despite this relatively low risk, it is noteworthy that ISF cases tend to exhibit a significantly high incidence of hospitalization. This suggests that although the immediate life-threatening aspect is relatively rare, the injury itself necessitates a considerable degree of medical care and observation due to its potentially severe nature, ultimately concluding that the risk of emergency neurosurgery or fatality is exceedingly low, yet it is accompanied by a notably high rate of hospitalization [6].

Despite the establishment of guidelines for TBI in children [7,8], there is room for research, as new evidence of ISF in the pediatric population has emerged since the publication of the last meta-analysis [6]. In this matter particularly, there is no robust current evidence demonstrating the requirement of acute neurosurgical intervention, hospitalizations after injury, and neuroimaging in ISF [9]. Hence, the authors conducted a single-arm update meta-analysis to unveil the state of the evidence concerning these factors.

2. Materials and Methods

2.1. Eligibility Criteria

Inclusion in this meta-analysis was restricted to studies that met all the following criteria (1) randomized or non-randomized studies; (2) report isolated pediatric skull fracture on computed tomography (CT) scan; (3) studies that report one of the interest outcomes; (4) studies reporting four or more patients. We excluded non-English papers, reviews, letters to the editor, abstracts, and commentaries from the initial assessment.

2.2. Search Strategy

We systematically searched for isolated pediatric skull fractures on PubMed, Cochrane, Web of Science, and Embase databases with the following terms: (Pediatric OR child) AND ("skull fracture" OR "head injury" OR "head trauma") AND ("surgical intervention" OR "neurosurgical intervention" OR "surgical treatment") AND ("conservative care" OR management OR "conservative management"). Due to the lack of randomized controlled trials, our sample is mostly composed of non-randomized studies. The references from all included studies, previous systematic reviews, and meta-analyses were also searched manually for any additional studies. Two authors (F.A. and L.B.P.) independently extracted the data following predefined search criteria.

2.3. Outcomes Definitions

Main outcomes were defined considering mortality, the necessity of acute neurosurgery intervention, repeated neuroimaging, and hospitalizations. Cases of ISFs were considered only if they were diagnosed through CT scanning.

2.4. Quality Assessment

Two authors (F.A and L.B.P) independently evaluated the study quality, and any differences in their assessments were resolved via consensus. ROBINS-I scale was employed to assess the studies. By utilizing this standardized assessment tool, our objective was to assess the methodological rigor and quality of the studies included in our analysis.

2.5. Statistical Analysis

This systematic review and meta-analysis were performed following the Cochrane Collaboration and the Preferred Reporting Items for Systematic Reviews and Meta-Analysis (PRISMA) statement guidelines [10]. Relative risk (RR) with 95% confidence intervals was used to compare outcomes in specific treatment scenarios. Cochran Q test and I^2 statistics were used to assess for heterogeneity; p-value inferior to 0.05 and $I^2 < 35\%$ were considered significant for heterogeneity. Review Manager was used for statistical analysis.

3. Results

3.1. Study Selection

We located a total of 4572 articles through our search efforts, with 1935 found in PubMed, 1616 in Embase, 994 in Web of Science, and 27 in Cochrane database. After the initial screening, where we assessed 3259 non-duplicate citations, we excluded 3228 articles based on title or abstract screening, leaving us with 31 articles for a full-text review. Subsequently, nine articles were excluded during the full-text screening and data extraction process. Next, three citations were manually added. Ultimately, we included 25 studies in our final analysis [9,11–34], as outlined in Figure 1.

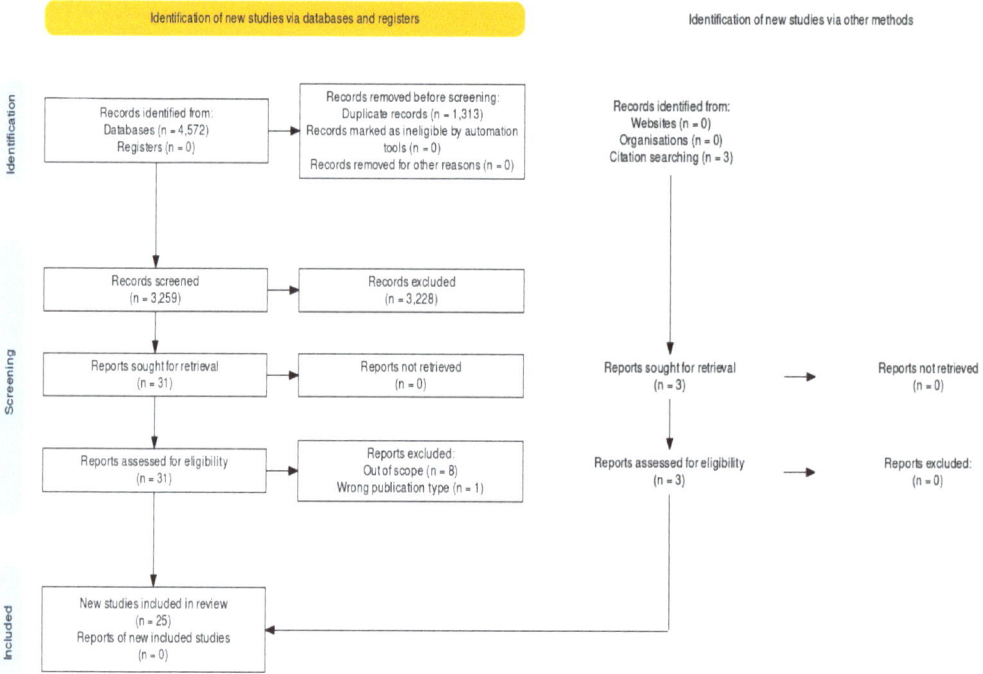

Figure 1. Prisma Flow Diagram.

3.2. Quality Assessment

Figure 2 uses a concise color-coded system based on the ROBINS-I scale to present the risk of bias among 25 studies. Green represents the two studies with "Low Risk of Bias", yellow delineates the eighteen studies with "Moderate Risk of Bias", and red highlights the five studies flagged for "Serious Risk of Bias".

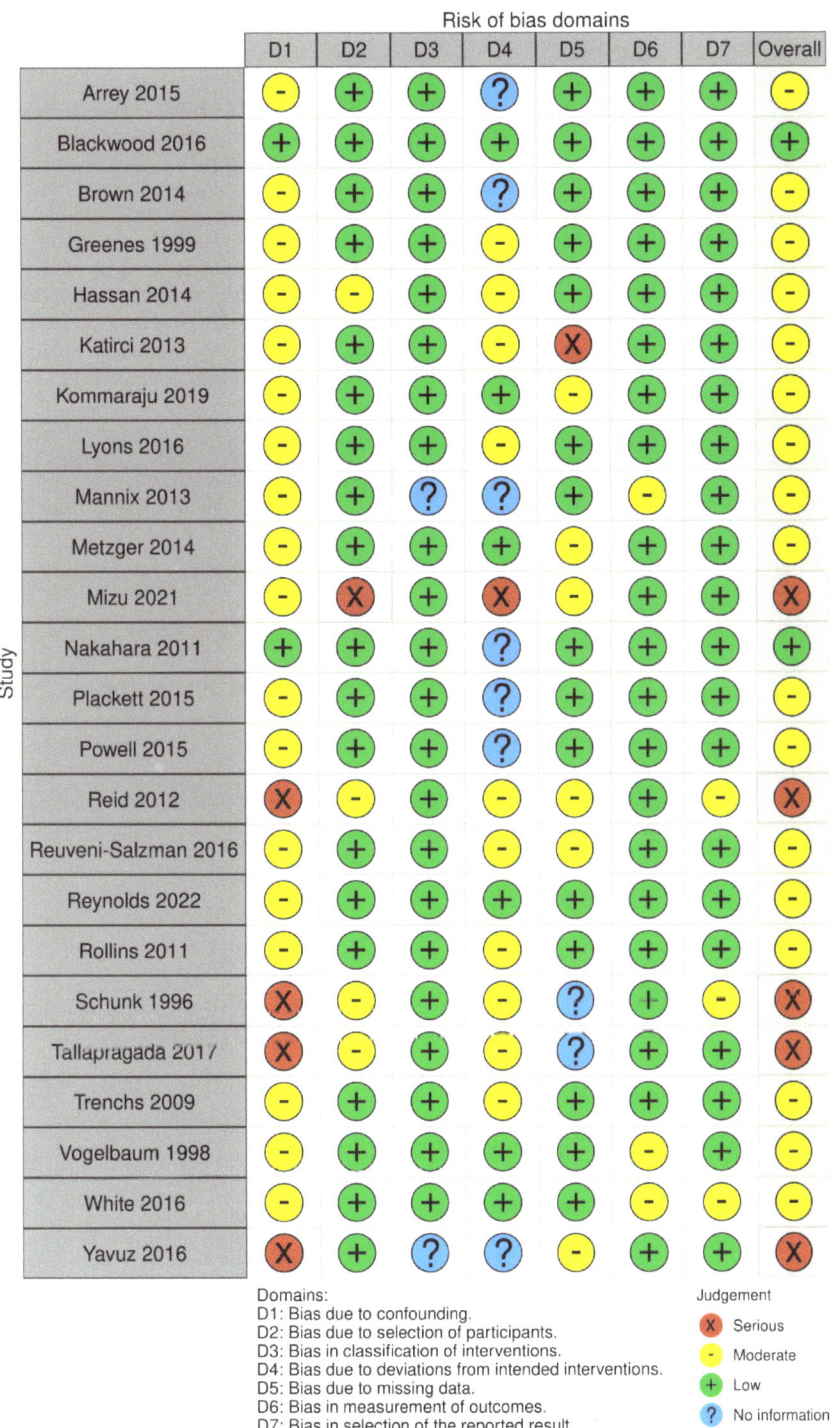

Figure 2. Quality assessment of the included studies employing the ROBINS-I scale [9,11–13,15–34].

3.3. Patient Baseline Characteristics

A total of 10,350 skull fractures from 25 studies were included, of which 7228 were ISFs identified after CT scanning. Within the selected reports, 18 (72%) were retrospective analysis of patients' characteristics and data. The United States of America (US) was the country in which most of the studies were established, encompassing 17 (68%) citations. From the included reports, twenty (80%) were initiated in this century; however, only five (20%) were conducted from 2010 onwards. Out of the total, four (16%) references were multicentric, with one being from Australia and the rest being from the US. One of these multicentric studies accounted for 44% of the included skull fractures. Except for Mannix et al. [20], all studies encompassed patients with equal or less than 18 years. Concerning the age of the patients, 16 (64%) studies included only patients with 15 years or less. When analyzing all of the reports, the initial Glasgow Coma Scale (GCS) score ranged from 13 to 15 in 2 (8%) and from 14 to 15 in 3 (12%) of them, whereas in 12 (48%) the GCS score was 15. A summary of the data can be examined in Table 1.

Table 1. Baseline characteristics of included studies.

Study and Year	Study Design	Single or Multicenter	Enrolment Period	Local of Research	No. of Any Skull Fracture	No. of Isolated Skull Fracture (%)	Age Range	Initial GCS Score
Arrey 2015 [11]	R	Single	2009–2013	US	326	326 (100)	<15 years	NR
Blackwood 2016 [12]	R	Single	2004–2014	US	71	71 (100)	<12 years	15
Brown 2014 [13]	R	Single	2010–2011	UK	6	3 (50)	<1 year	NR
Greenes 1997 [14]	P	Single	1992–1994	US	105	78 (74)	<23 months	NR
Greenes 1999 [15]	P	Single	1998–1998	US	86	63 (74)	<2 years	NR
Hassan 2014 [16]	R	Single	2007–2010	US	223	128 (73)	<5 years	15
Katirci 2013 [17]	R	Single	2009–2010	Turkey	152	127 (84)	≤18 years	13–15
Kommaraju 2019 [18]	R	Single	2005–2015	US	127	127 (100)	≤18 years	14–15
Lyons 2016 [19]	P	Single	2008–2015	US	320	300 (94)	≤18 years	14–15
Mannix 2013 [20]	R	Multicenter	2005–2011	US	4596	3915 (85)	<19 years	NR
Metzger 2014 [21]	P	Single	2010–2014	US	88	88 (100)	≤16 years	15
Mizu 2021 [22]	R	Single	2011–2019	Japan	79	37 (47)	≤15 years	15
Nakahara 2011 [23]	R	Single	2005–2007	Japan	38	4 (11)	<4 years	15
Plackett 2015 [24]	R	Multicenter	2010–2014	US	42	42 (100)	≤13 years	15
Powell 2015 [25]	P	Multicenter	2004–2006	US	350	350 (100)	≤18 years	14–15

Table 1. Cont.

Study and Year	Study Design	Single or Multicenter	Enrolment Period	Local of Research	No. of Any Skull Fracture	No. of Isolated Skull Fracture (%)	Age Range	Initial GCS Score
Reid 2012 [26]	R	Single	2003–2010	US	92	82 (89)	<2 years	15
Reuveni-Salzman 2016 [27]	R	Single	2006–2012	Israel	222	222 (100)	<14 years	15
Reynolds 2022 [9]	R	Single	2015–2017 and 2019–2020	US	244	244 (100)	≤18 years	NR
Rollins 2011 [28]	R	Single	2003–2008	US	1810	235 (13)	<14 years	15
Schunk 1996 [29]	R	Single	1992	US	79	43 (54)	<18 years	15
Tallapragada 2017 [30]	R	Multicenter	2009–2014	Australia	358	167 (47)	≤16 years	13–15
Trenchs 2009 [31]	P	Single	2004–2006	Spain	150	29 (19)	≤1 year	15
Vogelbaum 1998 [32]	R	Single	1993–1994	US	44	44 (100)	≤15 years	15
White 2016 [33]	R	Single	2005–2013	US	619	438 (71)	3.4 years (SD 4.1)	NR
Yavuz 2016 [34]	R	Single	1998–2000	Turkey	123	65 (53)	≤15 years	NR

Abbreviations: R—Retrospective; NR—Non reported, P—Prospecitve.

3.4. Outcomes from the Included Patients

In our sample, among the 7228 patients presenting ISFs confirmed by head CT, only two children underwent acute neurological surgery, representing virtually 0% of the patients. In contrast to the few patients who needed acute neurosurgery, a greater number of the children were hospitalized. In summary, 5351 (74%) of them were hospitalized. The length of their hospital stay did not exceed a period of time corresponding to 72 h, including an observation period and an eventual hospital admission. No deaths were reported in any of the 25 studies, despite the high number of hospitalized children and the two acute neurological procedures. Furthermore, only 10 studies provided useful data concerning the number of patients who underwent nonaccidental trauma evaluation. This amount, when reported, reached a total of 378 (5%) patients. Moreover, proceeding with the same rationale as Bressan et al. [6], the total number of patients that repeated neuroimaging varies in our whole study depending on the reported data of a single reference [33]. This reference does not specify the real number of patients with isolated nondisplaced linear skull fractures that repeated this imaging process, despite mentioning that 560 patients received a repeated CT. Thus, the data in this particular study is considered non reported. Hence, a total of 150 patients were identified as having repeated neuroimaging. Table 2 provides a greater view of the exposed data. Subsequently, a pooled analysis was performed.

Table 2. Outcomes from the included patients.

Study	No. Isolated Skull Fracture on CT	No. Acute Neurosurgery (%)	No. Hospitalized (%)	Length of Hospital Stay	No. Deaths (%)	No. Nonaccidental Trauma Evaluation * (%)	No. Repeated Neuroimaging (%)
Arrey 2015 [11]	326	0	271 (83)	<72 h	0	24 (7)	NR
Blackwood 2016 [12]	71	0	55 (77)	<72 h	0	0	3 (4)
Brown 2014 [13]	3	0	3 (100)	<72 h	0	NR	NR
Greenes 1997 [14]	78	0	78 (100)	<72 h	0	NR *	NR
Greenes 1999 [15]	63	0	24 (44)	<72 h	0	NR	NR
Hassan 2014 [16]	128	0	NR	<72 h	0	NR	NR
Katirci 2013 [17]	127	0	NR	<72 h	0	NR	NR
Kommaraju 2019 [18]	127	0	127 (100)	<72 h	0	NR	2
Lyons 2016 [19]	300	0	213 (71)	<72 h	0	99 (31)	NR
Mannix 2013 [20]	3.915	1 (0.03)	3069 (78)	<72 h	0	186 (6)	47 (1)
Metzger 2014 [21]	88	0	50 (57)	<72 h	0	10 (23)	2 (2)
Mizu 2021 [22]	37	0	28 (76)	<72 h	0	NR	17 (46)
Nakahara 2011 [23]	4	0	NR	<72 h	0	NR	NR
Plackett 2015 [24]	42	0	NR	<72 h	0	NR	NR
Powell 2015 [25]	350	0	201 (57)	<72 h	0	NR	62 (18)
Reid 2012 [26]	82	0	2 (2)	<72 h	0	2 (2)	NR
Reuveni-Salzman 2016 [27]	222	0	222 (100)	<72 h	0	2 (1)	4 (2)
Reynolds 2022 [9]	244	0	115	<72 h	0	NR	NR
Rollins 2011 [28]	235	0	177 (75)	<72 h	0	2 (1)	13 (6)
Schunk 1996 [29]	43	0	38 (88)	<72 h	0	NR	NR
Tallapragada 2017 [30]	167	1 (0.6)	167 (100)	<72 h	0	NR	NR
Trenchs 2009 [31]	29	0	29 (100)	<72 h	0	NR	0
Vogelbaum 1998 [32]	44	0	44 (100)	<72 h	0	22 (50)	NR
White 2016 [33]	438	0	438 (100)	<72 h	0	31 (7)	NR **
Yavuz 2016 [34]	65	0	NR	<72 h	0	NR	NR

Abbreviations: NR—Non reported. * In ten studies, 101 patients with any skull fracture were evaluated child abuse, being found a total of thirty patients; number not specified for the subgroup of patients with linear nondisplaced skull fractures. ** In this study, 560 patients of the total 619 (181 with an isolated depressed skull fracture and 438 with an isolated nondisplaced skull fracture) received a repeated CT, and no children had new CT findings. The maximum and minimum number of patients with an isolated nondisplaced linear skull fracture who could have received a repeated CT ranged between 438 and 379.

3.5. Acute Neurosurgical Intervention

From 7219 patients from 25 studies, two required acute neurosurgical intervention (0,0%). After common and random analysis, the risk was calculated to be 0% (95% CI: 0–0%; $I^2 = 0$%). The plot is available in Figure 3.

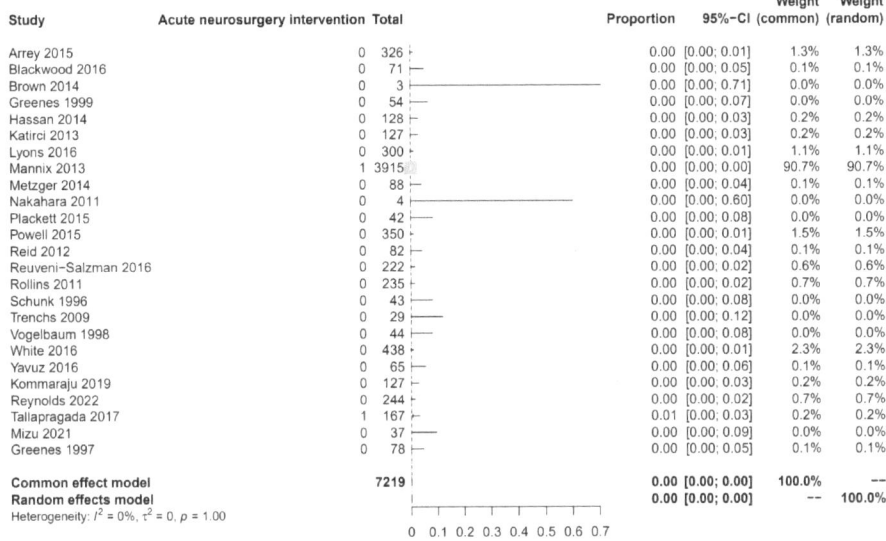

Figure 3. Patients who required acute neurosurgical intervention after an isolated skull fracture [9,11–34].

3.6. Hospitalization after Injury

A sum of 6853 patients from 20 studies analyzed the incidence of hospitalization to more complete exams evaluation after the injury. Due to increased heterogeneity, after a random analysis, the risk of hospitalization was calculated to be 78% (95% CI: 66–89%; $I^2 = 100$%). The most heterogeneous study was Reid et al. [26], in which only two patients out of eighty-two were hospitalized (2.4%). The statistics are depicted in Figure 4.

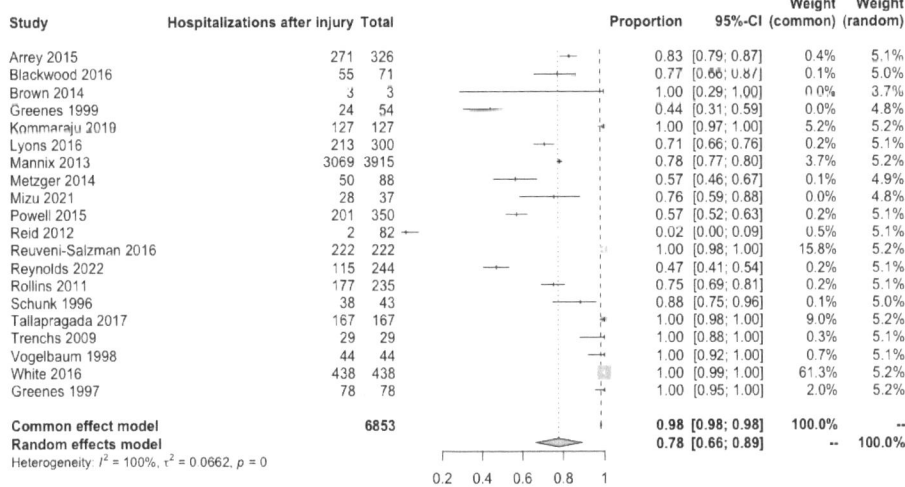

Figure 4. Patients who required hospitalization after an isolated skull fracture [9,11–15,18–22,25–34].

3.7. Repeated Neuroimaging

From nine studies with 5074 patients, neuroimaging was repeated in 150 patients (3%). Once again, due to high heterogeneity, after a random analysis the results came to a rate of 7% (95% CI: 0–15%; I^2 = 92%). Mizu et al. [22] contributed significantly to the present heterogeneity. The outcome is illustrated in Figure 5.

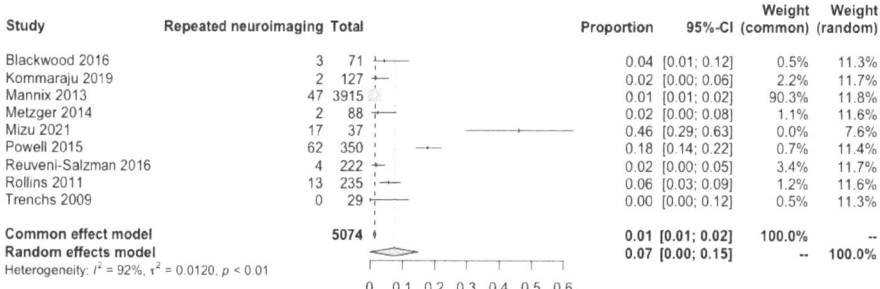

Figure 5. Patients who required repeated neuroimaging after an isolated skull fracture [12,18,20–22,25,27,28,31].

4. Discussion

The management of ISFs in children is a multifaceted process that involves weighing the necessity of surgical intervention. Traditionally, these fractures have been perceived as potentially warranting surgery in severe cases to prevent or address complications such as epidural or subdural hematomas and other intracranial injuries [35]. In contrast, conservative management entails close observation, neuroimaging, and follow-up, and it is typically preferred for asymptomatic or mildly symptomatic isolated fractures. This approach aligns with the principle of minimizing invasive procedures in pediatric patients [36]. The positive outcomes observed in our meta-analysis, which support the efficacy of conservative management for ISFs, contribute significantly to the ongoing discourse on the most appropriate approach to these cases. These findings underscore the importance of a thorough evaluation to determine whether surgical intervention or medical hospitalization is genuinely necessary. While an isolated skull fracture typically bears a low positive predictive value for adverse outcomes, an escalation in risk emerges if supplementary information from the patient's history, physical examination, laboratory results, additional imaging, or social work evaluation raises heightened concerns regarding the condition.

In our analysis, we highlight an exceptionally low incidence of acute neurosurgical intervention. Out of the 7219 patients analyzed, only two cases (0.0%) required such intervention, seen in Mannix et al. [20], and Tallapragada et al. [30] studies. This finding underscores the rarity of severe complications that necessitate surgical treatment in children with ISFs [37]. It suggests that a conservative approach, involving observation and non-operative management, is generally effective in managing these cases.

Because of these necessities, our study reports a notably high hospitalization rate among pediatric patients with ISFs. Approximately 78% of these patients were admitted to the hospital to receive a more complete evaluation of exams. The rationale behind this high hospitalization rate likely includes the need for close monitoring, repeated neurological assessments, and evaluation for potential complications, even though the incidence of surgical intervention is extremely low. While this cautious approach ensures the safety and thorough evaluation of these young patients, it also raises questions about the utilization of healthcare resources, the potential for over hospitalization in cases where conservative management may be more appropriate, when analyzing the amount spend annually for these scenarios [38], and the risk of iatrogenic damage caused by hospitalization itself [39].

Additionally, these discussions, advanced neuroimaging techniques play a pivotal role in assessing the extent and severity of injury, aiding in more informed decision-making, such as the PECARN Rule [40], developed to identify children at minimum risk of clinically significant TBI by diagnosing the extend and severity of the lesion. The ability to accurately diagnose and monitor these fractures using neuroimaging is an essential advancement [41]. The potential of emerging imaging technologies holds promise for future research and improving diagnostic accuracy [42]. Our study delves into the practice of repeating neuroimaging in pediatric patients with ISFs fractures, showing a routine repeat neuroimaging that does not consistently follow a homogeneous proportion across studies. The data suggests a repeat rate of 3%, which increases to 7% when accounting for high heterogeneity. This variation in practice reflects the lack of consensus on the necessity of repeat imaging, with some suggestions in the medical literature [43,44].

In summary, our analysis of the medical literature on pediatric skull fractures reveals a complex clinical landscape. Clinicians frequently recommend hospitalization for these cases at a notably high rate (78%), even though the ultimate need for neurosurgical intervention is relatively low. Moreover, there is substantial heterogeneity in the decision to repeat neuroimaging in our study. This variability may stem from unclear and non-uniform guidelines for managing such scenarios. We recognize the critical importance of decision-making in these situations and the absence of clear directives [45].

In light of these findings, data suggest a cautious approach among clinicians when contemplating surgical interventions and hospitalization. Emphasizing the significance of comprehensive clinical assessments and imaging becomes paramount in determining the appropriate course of action for each patient, and advocating to a conservative management unless there are clear clinical or neurological warning signs, and the skull imaging indicates no significant abnormalities.

5. Limitations

While our discussion has provided valuable insights into the management and outcomes of ISFs in pediatric patients, it is crucial to acknowledge several limitations that temper the interpretation of these findings.

The inherent heterogeneity in the data sources used for our meta-analysis is a notable concern. The included studies may have varied widely in terms of patient demographics, geographical locations, healthcare settings, and diagnostic criteria. This diversity can introduce variability in the results and may restrict the generalizability of our findings to a broader population of pediatric patients with ISFs.

Also, the potential for publication bias in meta-analyses cannot be overlooked. Studies with positive or statistically significant results are often more likely to be published than those with negative or non-significant findings. This bias could impact the overall outcomes of our analysis, potentially not fully representing the entirety of relevant research on this topic.

Another point of limitation is the quality of the included studies. Variability in study design, data collection methods, and reporting quality among the included studies could introduce biases or errors in our analysis. It is essential to recognize that the strength of our meta-analysis hinges on the quality of the underlying data.

Moreover, clinical heterogeneity among patients with ISFs is a complex issue that is difficult to fully account for in our analysis. Clinical factors such as the presence of associated injuries, neurological deficits, or other individual circumstances such as the pediatric population including more or less neonates may significantly influence the decision to pursue surgical intervention. These nuances may not be fully captured by the data we analyzed.

Furthermore, the temporal aspect must be considered. Our meta-analysis is based on data available up to a certain point in time. Clinical practices and guidelines can evolve over time, and new diagnostic technologies or approaches may have emerged since our data cutoff date, potentially impacting the management and outcomes of ISFs in children.

Ethical and cultural factors are also significant considerations. Our discussion does not delve into how these factors may influence clinical decision-making. Variations in healthcare practices and cultural norms can substantially impact whether surgical intervention is considered or favored in specific regions or healthcare settings.

Finally, the high rate of hospitalization that we observed in our analysis may not be universally applicable. Resource availability, healthcare infrastructure, and local practices can vary significantly across different regions and healthcare systems. The decision to hospitalize a child with an ISFs may be influenced by these contextual factors.

6. Conclusions

Our study delved into pediatric traumatic brain injuries, spotlighting ISFs. Out of 7228 children with such fractures confirmed via CT scans, an almost negligible number required immediate neurosurgical interventions, yet a significant 74% were hospitalized for up to 72 h. Notably, despite this high hospitalization rate, the mortality was zero, and repeat neuroimaging was uncommon.

This research is crucial in shedding light on the outcomes and implications of pediatric concerning ISFs. The apparent disparity between high hospitalization rates and the lack of severe outcomes necessitates further exploration—are these hospitalizations truly necessary? Future studies should prioritize understanding this dichotomy, employ rigorous randomized controlled trials, and assess the long-term impacts of these injuries, ultimately aiming to optimize treatment guidelines and observational protocols.

Author Contributions: Conceptualization, L.B.P. and R.B.; methodology, G.V.; software, F.F.A.; validation, L.B.P., R.B. and S.B.; formal analysis, L.B.P.; investigation, W.S.P.; resources, W.S.P.; data curation, L.d.B.O.; writing—original draft preparation, M.Y.F.; writing—review and editing, R.B.; visualization, L.B.P.; supervision, W.S.P.; project administration, L.B.P.; funding acquisition, W.S.P. All authors have read and agreed to the published version of the manuscript.

Funding: This research received no external funding. The APC was funded by the University of São Paulo.

Conflicts of Interest: The authors declare no conflict of interest.

References

1. Araki, T.; Yokota, H.; Morita, A. Pediatric Traumatic Brain Injury: Characteristic Features, Diagnosis, and Management. *Neurol. Med. Chir.* **2017**, *57*, 82–93. [CrossRef]
2. Smith, E.B.; Lee, J.K.; Vavilala, M.S.; Lee, S.A. Pediatric Traumatic Brain Injury and Associated Topics: An Overview of Abusive Head Trauma, Nonaccidental Trauma, and Sports Concussions. *Anesthesiol. Clin.* **2019**, *37*, 119–134. [CrossRef]
3. Ghajar, J.; Hariri, R.J. Management of pediatric head injury. *Pediatr. Clin. N. Am.* **1992**, *39*, 1093–1125. [CrossRef]
4. Stark, M.J.; Hodyl, N.A.; Belegar, V.K.K.; Andersen, C.C. Intrauterine inflammation, cerebral oxygen consumption and susceptibility to early brain injury in very preterm newborns. *Arch. Dis. Child. Fetal Neonatal Ed.* **2016**, *101*, F137–F142, Erratum in *Arch. Dis. Child. Fetal Neonatal Ed.* **2016**, *101*, F372. [CrossRef]
5. Ommaya, A.K.; Goldsmith, W.; Thibault, L. Biomechanics and neuropathology of adult and paediatric head injury. *Br. J. Neurosurg.* **2002**, *16*, 220–242. [CrossRef]
6. Bressan, S.; Marchetto, L.; Lyons, T.W.; Monuteaux, M.C.; Freedman, S.B.; Da Dalt, L.; Nigrovic, L.E. Systematic Review and Meta-Analysis of the Management and Outcomes of Isolated Skull Fractures in Children. *Ann. Emerg. Med.* **2018**, *71*, 714–724.e2. [CrossRef]
7. Kochanek, P.M.; Tasker, R.C.; Bell, M.J.; Adelson, P.D.; Carney, N.; Vavilala, M.S.; Selden, N.R.; Bratton, S.L.; Grant, G.A.; Kissoon, N.; et al. Management of Pediatric Severe Traumatic Brain Injury: 2019 Consensus and Guidelines-Based Algorithm for First and Second Tier Therapies. *Pediatr. Crit. Care Med.* **2019**, *20*, 269–279. [CrossRef]
8. Kochanek, P.M.; Tasker, R.C.; Carney, N.; Totten, A.M.; Adelson, P.D.; Selden, N.R.; Davis-O'reilly, C.; Hart, E.L.; Bell, M.J.; Bratton, S.L.; et al. Guidelines for the Management of Pediatric Severe Traumatic Brain Injury, Third Edition: Update of the Brain Trauma Foundation Guidelines, Executive Summary. *Neurosurgery* **2019**, *84*, 1169–1178. [CrossRef]
9. Reynolds, R.A.; Kelly, K.A.; Ahluwalia, R.; Zhao, S.; Vance, E.H.; Lovvorn, H.N.; Hanson, H.; Shannon, C.N.; Bonfield, C.M. Protocolized management of isolated linear skull fractures at a level 1 pediatric trauma center. *J. Neurosurg. Pediatr.* **2022**, 1–8, ahead of print. [CrossRef]
10. Page, M.J.; McKenzie, J.E.; Bossuyt, P.M.; Boutron, I.; Hoffmann, T.C.; Mulrow, C.D. The PRISMA 2020 statement: An updated guideline for reporting systematic reviews. *BMJ* **2021**, *372*, n71. [CrossRef]
11. Arrey, E.N.; Kerr, M.L.; Fletcher, S.; Cox Jr, C.S.; Sandberg, D.I. Linear nondisplaced skull fractures in children: Who should be observed or admitted? *J. Neurosurg. Pediatr.* **2015**, *16*, 703–708. [CrossRef] [PubMed]

12. Blackwood, B.P.; Bean, J.F.; Sadecki-Lund, C.; Helenowski, I.B.; Kabre, R.; Hunter, C.J. Observation for isolated traumatic skull fractures in the pediatric population: Unnecessary and costly. *J. Pediatr. Surg.* **2016**, *51*, 654–658. [CrossRef] [PubMed]
13. Brown, C.W.; Akbar, S.P.; Cooper, J.G. Things that go bump in the day or night: The aetiology of infant head injuries presenting to a Scottish Paediatric Emergency Department. *Eur. J. Emerg. Med.* **2014**, *21*, 447–450. [CrossRef]
14. Greenes, D.S.; Schutzman, S.A. Infants with isolated skull fracture: What are their clinical characteristics, and do they require hospitalization? *Ann. Emerg. Med.* **1997**, *30*, 253–259. [CrossRef] [PubMed]
15. Greenes, D.S.; Schutzman, S.A. Clinical indicators of intracranial injury in head-injured infants. *Pediatrics* **1999**, *104 Pt 1*, 861–867. [CrossRef]
16. Hassan, S.F.; Cohn, S.M.; Admire, J.; Nunez-Cantu, O.; Arar, Y.; Myers, J.G.; Dent, D.L.; Eastridge, B.J.; Cestero, R.F.; Gunst, M.; et al. Natural history and clinical implications of nondepressed skull fracture in young children. *J. Trauma Acute Care Surg.* **2014**, *77*, 166–169. [CrossRef]
17. Katirce, Y.; Ocak, T.; Karamercan, M.A.; Kocaşaban, D.; Yurdakul, M.S.; Başpınar, I.; Coşkun, F. Compliance with Catch Rules in Administering Computerized Tomography Scans to Children Admitted to the Emergency Department with Minor Head Trauma. *Acta Med. Mediterr.* **2013**, *29*, 717.
18. Kommaraju, K.; Haynes, J.H.; Ritter, A.M. Evaluating the Role of a Neurosurgery Consultation in Management of Pediatric Isolated Linear Skull Fractures. *Pediatr. Neurosurg.* **2019**, *54*, 21–27. [CrossRef]
19. Lyons, T.W.; Stack, A.M.; Monuteaux, M.C.; Parver, S.L.; Gordon, C.R.; Gordon, C.D.; Proctor, M.R.; Nigrovic, L.E. A QI Initiative to Reduce Hospitalization for Children with Isolated Skull Fractures. *Pediatrics* **2016**, *137*, e20153370. [CrossRef]
20. Mannix, R.; Monuteaux, M.C.; Schutzman, S.A.; Meehan, W.P., 3rd; Nigrovic, L.E.; Neuman, M.I. Isolated skull fractures: Trends in management in US pediatric emergency departments. *Ann. Emerg. Med.* **2013**, *62*, 327–331. [CrossRef]
21. Metzger, R.R.; Smith, J.; Wells, M.; Eldridge, L.; Holsti, M.; Scaife, E.R.; Barnhart, D.C.; Rollins, M.D. Impact of newly adopted guidelines for management of children with isolated skull fracture. *J. Pediatr. Surg.* **2014**, *49*, 1856–1860. [CrossRef] [PubMed]
22. Mizu, D.; Matsuoka, Y.; Huh, J.Y.; Onishi, M.; Ariyoshi, K. Head CT findings and deterioration risk in children with head injuries and Glasgow Coma Scales of 15. *Am. J. Emerg. Med.* **2021**, *50*, 399–403. [CrossRef] [PubMed]
23. Nakahara, K.; Shimizu, S.; Utsuki, S.; Oka, H.; Kitahara, T.; Kan, S.; Fujii, K. Linear fractures occult on skull radiographs: A pitfall at radiological screening for mild head injury. *J. Trauma* **2011**, *70*, 180–182. [CrossRef]
24. Plackett, T.P.; Asturias, S.; Tadlock, M.; Wright, F.; Ton-That, H.; Demetriades, D.; Esposito, T.; Inaba, K. Re-evaluating the need for hospital admission and observation of pediatric traumatic brain injury after a normal head CT. *J. Pediatr. Surg.* **2015**, *50*, 1758–1761. [CrossRef] [PubMed]
25. Powell, E.C.; Atabaki, S.M.; Wootton-Gorges, S.; Wisner, D.; Mahajan, P.; Glass, T. Isolated linear skull fractures in children with blunt head trauma. *Pediatrics* **2015**, *135*, e851–e857. [CrossRef] [PubMed]
26. Reid, S.R.; Liu, M.; Ortega, H.W. Nondepressed linear skull fractures in children younger than 2 years: Is computed tomography always necessary? *Clin. Pediatr.* **2012**, *51*, 745–749. [CrossRef]
27. Reuveni-Salzman, A.; Rosenthal, G.; Poznanski, O.; Shoshan, Y.; Benifla, M. Evaluation of the necessity of hospitalization in children with an isolated linear skull fracture (ISF). *Child's Nerv. Syst.* **2016**, *32*, 1669–1674. [CrossRef]
28. Rollins, M.D.; Barnhart, D.C.; Greenberg, R.A.; Scaife, E.R.; Holsti, M.; Meyers, R.L.; Mundorff, M.B.; Metzger, R.R. Neurologically intact children with an isolated skull fracture may be safely discharged after brief observation. *J. Pediatr. Surg.* **2011**, *46*, 1342–1346. [CrossRef]
29. Schunk, J.E.; Rodgerson, J.D.; Woodward, G.A. The utility of head computed tomographic scanning in pediatric patients with normal neurologic examination in the emergency department. *Pediatr. Emerg. Care* **1996**, *12*, 160–165. [CrossRef]
30. Tallapragada, K.; Peddada, R.S.; Dexter, M. Paediatric mild head injury: Is routine admission to a tertiary trauma hospital necessary? *ANZ J. Surg.* **2018**, *88*, 202–206. [CrossRef]
31. Trenchs, V.; Curcoy, A.I.; Castillo, M.; Badosa, J.; Luaces, C.; Pou, J.; Navarro, R. Minor head trauma and linear skull fracture in infants: Cranial ultrasound or computed tomography? *Eur. J. Emerg. Med.* **2009**, *16*, 150–152. [CrossRef] [PubMed]
32. Vogelbaum, M.A.; Kaufman, B.A.; Park, T.S.; Winthrop, A.L. Management of uncomplicated skull fractures in children: Is hospital admission necessary? *Pediatr. Neurosurg.* **1998**, *29*, 96–101. [CrossRef]
33. White, I.K.; Pestereva, E.; Shaikh, K.A.; Fulkerson, D.H. Transfer of children with isolated linear skull fractures: Is it worth the cost? *J. Neurosurg. Pediatr.* **2016**, *17*, 602–606. [CrossRef] [PubMed]
34. Yavuz, M.S.; Asirdizer, M.; Cetin, G.; Günay Balci, Y.; Altinkok, M. The correlation between skull fractures and intracranial lesions due to traffic accidents. *Am. J. Forensic Med. Pathol.* **2003**, *24*, 339–345. [CrossRef]
35. Teasdale, G.M.; Murray, G.; Anderson, E.; Mendelow, A.D.; MacMillan, R.; Jennett, B.; Brookes, M. Risks of acute traumatic intracranial haematoma in children and adults: Implications for managing head injuries. *BMJ* **1990**, *300*, 363–367. [CrossRef] [PubMed]
36. Lerwick, J.L. Minimizing pediatric healthcare-induced anxiety and trauma. *World J. Clin. Pediatr.* **2016**, *5*, 143–150. [CrossRef]
37. Hassan, S.; Alarhayema, A.Q.; Cohn, S.M.; Wiersch, J.C.; Price, M.R. Natural History of Isolated Skull Fractures in Children. *Cureus* **2018**, *10*, e3078. [CrossRef]
38. Schutzman, S.A.; Greenes, D.S. Pediatric minor head trauma. *Ann. Emerg. Med.* **2001**, *37*, 65–74. [CrossRef]

39. Walsh, K.E.; Landrigan, C.P.; Adams, W.G.; Vinci, R.J.; Chessare, J.B.; Cooper, M.R.; Hebert, P.M.; Schainker, E.G.; McLaughlin, T.J.; Bauchner, H. Effect of computer order entry on prevention of serious medication errors in hospitalized children. *Pediatrics* **2008**, *121*, e421–e427. [CrossRef]
40. Gambacorta, A.; Moro, M.; Curatola, A.; Brancato, F.; Covino, M.; Chiaretti, A.; Gatto, A. PECARN Rule in diagnostic process of pediatric patients with minor head trauma in emergency department. *Eur. J. Pediatr.* **2022**, *181*, 2147–2154. [CrossRef]
41. Mulroy, M.H.; Loyd, A.M.; Frush, D.P.; Verla, T.G.; Myers, B.S.; Bass, C.R. Evaluation of pediatric skull fracture imaging techniques. *Forensic Sci. Int.* **2012**, *214*, 167–172. [CrossRef] [PubMed]
42. Jeong, T.S.; Yee, G.T.; Kim, K.G.; Kim, Y.J.; Lee, S.G.; Kim, W.K. Automatically Diagnosing Skull Fractures Using an Object Detection Method and Deep Learning Algorithm in Plain Radiography Images. *J. Korean Neurosurg. Soc.* **2023**, *66*, 53–62. [CrossRef]
43. Chateil, J.F. Head trauma in children—How to image? *Pediatr. Radiol.* **2011**, *41* (Suppl. S1), 149–150. [CrossRef]
44. O'Brien Sr, W.T.; Caré, M.M.; Leach, J.L. Pediatric Emergencies: Imaging of Pediatric Head Trauma. *Semin. Ultrasound CT MR.* **2018**, *39*, 495–514. [CrossRef] [PubMed]
45. Easter, J.S.; Bakes, K.; Dhaliwal, J.; Miller, M.; Caruso, E.; Haukoos, J.S. Comparison of PECARN, CATCH, and CHALICE rules for children with minor head injury: A prospective cohort study. *Ann. Emerg. Med.* **2014**, *64*, 145–152.e1525. [CrossRef] [PubMed]

Disclaimer/Publisher's Note: The statements, opinions and data contained in all publications are solely those of the individual author(s) and contributor(s) and not of MDPI and/or the editor(s). MDPI and/or the editor(s) disclaim responsibility for any injury to people or property resulting from any ideas, methods, instructions or products referred to in the content.

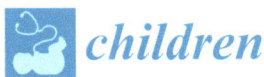

Article

Clinical Patterns and Treatment of Pediatric Facial Fractures: A 10-Year Retrospective Romanian Study

Raluca Iulia Juncar [1], Abel Emanuel Moca [1,*], Mihai Juncar [1], Rahela Tabita Moca [2] and Paul Andrei Țenț [1]

[1] Department of Dentistry, Faculty of Medicine and Pharmacy, University of Oradea, 10 Piața 1 Decembrie Street, 410073 Oradea, Romania
[2] Doctoral School of Biomedical Sciences, University of Oradea, 1 Universității Street, 410087 Oradea, Romania
* Correspondence: abelmoca@yahoo.com

Abstract: Pediatric facial fractures have different clinical patterns and require different therapeutic approaches in comparison with those of facial fractures that occur among adults. The aim of this study was to describe the main clinical characteristics of pediatric facial fractures (such as fracture location, fracture pattern, treatment, complications and evolution) in a group of pediatric patients from NW Romania. This research was a retrospective study that was conducted for 10 years in a tertiary hospital for oral and maxillofacial surgery from NW Romania. A total of 142 pediatric patients were included in this study, with ages between 0 and 18 years. Mandibular (66.2%), midface (25.4%) and combined fractures (8.5%) were identified, and patients from the 13–18 years age group were more frequently affected by facial fractures (78.9%). Most of the diagnosed fractures among all three types of fractures were total fractures, and most mandibular (92.6%) and midface (80.6%) fractures were without displacement. Hematomas, lacerations and abrasions were identified as associated lesions. Patients with associated lesions were more frequently associated with combined fractures or midface fractures than mandibular fractures. The instituted treatment was, in general, orthopedic, for all three types of fractures (mandibular—86.2%; midface—91.7%; combined—66.7%). Most fractures, mandibular (96.8%), midface (100%) and combined (91.7%) fractures, had a favorable evolution. Most fractures did not present any complications at the follow-up. Pediatric facial fractures have unique patterns and must be treated with caution, considering the particularities of pediatric facial anatomy.

Keywords: pediatric facial fractures; clinical patterns; treatment; Romania

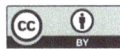

Citation: Juncar, R.I.; Moca, A.E.; Juncar, M.; Moca, R.T.; Țenț, P.A. Clinical Patterns and Treatment of Pediatric Facial Fractures: A 10-Year Retrospective Romanian Study. *Children* **2023**, *10*, 800. https://doi.org/10.3390/children10050800

Academic Editors: Christiaan J. A. van Bergen and Cinzia Maspero

Received: 25 February 2023
Revised: 19 April 2023
Accepted: 27 April 2023
Published: 28 April 2023

Copyright: © 2023 by the authors. Licensee MDPI, Basel, Switzerland. This article is an open access article distributed under the terms and conditions of the Creative Commons Attribution (CC BY) license (https://creativecommons.org/licenses/by/4.0/).

1. Introduction

Facial fractures are frequently encountered in emergency departments [1], and they are traumas that can cause disabilities [2]. For the proper treatment of facial fractures, interdisciplinary collaboration is needed, involving teams of plastic surgeons and maxillofacial surgeons [2]. Although they are less common among children, and more frequent among adults [3], pediatric facial fractures may have a negative impact on children's development [4], are frequently associated with severe injuries and can cause morbidity and disability [5]. In order to reduce the negative effects and to achieve an optimal therapeutic result, it is necessary that the initial evaluation is thorough, the established diagnosis is correct and the treatment is instituted immediately [4].

Pediatric facial fractures have a relatively low incidence, ranging from 4.6% [6] to 14.7% [7] among patients under the age of 18, and have a complex etiology, which varies depending on the age of the child, but accidents occurring during the playing of different sports [8], traffic accidents [9] and fall injuries [10] are among the etiological factors that are most frequently incriminated. Despite the relatively low incidence, pediatric facial fractures have a significant morbidity [6] because due to the anatomical particularities of the pediatric patient [11], the force required to produce a pediatric facial fracture is much higher than the one required to produce a similar fracture in adult patients [7]. Pediatric facial fractures must be treated differently to those that occur among adult patients, both due to the different anatomy of the child, but also due to the impact on future growth and development [12]. In early childhood, the midface is protected by the mandible and the forehead, which can be more prominent. This characteristic makes midface fractures rarer until the age of six [5], but as the child grows, the midface becomes more prominent, and the incidence of midface fractures also increases [12]. Pediatric facial fractures generally occur without displacement due to them having flexible sutures and a more flexible facial skeleton. The strength of the mandible and maxilla is also increased by unerupted permanent teeth [13]. Pneumatization and the development of the paranasal sinuses ensure additional resistance to fractures among children. The ethmoid and maxillary sinuses begin to develop in utero, and at birth, the maxillary sinuses appear as small sacs in the mesenchyme of the lateral nasal wall [14]. The ethmoid sinuses almost reach their final size at the age of 12 years, and the maxillary sinuses mature at 9 years of age [15]. The sphenoid bone begins to pneumatize at the third year of life, and the development of the nose and paranasal sinuses continues until they reach their final size, around the age of 18 [14].

These anatomical particularities also influence diagnosis because pediatric facial fractures have distinct imaging characteristics [16]. Two-dimensional radiography offers limited information that can be used for the diagnosis of pediatric facial fractures, especially for midface and condylar fractures, but panoramic radiography is useful for the initial imaging evaluation when a fracture in the body of the mandible is suspected [16]. The best imaging modality for the diagnosis of facial fractures is computed tomography (CT), which allows the precise visualization of anatomical details necessary for the treatment of fractures [16], and in children, the specificity and sensitivity of head and face CT for detecting facial fractures is high: up to 100% [17]. However, small children are often uncooperative, and the imaging examination can only be performed under sedation [18]. In addition, CT requires a higher dose of radiation [16]. Due to these disadvantages, the diagnosis of pediatric facial fractures is often based solely on clinical examination [19].

The treatment of pediatric facial fractures varies based on the confirmed diagnosis and must account for children's and adolescents' active growth [20]. Generally, some principles of the reduction and stabilization of oral and maxillofacial fractures that apply to adults can also be applied to pediatric patients [20], but the different anatomical characteristics of children, as well as their active growth, must be considered when opting for a certain therapeutic approach [21]. In children, a conservative treatment is generally preferred, but when the fractures are severe, rigid fixation can be used for short periods of time in order not to compromise the developing dentition or skeletal growth [20]. The clinical characteristics of pediatric facial fractures differ among the various populations studied [22], and knowledge of these characteristics is essential in order to ensure a good prevention and an optimal therapeutic management. The authors were unable to find a publication that described the clinical features of pediatric facial fractures in the area that was researched up until the time this research was conducted.

The aim of this study was to describe the main clinical patterns of pediatric facial fractures (such as fracture location, fracture pattern, treatment, complications, evolution) among a sample of children and adolescents from NW Romania.

2. Materials and Methods
2.1. Ethical Considerations

The study was authorized by the University of Oradea's Ethics Committee (IRB No. 3402/15.04.2018) and was carried out in accordance with the guidelines outlined in the 2008 Declaration of Helsinki and its following amendments. The legal guardians of the minors who participated in the study signed consent forms allowing the anonymous use of their medical information. Patients aged 18 had the possibility to complete a consent form, allowing the anonymous use of their medical data.

2.2. Participants and Data Collection

In order to complete this retrospective study, the medical records of patients admitted to a tertiary hospital for oral and maxillofacial surgery in the north-west region of Romania were analyzed. The analyzed medical files belonged to patients who were admitted between 1 January 2002 and 31 December 2011 (a period of 10 years). All medical records were verified impartially by two authors to prevent a bias occurring (R.I.J. and A.E.M.), and all the collected data were centralized using Microsoft Excel software. It must be emphasized that not all the patients admitted in this hospital needed surgery, but the specific focus of the hospital is oral and maxillofacial surgeries.

Data were extracted from the medical records of patients hospitalized during the mentioned period, and the following variables were analyzed: type of facial fracture (maxillary, mandibular and combined); fracture amplitude (total and fissure); fracture displacement (with displacement and without displacement); associated lesions (hematoma, laceration and abrasion); type of treatment instituted (orthopedic, cerclage, osteosynthesis plates and combined); treatment evolution (favorable and unfavorable); complications after treatment (absent, osteitis and vicious consolidation). The ages of the patients (0–6 years, 7–12 years and 13–18 years) and their living environments (urban and rural) were also considered.

The following criteria were required for patients to be included in the study: patients aged 18 years or less; patients who had at least one facial fracture line at the time of admission; patients who had undergone imaging that confirmed the presence and trajectory of the fracture line; patients who benefited from fracture treatment in the host institution; patients who were followed-up for at least 8 weeks after intervention and treatment.

The following exclusion criteria were considered: patients aged 19 years or more; patients who did not have facial fractures; patients who did not undergo imaging to confirm the fracture line and its trajectory; patients who were initially treated in another hospital; patients who were followed-up for less than 8 weeks after treatment; patients who did not have complete information in the medical records. Patients for whom the consent for the anonymous use of medical data was not signed were also excluded.

2.3. Statistical Analysis

Microsoft Office Excel/Word 2013 (Microsoft, Redmond, WA, USA) and IBM SPSS Statistics 25 (IBM, Chicago, IL, USA) were used for the statistical analysis. Quantitative variables were reported as means with standard deviations or medians with interpercentile ranges, and Mann–Whitney U/Kruskal–Wallis H tests were used to compare the groups. Fisher's Exact Tests were used to compare qualitative variables that were stated in absolute forms or as percentages. Data from the contingency tables were detailed using Z-tests with a Bonferroni correction.

3. Results

During the investigated period of time, 12,645 patients were admitted in the host institution, but after applying the inclusion and exclusion criteria, 142 patients remained in the study (Figure 1).

The final sample consisted, therefore, of 142 patients, divided into three age categories, as follows: 0–6 years ($n = 8$), 7–12 years ($n = 22$) and 13–18 years ($n = 112$) (Figure 2). Fifty-five patients were from a rural environment, and eighty-seven were from an urban environment (Figure 3). Ninety-four patients had a mandibular fracture, thirty-six had a midface fracture and twelve had a combined fracture (Figure 4).

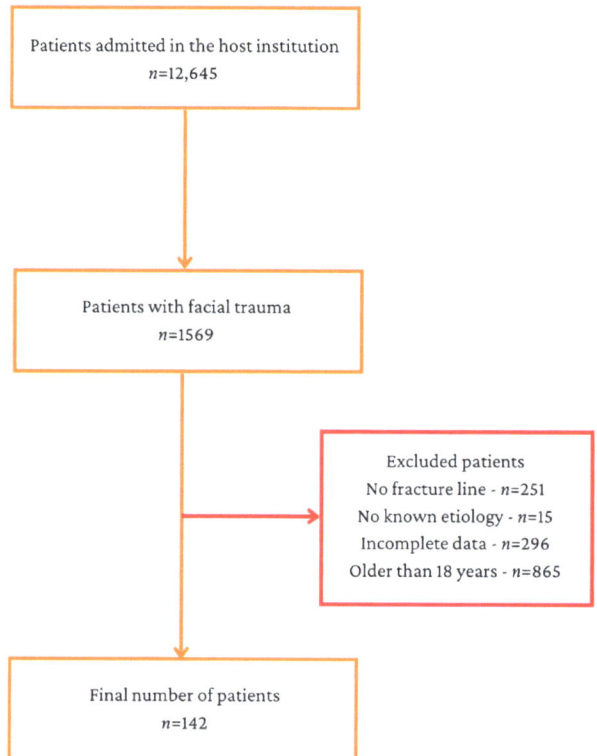

Figure 1. Study flowchart.

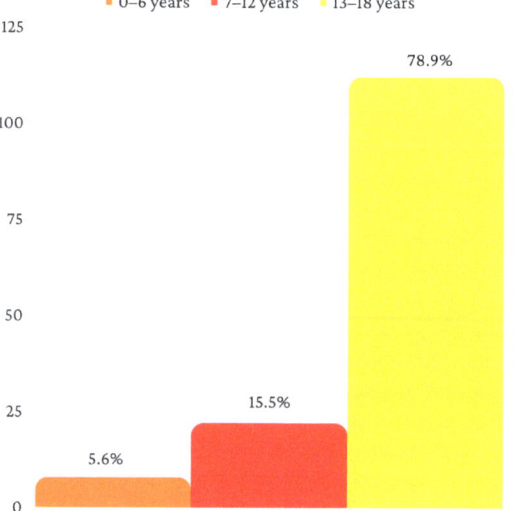

Figure 2. Distribution according to age.

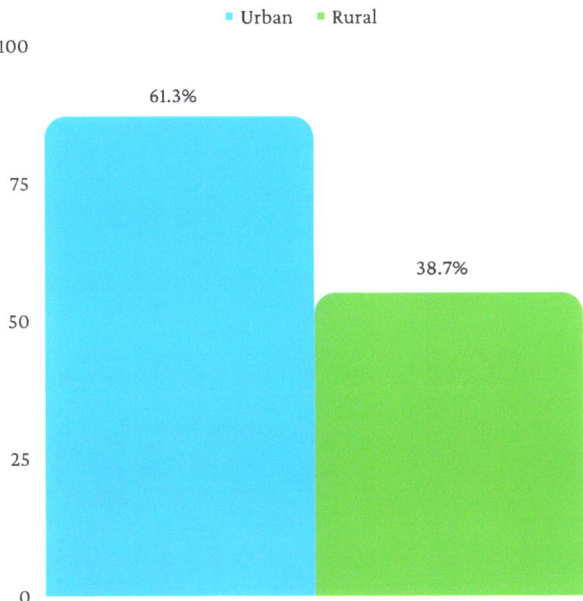

Figure 3. Distribution according to living environment.

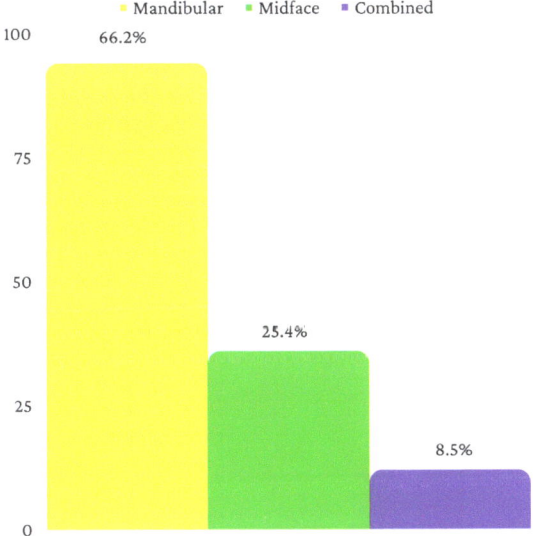

Figure 4. Distribution according to type of fracture.

The mean age of the patients was 14.93 ± 3.75 years, with a median of 17 years.

Data in Table 1 show the distribution of patients according to the type of fracture and age/living environment. In the studied sample, mandibular fractures predominated in the 13–18 age group (84%), the proportion of which is similar to those of midface (69.4%) and combined (66.7%) fractures. However, in the 7–12 years age group, nine midface fractures (25% of all fractures) and four combined fractures (33.3% of the total number of combined fractures) were recorded. Among the patients from a rural environment, midface fractures were most frequently identified (52.8%), while among the patients from an urban environment, mandibular fractures accounted for more than half of the total number of patients living in an urban environment (62.8%). Patients living in the urban environment were more frequently associated with combined fractures than midface fractures (91.7% vs. 47.2%), while patients living in the rural environment were more frequently associated with midface fractures than combined fractures (52.8% vs. 8.3%).

Table 1. Type of fracture and age/age group/living environment.

Fracture (n, %)	Mandibular	Midface	Combined	
Age				p *
Mean ± SD	15.32 ± 3.63	14.02 ± 4.01	14.58 ± 3.75	0.139
Median (IQR)	17 (14–18)	16 (10.25–17)	16 (10.25)–18	
Age Group				p **
0–6 years	6 (6.4%)	2 (5.6%)	0 (0%)	
7–12 years	9 (9.6%)	9 (25%)	4 (33.3%)	0.067
13–18 years	79 (84%)	25 (69.4%)	8 (66.7%)	
Living environment				p **
Rural	35 (37.2%)	19 (52.8%)	1 (8.3%)	0.017
Urban	59 (62.8%)	17 (47.2%)	11 (91.7%)	

n—number; %—percentage; * Kruskal–Wallis H Test; ** Fisher's Exact Test.

Data in Table 2 show the locations of mandibular fractures. Fractures of the mandibular angle (50%) were most frequently diagnosed, followed by lateral fractures (34%), subcondylar fractures (33%) and paramedian fractures (28.70%). Only a small number of patients had fractures of the vertical ramus, median fractures or coronoid fractures.

Table 2. Location of the mandibular fractures.

Fracture Location	No.	Percentage *
Mandibular angle	47	50%
Lateral	32	34%
Subcondylar	31	33%
Paramedian	27	28.70%
Vertical ramus	3	3.20%
Median	2	2.10%
Coronoid	2	2.10%

* out of the total number of mandibular fractures.

Data in Table 3 show the locations of the midface fractures. Disjunctions of the malar bone were the most frequent ones (47.2%), followed by alveolar fractures (30.6%) and nasal fractures (22.2%). Le Fort I, II and III fractures were identified in six patients, while orbital floor fractures were diagnosed in five patients.

Table 3. Location of the midface fractures.

Fracture Location	No.	Percentage *
Disjunction of the malar bone	17	47.2%
Alveolar	11	30.6%
Nasal	8	22.2%
Orbital floor	5	13.9%
Le Fort I	2	5.6%
Le Fort II	2	5.6%
Le Fort III	2	5.6%
Malar dysfunction	17	47.2%

* out of the total number of mandibular fractures.

Most of the patients had total mandibular fractures ($n = 93$, 98.9%), midface fractures ($n = 30$, 83.3%) and combined fractures ($n = 11$, 91.7%). Patients with fissures were more frequently associated with midface fractures than they were with mandibular fractures (16.7% vs. 1.1%), while patients with total fractures were more frequently associated with mandibular fractures than they were with midface fractures (98.9% vs. 83.3%). Most mandibular fractures ($n = 87$, 92.6%) and midface fractures ($n = 29$, 80.6%) were without displacement, but for combined fractures, the distribution between displaced and non-displaced fractures was equal. Patients with displaced fractures were more frequently associated with combined fractures than they were with mandibular fractures (50% vs. 7.4%) (Table 4).

Table 4. Type of fracture and amplitude/displacement.

Fracture (n, %)	Mandibular	Midface	Combined	p *
		Amplitude		
Fissure	1 (1.1%)	6 (16.7%)	1 (8.3%)	0.002
Total	93 (98.9%)	30 (83.3%)	11 (91.7%)	
		Displacement		
No	87 (92.6%)	29 (80.6%)	6 (50%)	0.001
Yes	7 (7.4%)	7 (19.4%)	6 (50%)	

n—number; %—percentage; * Fisher's Exact Test.

Data in Table 5 show the distribution of patients according to the type of fracture and the presence of associated lesions. Most patients diagnosed with a mandibular fracture (76.6%) did not present any hematoma, but they presented lacerations (83%) or abrasions (77.7%). A total of 80.6% of the patients diagnosed with midface fractures had an associated hematoma, and 91.7% of the patients diagnosed with combined fractures had an associated hematoma. The observed associations were statistically significant, and Z tests with Bonferroni correction detailed the following: patients with hematomas were more frequently associated with combined fractures or midface fractures than they were with mandibular fractures (91.7%/80.6% vs. 23.4%); patients with lacerations were more frequently associated with combined fractures or midface fractures than they were with mandibular fractures (58.3%/47.2% vs. 17%); patients with abrasions were more frequently associated with combined fractures or midface fractures than they were with mandibular fractures (83.3%/44.4% vs. 22.3%).

Table 5. Type of fracture and associated lesions.

Fracture (n, %)	Mandibular	Midface	Combined	p *
		Hematoma		
No	72 (76.6%)	7 (19.4%)	1 (8.3%)	<0.001
Yes	22 (23.4%)	29 (80.6%)	11 (91.7%)	
		Laceration		
No	78 (83%)	19 (52.8%)	5 (41.7%)	<0.001
Yes	16 (17%)	17 (47.2%)	7 (58.3%)	
		Abrasion		
No	73 (77.7%)	20 (55.6%)	2 (16.7%)	<0.001
Yes	21 (22.3%)	16 (44.4%)	10 (83.3%)	

n—number; %—percentage; * Fisher's Exact Test.

The instituted treatment was, in general, orthopedic, for all three types of fractures (mandibular—86.2%; midface—91.7%; combined—66.7%). Most patients had favorable evolutions of mandibular ($n = 91$, 96.8%), midface ($n = 36$, 100%) and combined ($n = 11$, 91.7%) fractures. Most fractures did not present any complications at the follow-up. According to the Fisher's Exact Test, the associations between treatment choice, evolution and complications were not statistically significant (Table 6).

Table 6. Type of fracture and treatment/evolution/complications.

Fracture (n, %)	Mandibular	Midface	Combined	p *
Treatment				
Orthopedic	81 (86.2%)	33 (91.7%)	8 (66.7%)	0.085
Osteosynthesis plates	1 (1.1%)	1 (2.8%)	0 (0%)	
Cerclage	5 (5.3%)	0 (0%)	0 (0%)	
Combined	7 (7.4%)	2 (5.6%)	4 (33.3%)	
Evolution				
Favorable	91 (96.8%)	36 (100%)	11 (91.7%)	0.229
Unfavorable	3 (3.2%)	0 (0%)	1 (8.3%)	
Complications				
No complications	91 (96.8%)	36 (100%)	11 (91.7%)	0.124
Osteitis	3 (3.2%)	0 (0%)	0 (0%)	
Vicious consolidation	0 (0%)	0 (0%)	1 (8.3%)	

n—number; %—percentage; * Fisher's Exact Test.

4. Discussion

The clinical patterns of pediatric facial fractures are diverse, are influenced by a multitude of factors, can have different degrees of severity and various locations and can cause complications [23,24]. It was initially assumed that age, gender and living environment could have an impact on the clinical patterns of pediatric facial fractures among the analyzed sample of children and adolescents, and these variables were investigated. The different locations of mandibular and midface fractures, as well as the amplitude and the displacement of fracture fragments, were considered to be important for drawing valid conclusions regarding the clinical characteristic of pediatric facial fractures. Knowing about the various treatment approaches, the short-term evolution and the possible complications helped to outline a clear picture regarding the morbidity of these fractures.

Age has a great influence on the clinical characteristics of pediatric facial fractures [23]. The patients included in this study were distributed in three different age groups, 0–6 years, 7–12 years and 13–18 years, respectively. This type of age distribution was preferred because it includes three important stages of development (preschool, school and adolescence) [23]. At the same time, the distribution of the three age groups respects the chronology of primary, mixed and permanent dentition. Primary teeth begin to erupt immediately after birth [25], with the stage of deciduous dentition ending at the age of six, when permanent teeth begin to erupt [26]. With the onset of the eruption of permanent teeth, the stage of mixed dentition begins, which ends when all permanent teeth have been exfoliated and the second permanent molars erupt, which usually occurs at the age of 12 [26]. After all primary teeth have been exfoliated, the growth of permanent dentition begins [26]. In the current study, the most frequently affected patients were included in the 13–18 years age group, which is a situation that was similar to studies from other populations [27,28]. Ferreira et al. (2016) reviewed a total of 2071 pediatric facial fractures among a sample of 1416 patients. They divided the patients into six different age group, as follows: 0–3 years, 4–6 years, 7–9 years, 10–12 years, 13–15 years and 16–18 years. Eight hundred and seventy-nine patients (62%) belonged to the last two age groups (13–15 years and 16–18 years) [27]. Hoppe et al. (2014) investigated a sample of 285 patients with pediatric facial fractures. They distributed the patients into four different age groups, as follows: 0–2 years, 3–8 years, 9–14 years and 15–18 years. Most fractures were identified in the last age group (15–18 years).

The patients were also distributed according to the living environment, urban or rural ones, because it has been demonstrated that the living environment and environmental circumstances influence different aspects of pediatric trauma [29]. Fractures have a higher incidence among patients living in urban environments, which is probably due to the higher population density and a greater exposure to different sports [30], but also due to the high degree of community violence in the urban environment [31]. In this study, a predilection for fractures occurring among patients living in the urban environment was observed, as well, with more than half of the patients included in this study sample living in an urban environment.

Regarding the location, fractures can involve the mandible, the midface or they can be combined. The literature usually identifies pediatric mandibular fractures as the most common pediatric facial fractures [32,33]. The mandible is a U-shaped bone that has 13 muscle attachments for muscles that perform numerous functions. The innervation of the mandible is provided by the lower alveolar nerve and its branches [34]. Iida and Matsuya (2002) identified, among a sample of 174 pediatric patients from Osaka, that 56% of facial fractures involved the mandible. The most frequent locations of mandibular fractures were condylar fractures, followed by fractures in the canine region and mandibular angle fractures. Eleven percent of patients were diagnosed with midface fractures [32]. Mukhopadhyay S. (2018) identified 131 mandibular fractures among a sample of 89 children. The most frequent locations were the condylar region, the angle of the mandible, the parasymphysis, the body of the mandible and the symphysis [33]. In this study, mandibular fractures were the most frequent ones, as well, but the preferred locations were slightly different compared to those in the previously cited studies. Thus, in this study, most mandibular fractures occurred at the level of the mandibular angle, followed by lateral mandibular fractures, and only then by subcondylar fractures. The predominance of mandibular fractures is most likely due to the prominent position of the mandible in the facial skeleton [35]. Pediatric mandibular fractures are, in general, without displacement or with minimal displacement due to the high elasticity of the cortical bone [36]. This is in agreement with this study, where most mandibular fractures were not displaced.

Hematomas are among the associated lesions that are most frequently identified after facial fractures. They are produced by the extravasation of blood from the marrow into tissue spaces [37]. In the present study, hematomas were most frequently associated with midface and combined fractures. Chapman et al. (2009) reported orbital hematomas as frequent complications in fractures involving the orbital roof [38], and Ferreira et al. (2015) identified an association between midface and combined fractures and associated lesions such as hematomas or abrasions [39]. The results are similar to this study, where associated injuries such as hematomas, lacerations and abrasions were identified especially in midface and combined fractures.

The treatment of pediatric facial fractures offers various possibilities, and researchers must take into account the age of the child. Among younger children, non-surgical treatments are preferred due to their higher healing and remodeling capacity, but also in order to avoid the impairment of future craniofacial growth [7,40]. Along with the increase in age and severity of the fracture, the need for surgical interventions in the management of pediatric facial fractures also increases [41]. Among pediatric patients, open reduction and internal fixation increase the risk of intramaxillary teeth injuries, developmental disorders and the need for future surgical reinterventions [5], but the development of bio-resorbable plates has been proven to be effective in reducing the risks of the surgical management of pediatric facial fractures [42]. In this study, most of the mandibular, midface and combined fractures were treated conservatively and orthopedically, with favorable evolution. The high osteogenic potential of pediatric patients is one of the factors responsible for the favorable evolution of these fractures [43].

In a previously published paper, the authors aimed to identify the main etiology among this sample of patients and offered information regarding the epidemiology (age, gender, living environment, fracture line and associated soft tissue lesions) [44]. However, due to the large amount of information, it was considered that addressing all issues related to pediatric facial fractures in a single manuscript would make the reading experience hard and redundant. Clinical patterns, treatment, evolution and complications were, therefore, not presented in the first article. Although the sample remains the same, this paper presented a large amount of information regarding the aforementioned issues, which helps in understanding the different fracture patterns, their treatment approach and evolution. Etiology was not discussed since it was presented in the previous paper. It is the authors' opinion that the present study provides valuable information regarding the clinical patterns of pediatric facial fractures in the investigated region. This information can be used for establishing predictable therapeutic protocols, but also for rapidly and correctly diagnosing pediatric facial fractures. The implementation of pediatric facial fracture prevention programs can also take into account the information presented in this study.

However, the study also has some limitations. The retrospective nature of this research may determine that the data recorded at the time of admission, as well as the data recorded at the follow-up, may be incorrect or incomplete. The unicentric approach used limits the number of cases to a single oral and maxillofacial surgery center, which makes it possible for cases registered and treated in other institutions to present differences among the investigated characteristics. Another limitation is the absence of a long-term follow-up, since in this study, only post-fracture healing was evaluated. The small number of children diagnosed with pediatric facial fractures can also be considered as a limitation.

5. Conclusions

Most pediatric facial fractures were recorded in the 13–18 years age group. Mandibular and combined fractures predominated among patients living in an urban environment, and midface fractures predominated among patients living in a rural environment. Most fractures were total fractures, but without the displacement of fractured fragments. Most patients with associated lesions such as hematomas, lacerations and abrasions were more frequently associated with midface or combined fractures than they were with mandibular fractures. For the majority of patients, the instituted treatment had a favorable evolution, without complications at the follow-up.

Author Contributions: Conceptualization, R.I.J. and P.A.Ț.; methodology, R.I.J.; software, R.T.M.; validation, A.E.M. and M.J.; formal analysis, P.A.Ț.; investigation, R.I.J.; resources, A.E.M. and M.J.; data curation, A.E.M.; writing—original draft preparation, R.I.J.; writing—review and editing, P.A.Ț. and A.E.M.; visualization, A.E.M. and R.T.M.; supervision, P.A.Ț.; project administration, M.J.; funding acquisition, M.J. All authors contributed equally to this manuscript. All authors have read and agreed to the published version of the manuscript.

Funding: This research received no external funding.

Institutional Review Board Statement: The study was conducted in accordance with the Declaration of Helsinki, and approved by the Ethics Committee of the University of Oradea (IRB No. 3402/15.04.2018). The approval date is 15 April 2018.

Informed Consent Statement: Informed consent was obtained from all subjects involved in the study.

Data Availability Statement: The data presented in this study are available on request from the corresponding authors. The data are not publicly available due to privacy reasons.

Conflicts of Interest: The authors declare no conflict of interest.

References

1. Gómez Roselló, E.; Quiles Granado, A.M.; Artajona Garcia, M.; Juanpere Martí, S.; Laguillo Sala, G.; Beltrán Mármol, B.; Pedraza Gutiérrez, S. Facial fractures: Classification and highlights for a useful report. *Insights Imaging* **2020**, *11*, 49. [CrossRef] [PubMed]
2. Lalloo, R.; Lucchesi, L.R.; Bisignano, C.; Castle, C.D.; Dingels, Z.V.; Fox, J.T.; Hamilton, E.B.; Liu, Z.; Roberts, N.L.S.; Sylte, D.O.; et al. Epidemiology of facial fractures: Incidence, prevalence and years lived with disability estimates from the Global Burden of Disease 2017 study. *Inj. Prev.* **2020**, *26 (Suppl. S1)*, i27–i35. [CrossRef]
3. Juncar, M.; Tent, P.A.; Juncar, R.I.; Harangus, A.; Mircea, R. An epidemiological analysis of maxillofacial fractures: A 10-year cross-sectional cohort retrospective study of 1007 patients. *BMC Oral Health* **2021**, *21*, 128. [CrossRef] [PubMed]
4. Cole, P.; Kaufman, Y.; Hollier, L.H., Jr. Managing the pediatric facial fracture. *Craniomaxillofac. Trauma Reconstr.* **2009**, *2*, 77–83. [CrossRef]
5. Braun, T.L.; Xue, A.S.; Maricevich, R.S. Differences in the Management of Pediatric Facial Trauma. *Semin. Plast. Surg.* **2017**, *31*, 118–122. [CrossRef] [PubMed]
6. Imahara, S.D.; Hopper, R.A.; Wang, J.; Rivara, F.P.; Klein, M.B. Patterns and outcomes of pediatric facial fractures in the United States: A survey of the National Trauma Data Bank. *J. Am. Coll. Surg.* **2008**, *207*, 710–716. [CrossRef]

7. Vyas, R.M.; Dickinson, B.P.; Wasson, K.L.; Roostaeian, J.; Bradley, J.P. Pediatric facial fractures: Current national incidence, distribution, and health care resource use. *J. Craniofac. Surg.* **2008**, *19*, 339–349. [CrossRef] [PubMed]
8. Dobitsch, A.A.; Oleck, N.C.; Liu, F.C.; Halsey, J.N.; Hoppe, I.C.; Lee, E.S.; Granick, M.S. Sports-Related Pediatric Facial Trauma: Analysis of Facial Fracture Pattern and Concomitant Injuries. *Surg. J.* **2019**, *5*, e146–e149. [CrossRef]
9. Montovani, J.C.; de Campos, L.M.; Gomes, M.A.; de Moraes, V.R.; Ferreira, F.D.; Nogueira, E.A. Etiology and incidence facial fractures in children and adults. *Braz. J. Otorhinolaryngol.* **2006**, *72*, 235–241. [CrossRef]
10. Gassner, R.; Tuli, T.; Hächl, O.; Moreira, R.; Ulmer, H. Craniomaxillofacial trauma in children: A review of 3385 cases with 6060 injuries in 10 years. *J. Oral Maxillofac. Surg.* **2004**, *62*, 399–407. [CrossRef]
11. Andrew, T.W.; Morbia, R.; Lorenz, H.P. Pediatric Facial Trauma. *Clin. Plast. Surg.* **2019**, *46*, 239–247. [CrossRef] [PubMed]
12. Grunwaldt, L.; Smith, D.M.; Zuckerbraun, N.S.; Naran, S.; Rottgers, S.A.; Bykowski, M.; Kinsella, C.; Cray, J.; Vecchione, L.; Saladino, R.A.; et al. Pediatric facial fractures: Demographics, injury patterns, and associated injuries in 772 consecutive patients. *Plast. Reconstr. Surg.* **2011**, *128*, 1263–1271. [CrossRef] [PubMed]
13. Totonchi, A.; Sweeney, W.M.; Gosain, A.K. Distinguishing anatomic features of pediatric facial trauma. *J. Craniofac. Surg.* **2012**, *23*, 793–798. [CrossRef] [PubMed]
14. Adibelli, Z.H.; Songu, M.; Adibelli, H. Paranasal sinus development in children: A magnetic resonance imaging analysis. *Am. J. Rhinol. Allergy.* **2011**, *25*, 30–35. [CrossRef]
15. Shah, R.K.; Dhingra, J.K.; Carter, B.L.; Rebeiz, E.E. Paranasal sinus development: A radiographic study. *Laryngoscope* **2003**, *113*, 205–209. [CrossRef]
16. Alcalá-Galiano, A.; Arribas-García, I.J.; Martín-Pérez, M.A.; Romance, A.; Montalvo-Moreno, J.J.; Juncos, J.M. Pediatric facial fractures: Children are not just small adults. *Radiographics* **2008**, *28*, 441–461. [CrossRef]
17. Ryu, J.; Yun, S.J.; Lee, S.H.; Choi, Y.H. Screening of pediatric facial fractures by brain computed tomography: Diagnostic performance comparison with facial computed tomography. *Pediatr. Emerg. Care* **2020**, *36*, 1259. [CrossRef]
18. Goldwasser, T.; Bressan, S.; Oakley, E.; Arpone, M.; Babl, F.E. Use of sedation in children receiving computed tomography after head injuries. *Eur. J. Emerg. Med.* **2015**, *22*, 413–418. [CrossRef]
19. Nguyen, B.N.; Edwards, M.J.; Srivatsa, S.; Wakeman, D.; Claderon, T.; Lamoshi, A.; Wallenstein, K.; Fabiano, T.; Cantor, B.; Bass, K.; et al. Clinical and radiographic predictors of the need for facial CT in pediatric blunt trauma: A multi-institutional study. *Trauma Surg. Acute Care Open* **2022**, *7*, e000899. [CrossRef]
20. Siy, R.W.; Brown, R.H.; Koshy, J.C.; Stal, S.; Hollier, L.H., Jr. General management considerations in pediatric facial fractures. *J. Craniofac. Surg.* **2011**, *22*, 1190–1195. [CrossRef]
21. Ferreira, P.; Marques, M.; Pinho, C.; Rodrigues, J.; Reis, J.; Amarante, J. Midfacial fractures in children and adolescents: A review of 492 cases. *Br. J. Oral Maxillofac. Surg.* **2004**, *42*, 501–505. [CrossRef] [PubMed]
22. Zimmermann, C.E.; Troulis, M.J.; Kaban, L.B. Pediatric facial fractures: Recent advances in prevention, diagnosis and management. *Int. J. Oral Maxillofac. Surg.* **2006**, *35*, 2–13. [CrossRef]
23. Segura-Palleres, I.; Sobrero, F.; Roccia, F.; de Oliveira Gorla, L.F.; Pereira-Filho, V.A.; Gallafassi, D.; Faverani, L.P.; Romeo, I.; Bojino, A.; Copelli, C. Characteristics and age-related injury patterns of maxillofacial fractures in children and adolescents: A multicentric and prospective study. *Dent. Traumatol.* **2022**, *38*, 213–222. [CrossRef]
24. Chao, M.T.; Losee, J.E. Complications in pediatric facial fractures. *Craniomaxillofac. Trauma Reconstr.* **2009**, *2*, 103–112. [CrossRef] [PubMed]
25. Burgueño Torres, L.; Mourelle Martínez, M.R.; de Nova García, J.M. A study on the chronology and sequence of eruption of primary teeth in Spanish children. *Eur. J. Paediatr. Dent.* **2015**, *16*, 301–304. [PubMed]
26. Lynch, R.J. The primary and mixed dentition, post-eruptive enamel maturation and dental caries: A review. *Int. Dent. J.* **2013**, *63* (Suppl. S2), 3–13. [CrossRef]
27. Ferreira, P.C.; Barbosa, J.; Braga, J.M.; Rodrigues, A.; Silva, Á.C.; Amarante, J.M. Pediatric Facial Fractures: A Review of 2071 Fractures. *Ann. Plast. Surg.* **2016**, *77*, 54–60. [CrossRef]
28. Hoppe, I.C.; Kordahi, A.M.; Paik, A.M.; Lee, E.S.; Granick, M.S. Age and sex-related differences in 431 pediatric facial fractures at a level 1 trauma center. *J. Craniomaxillofac. Surg.* **2014**, *42*, 1408–1411. [CrossRef]
29. Marek, A.P.; Nygaard, R.M.; Cohen, E.M.; Polites, S.F.; Sirany, A.E.; Wildenberg, S.E.; Elsbernd, T.A.; Murphy, S.; Dean Potter, D.; Zielinski, M.D.; et al. Rural versus urban pediatric non-accidental trauma: Different patients, similar outcomes. *BMC Res. Notes* **2018**, *11*, 519. [CrossRef]
30. Hedström, E.M.; Waernbaum, I. Incidence of fractures among children and adolescents in rural and urban communities—Analysis based on 9965 fracture events. *Inj. Epidemiol.* **2014**, *1*, 14. [CrossRef]
31. Pittman, S.K.; Farrell, A.D. Patterns of community violence exposure among urban adolescents and their associations with adjustment. *Am. J. Community Psychol.* **2022**, *70*, 265–277. [CrossRef] [PubMed]
32. Iida, S.; Matsuya, T. Paediatric maxillofacial fractures: Their aetiological characters and fracture patterns. *J. Craniomaxillofac. Surg.* **2002**, *30*, 237–241. [CrossRef] [PubMed]
33. Mukhopadhyay, S. A retrospective study of mandibular fractures in children. *J. Korean Assoc. Oral Maxillofac. Surg.* **2018**, *44*, 269–274. [CrossRef]
34. Panesar, K.; Susarla, S.M. Mandibular Fractures: Diagnosis and Management. *Semin. Plast. Surg.* **2021**, *35*, 238–249. [CrossRef]

35. Gadicherla, S.; Sasikumar, P.; Gill, S.S.; Bhagania, M.; Kamath, A.T.; Pentapati, K.C. Mandibular Fractures and Associated Factors at a Tertiary Care Hospital. *Arch. Trauma Res.* **2016**, *5*, e30574. [CrossRef] [PubMed]
36. Pickrell, B.B.; Serebrakian, A.T.; Maricevich, R.S. Mandible Fractures. *Semin. Plast. Surg.* **2017**, *31*, 100–107. [CrossRef] [PubMed]
37. Niazi, K.T.; Raja, D.K.; Prakash, R.; Balaji, V.R.; Manikandan, D.; Ulaganathan, G.; Yoganandha, R. Massive expanding hematoma of the chin following blunt trauma. *J. Pharm. Bioallied Sci.* **2016**, *8* (Suppl. S1), S182–S184. [CrossRef]
38. Chapman, V.M.; Fenton, L.Z.; Gao, D.; Strain, J.D. Facial fractures in children: Unique patterns of injury observed by computed tomography. *J. Comput. Assist. Tomogr.* **2009**, *33*, 70–72. [CrossRef]
39. Ferreira, P.C.; Barbosa, J.; Amarante, J.M.; Carvalho, J.; Rodrigues, A.G.; Silva, Á.C. Associated injuries in pediatric patients with facial fractures in Portugal: Analysis of 1416 patients. *J. Craniomaxillofac. Surg.* **2015**, *43*, 437–443. [CrossRef]
40. Kim, S.H.; Lee, S.H.; Cho, P.D. Analysis of 809 facial bone fractures in a pediatric and adolescent population. *Arch. Plast. Surg.* **2012**, *39*, 606–611. [CrossRef]
41. Mckenzie, J.; Nguyen, E. Minimally Invasive Surgical Management of Complex Pediatric Facial Fractures. *Craniomaxillofac. Trauma Reconstr. Open* **2021**, *6*, 24727512211022601. [CrossRef]
42. Singh, G.; Mohammad, S.; Chak, R.K.; Lepcha, N.; Singh, N.; Malkunje, L.R. Bio-resorbable plates as effective implant in paediatric mandibular fracture. *J. Maxillofac. Oral Surg.* **2012**, *11*, 400–406. [CrossRef] [PubMed]
43. Naik, P. Remodelling in Children's Fractures and Limits of Acceptability. *Indian J. Orthop.* **2021**, *55*, 549–559. [CrossRef]
44. Țenț, P.A.; Juncar, R.I.; Moca, A.E.; Moca, R.T.; Juncar, M. The Etiology and Epidemiology of Pediatric Facial Fractures in North-Western Romania: A 10-Year Retrospective Study. *Children* **2022**, *9*, 932. [CrossRef] [PubMed]

Disclaimer/Publisher's Note: The statements, opinions and data contained in all publications are solely those of the individual author(s) and contributor(s) and not of MDPI and/or the editor(s). MDPI and/or the editor(s) disclaim responsibility for any injury to people or property resulting from any ideas, methods, instructions or products referred to in the content.

MDPI AG
Grosspeteranlage 5
4052 Basel
Switzerland
Tel.: +41 61 683 77 34

Children Editorial Office
E-mail: children@mdpi.com
www.mdpi.com/journal/children

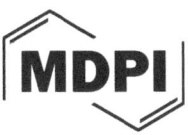

Disclaimer/Publisher's Note: The statements, opinions and data contained in all publications are solely those of the individual author(s) and contributor(s) and not of MDPI and/or the editor(s). MDPI and/or the editor(s) disclaim responsibility for any injury to people or property resulting from any ideas, methods, instructions or products referred to in the content.

www.ingramcontent.com/pod-product-compliance
Lightning Source LLC
LaVergne TN
LVHW072356090526
838202LV00019B/2556